Cosmetology and Dermatology

Cosmetology and Dermatology

Edited by **Deb Willis**

hayle
medical

New York

Published by Hayle Medical,
30 West, 37th Street, Suite 612,
New York, NY 10018, USA
www.haylemedical.com

Cosmetology and Dermatology
Edited by Deb Willis

International Standard Book Number: 978-1-63241-410-6 (Hardback)

Printed in the United States of America.

Contents

Preface

Every book is a source of knowledge and this one is no exception. The idea that led to the conceptualization of this book was the fact that the world is advancing rapidly; which makes it crucial to document the progress in every field. I am aware that a lot of data is already available, yet, there is a lot more to learn. Hence, I accepted the responsibility of editing this book and contributing my knowledge to the community.

Cosmetology and dermatology are often considered similar branches of medical science though both have different approaches and uses. Both these branches do overlap at the point of cosmetic surgery. Cosmetology refers to the practice of beautifying a person's appearance. It incorporates providing care and beauty treatments for nails, hair and skin. On the other hand, dermatology deals with treating diseases related to skin, hair or nails. This book will cover both of these topics and explain in detail their integrated applications. It is compiled in such a manner, that it will provide in-depth knowledge about the theory and practice of these fields. Those in search of information to further their knowledge will be greatly assisted by this book. It is a ripe text for cosmetologists, dermatologists, professional researchers and students associated with cosmetology and dermatology at various levels.

While editing this book, I had multiple visions for it. Then I finally narrowed down to make every chapter a sole standing text explaining a particular topic, so that they can be used independently. However, the umbrella subject sinews them into a common theme. This makes the book a unique platform of knowledge.

I would like to give the major credit of this book to the experts from every corner of the world, who took the time to share their expertise with us. Also, I owe the completion of this book to the never-ending support of my family, who supported me throughout the project.

Editor

Epidemiological and Clinical Aspects of Skin Bleaching in Secondary School in Bohicon, Benin

F. Atadokpédé[1], H. Adégbidi[1], C. Koudoukpo[2], J. Téclessou[1], C. Aholoukpé[1], B. Degboé[1], F. do Ango-Padonou[1], H. Yedomon[1]

[1]Faculté des Sciences de la Santé, Cotonou, Bénin
[2]Faculté de Médecine, Université de Parakou, Parakou, Bénin
Email: fatadokpede2009@yahoo.fr

Abstract

Skin bleaching is a public health problem in West Africa most studied in general population. We conducted a cross-sectional survey to evaluate the prevalence of the phenomenon in secondary schools in central Benin. The prevalence of voluntary depigmentation (VD) was 36.6%. The sex ratio was 0.49. Gender was statistically associated with VD (p value < 0.000). Bleaching products used were often hydroquinone (42.2%), and corticosteroid (22.7%). The mean duration of the practice was 20 months. Products were applied over all body twice a day in most students. The main dermatological complications of the practice were discoloration (32.2%), stretch marks (20%), acne (18.5%), and fungal infections (13.1%). Parents funded and chose the bleaching products in most cases. This was the first survey conducted in secondary schools in West Africa targeted voluntary depigmentation. The high prevalence of the practice raises some questions, among them the core values of West African societies.

Keywords

Skin Bleachning, Schools, Benin

1. Introduction

Voluntary depigmentation (VD) is a practice of using drugs or any other products with a depigmenting potential for cosmetic purposes. The aim of this practice is to obtain a reduction of the physiological skin pigmentation. Reported in the literature in the late sixties, the VD seems to have developed in the modern era with the marketing of topical steroids and compounds with hydroquinone. This is a relatively old and widespread practice in Black Africa. The term voluntary depigmentation is often used in the literature to put special emphasis on its intentional aspect.

VD is a female practice in Africa with prevalence ranging from 25% to 67% [1]-[4] in West Africa. This social phenomenon has mainly been described in adults. Studies on the VD in school are rare. The objective of this study was to investigate the epidemiological and clinical aspects of VD in school in central Benin.

2. Population and Methods

We conducted a descriptive and analytical cross-sectional study on a sample of students in public and private Colleges of General Education (CEG) in Bohicon, a city in central Benin. Students aged at least 15 years were included.

The town has 6 public and 9 private colleges. A college was used for pre-test and the other for the actual survey. We used a random sampling method in three steps:

-In the first stage a simple random sampling without replacement of 40% for public institutions and 60% for private institutions was conducted;

-In the second step, 50% of classes in selected schools were drawn by simple random sampling without replacement;

-In the third step, the selection of students was done by systematic random sampling. The sampling interval is calculated by dividing the total number of pupils in classes used by the sample size. We used the random number table for the selection of the first student. The other students were drawn systematically by adding the sampling interval to the random number selected.

Students selected were subjected to a pre-questionnaire and were examined by a dermatologist.

The data were recorded and analyzed using Epi Info 3.5.1.

The following statistical tests were used for the description of variables: mean, standard deviation, extreme values, proportion, chi-square test.

The ethical rules were followed by requesting a free and informed consent of the students, an administrative authorization to college principals and parental permission.

3. Results

Based on sampling, 429 students were selected and all agreed to participate in the study.

Of the 429 students surveyed and examined 157 practiced voluntary depigmentation. The prevalence of VD was 36.6% among school students in Bohicon.

Sixty-six point nine percent (66.9%) of students practicing VD were female and 33.1% male. The sex ratio was 0.49. Female gender was statistically associated with the VD in students (p value < 0.000).

The average age of students who practiced voluntary depigmentation was 18 years with a range of 18 to 27 years.

Thirty-eight point two percent (38.2%) of students practicing VD were in high school, 36.9% (p = 0.29) were in first class and 24.8% (p = 0.02) in twelfth grade.

Voluntary depigmentation was also common among students living in monogamous households (43.3%) than in polygamous households (42.7%). Only 14% of students living in homes whose parents are divorced or widowed practiced VD.

In our study, 86.6% of students practicing VD were Christians, 7% were Muslims and 6.4% practiced other religions.

3.1. Bleaching Agents Used by Students

Products containing hydroquinone were the most used (42.0%) followed by corticosteroids (22.7%) (**Table 1**).

3.2. Description of the Practice and Motivation

The average duration of use of bleaching agents among students was 20 months with a range of 1 - 98 months. The products were applied all over the body by 82.9% of females (**Table 2**).

Application was twice daily in 76.2% of women and 53.8% of men. It was daily in 25% of men and 21.9% of

Table 1. Skin bleaching products used by school children in central Benin.

Products	Proportion (%)
Hydroquinone	42.0
Corticosteroid	22.3
Mercury compounds	19.7
Fruit acids	13.6
Others	2.3
Total	100

Table 2. Areas of application of skin bleaching products by school children in central Benin.

Areas of application	Sex	
	Male (%)	Female (%)
Face	21 (40.4)	18 (17.1)
All body	31 (59.6)	87 (82.9)
Total	**52 (100)**	**105 (100)**

women. A weekly application was made in 21.1% of men and 1.9% of women. The mean monthly cost of products was 2.6 US dollars with a range of 0.7 dollars to 10 dollars. It was supported by parents (70.1%), friends (26.8%), and others (3.1). The choice of depigmenting cosmetics was made by the parents in 52.2% of cases, by the students themselves in 33.8% of cases and by friends in 14% of cases.

Motivations at the beginning of practice were aesthetic in 78.1% of girls and those evoked to continue the practice were looking for light-skin at 76.2% (**Table 3**).

The attitude of parents and friends in relation to the practice was encouraging in 57.6% of girls and 44.3% boys. However, 32.4% of parents of girls and 40% of parents of boys were indifferent. The opposition of parents to voluntary depigmentation was noted in 10% of cases in girls and 15.7% of boys.

3.3. Dermatological Complications

Discolorations were observed in 32.3% of students practicing VD (**Table 4**).

Superficial fungal infections were the most frequent infectious complications. They sat on the cheeks, arms, legs or internal surfaces of the body.

3.4. Knowledge of the Dangers of Depigmentation by Students

The assessment of knowledge of users showed that 98.7% of students were unaware of the harmful effects of the practice.

4. Discussion

After our investigation, we were able to determine the epidemiological profile of the VD in schools in Bohicon.

The method based on random sampling of school population allows us to say that our results are valid.

The prevalence of VD was high in school in central Benin since it concerned 36.6% of students of public and private schools. To our knowledge this is the first study assessing the prevalence of VD in schools in West Africa. Other studies in the general population in West Africa reported a high prevalence of the phenomenon:

-5% in the study by Mahe [1] involving 210 adult women in the general population in Mali;

-58.7% in the study of Nnoruka [5] in the general adult population in Nigeria;

-59% of the 910 women in the study by Pitche [3] in Togo;

-67% of women in the investigation by Wone in Dakar [4].

Table 3. Motivations of voluntary depigmentation among school children in Benin.

Motivations	Sex	
	Male	Female
Motivations at the beginning		
Skin defect	20 (38.5)	23 (21.9)
Aesthetic	32 (61.5)	83 (78.1)
Motivations to continue		
Search for light skin	13 (52.0)	27 (76.2)
Effectiveness	07 (28.0)	09 (01.9)
Fear to become black again	05 (20.0)	09 (21.9)
Motivations to stop		
Health disorders	13 (48.1)	31 (51.7)
Lack of efficacy	09 (33.3)	14 (23.3)
Opposition of parents	05 (18.5)	15 (25.0)

Table 4. Skin disorders observed among school children practicing voluntary depigmentation.

Skin disorders	Number	Proportion (%)
Dyschromia	42	32.3
Stretch marks	26	20.0
Acne	24	18.5
Superficial mycosis	17	13.1
Skin atrophy	17	13.1
Contact dermatitis	04	3.0
Total	130	100

Voluntary depigmentation was particularly marked among women in West Africa and various studies have targeted this population [3] [6] [7]. Sixty-six point nine percent (66.9%) of students practicing VD in our study were female, reflecting the predominance of the practice in teenager. However, the VD was also observed in 26.7% of men according to a Nigerian study [8]. The practice has also been reported in men in Congo and South Africa [9] [10]. In our study DV was noted in 33.1% of boys. A search for identity or a desire for seduction in this transition period between adolescence and adulthood may explain the VD in students.

The depigmenting cosmetics principles identified in our study are hydroquinone, steroids and mercury compounds. These products have been reported in previous studies [2] [3] [8]. Normaly these products are for medical use but they are diverted for use as cosmetics. In our study, hydroquinone was the most used (42.0%). In the opposite mercury compounds were widely used in the study by Pitché *et al.* in Togo [3], while products with hydroquinone were the most used in the study by Traoré *et al.* in Burkina Faso [2]. The market availability and the supposed effectiveness of skin-lightening products influence the use of bleaching agents by country.

The practice was for most students a twice-daily application all over the body. The same technique was noted in other studies [1] [3]. Some students preferred product application on the face. This could be related to a search for a more perfect complexion in this open area. The mean monthly cost of the products used by the students was 2.6 US dollars. At this cost, depigmenting cosmetics can be affordable for all and making high prevalence of VD in teenager and maintaining its sustainability.

The bleaching agents were funded in 70.1% of cases by the parents and the parents were involved in product choice in 52.2% of cases. It could be parents themselves practicing VD and therefore using these depigmenting cosmetic products for their children since infancy. Parents of students are heavily involved in practice by funding or by providing cosmetic depigmenting to their children. This calls into question the voluntary nature of the practice for these students who are still under the authority of parents.

Voluntary depigmentation is motivated initially by a desire to lighten the skin or correct a defect of the skin. These motivations are almost identical to those given in the literature [2] [11]. The practice is in progress because of effectiveness of bleaching agents and fear to become black again. Users seem therefore become dependent on these products as a drug [12]. But the onset of skin complications and the opposition of parents drive to stop the practice. Dyschromias represented 32.2% of the cutaneous complications observed in our study. These discolorations were also noted in 70.80% of women in Togo [3]. This pigmentary disorder is a real cosmetic problem for practitioners of VD because of the contrast between clear complexion and black complexion. This is double skin pigmentation with alternating areas of hyperpigmentation and hypopigmentation in the same individual. This dual pigmentation may be due to non-uniform application of the products on the body but also to the presence of physiologically pigmented or previously traumatized and resistant regions. These discolorations may cause a vicious circle with a determination to make them disappear by multiplying the applications or by combining different products. Acne and stretch marks are skin diseases frequently encountered during adolescence which makes it difficult to establish a cause and effect relationship between these conditions and the VD at this age. Nevertheless, 20% of students practicing VD had stretch marks in our study. The frequency of acne in students practicing VD in our study was 18.5%. This frequency is comparable to that seen in Senegal (19.5%) [13] but lower than that recorded in Togo (16.17%) [3].

The infections encountered in our study were fungal infections (13.1%). These are the most common infections in adults practicing VD. Sometimes unusual facial locations were also described by Mahé *et al.* [14]. Although our investigation related to high school students, 98.7% were unaware of the complications associated with the use of these products.

5. Conclusion

Voluntary depigmentation in schools in central Benin is a real public health problem. It also poses a problem of loss of core values in favor of artificial values. It is urgent that a true youth outreach program has been settled up to fight against this scourge, which could play a role in poor academic performance. The authors declare no conflict of interest.

References

[1]   Mahe, A., Blanc, L., Halna, J.M., Keita, S., Sanogo, T. and Bobin, P. (1993) An Epidemiologic Survey on the Cosmetic Use of Bleaching Agents by the Women of Bamako, Mali. *Annales de Dermatologie et de Vénéréologie*, **120**, 870-873.

[2]   Traoré, A., Kadeba, J.C. and Niamba, P. (2005) Use of Cutaneous Depigmenting Products by Women in Two Towns in Burkina Faso: Epidemiologic Data, Motivations, Products and Side Effects. *International Journal of Dermatology*, **44**, 30-32. http://dx.doi.org/10.1111/j.1365-4632.2005.02807.x

[3]   Pitché, P., Afanou, A., Amanga, Y. and Tchangai-Walla, K. (1998) Les pratiques cosmétiques dépigmentantes des femmes à Lomé (Togo). *Medecine d'Afrique Noire*, **45**, 709-713.

[4]   Wone, I., Tal-Dia, A., Diallo, O.F., Badiane, M., Touré, K. and Diallo, I. (2000) Prévalence de l'utilisation de produits cosmétiques dépigmentants dans deux quartiers à Dakar (Sénégal). *Dakar Médical*, **45**, 154-157.

[5]   Nnoruka, E. and Okoye, O. (2006) Tropical Steroid Abuse: Its Use as a Depigmenting Agent. *Journal of the National Medical Association*, **98**, 934-939.

[6]   Del Giudice, P. and Yves, P. (2002) The Widespread Use of Skin Lightening Creams in Senegal: A Persistent Public Health Problem in West Africa. *International Journal of Dermatology*, **41**, 69-72. http://dx.doi.org/10.1046/j.1365-4362.2002.01335.x

[7]   Morand, J.J., Ly, F., Lightburn, E. and Mahé, A. (2007) Complications de la dépigmentation cosmétique en Afrique. *Medecine Tropicale*, **67**, 627-634.

[8]   Adebajo, S.B. (2002) An Epidemiological Survey of the Use of Cosmetic Skin Lightening Cosmetics among Traders in Lagos Nigeria. *West African Journal of Medicine*, **21**, 51-55.

[9]   Hardwick, N., Van Gelger, L.W., Van der Merwe, C.A. and Van der Merwe, M.P. (1989) Exogenous Ochronosis: An Epidemiological Study. *British Journal of Dermatology*, **120**, 229-238. http://dx.doi.org/10.1111/j.1365-2133.1989.tb07787.x

[10] Didillon, H. and Bounsana, D. (1986) Modifier la couleur de sa peau: Mode ou complexe? Acte du colloque de Brazzaville, Karthala, 255-283.

[11] Muchadeyi, E., Thompson, S. and Baker, N. (1983) A Survey of the Constituents, Availability and Use of Skin Lightening Creams in Zimbabwe. *Central African Journal of Medicine*, **29**, 225-227.

[12] Ly, F., Mahé-Vasseur, P., Agne El Fecky, A. and Verschoore, M. (2007) Enquête qualitative sur la dépigmentation artificielle de la peau noire: Essai d'analyse anthropologique et psychosociale en contexte sénégalais. *Annales de Dermatologie et de Vénéréologie*, **134**, 21-22.

[13] Raynaud, E., Cellier, C. and Perret, J.L. (2001) Dépigmentation cutanée à visée cosmétique: Enquête de prévalence et effets indésirables dans une population féminine Sénégalaise. *Annales de Dermatologie et de Vénéréologie*, **128**, 720-724.

[14] Mahe, A., Ly, F., Aymard, G. and Dangou, J.M. (2003) Skin Diseases Associated with the Cosmetic Use of Bleaching Products in Women from Dakar, Sénégal. *British Journal of Dermatology*, **148**, 493-500. http://dx.doi.org/10.1046/j.1365-2133.2003.05161.x

Antioxidant, Collagen Synthesis Activity *in Vitro* and Clinical Test on Anti-Wrinkle Activity of Formulated Cream Containing *Veronica officinalis* Extract

Ha Youn Lee[1], Amal Kumar Ghimeray[1], Jun Hwan Yim[2], Moon Sik Chang[1*]

[1]R & D Center, Naturalsolution Co., Ltd., Incheon, Republic of Korea
[2]Free International City Development Center (Jeju Branch), Jeju-Do, Republic of Korea
Email: [*]justin0510@naturalsolution.co.kr

Abstract

In this study, our objective was to evaluate the antioxidant, cytotoxicity and collagen synthesis activity *in vitro* and also to test the anti-wrinkle effect of formulated cream containing *Veronica officinalis* extract *in vivo*. Antioxidant evaluation was based on the scavenging activity of free radicles (DPPH) and procollagen type 1 protein (P1P) synthesis test was performed in fibroblast cell. Clinical anti-wrinkle activity was performed on female subjects in placebo-controlled trail. Verbascoside (an isolated compound) showed higher (IC_{50} value of 36.24 ± 1.81 µg/ml) free radicle inhibition activity but weaker collagen synthesis activity. The ethanolic extract showed good inhibition to DPPH free radicals and also showed a significant effect in collagen synthesis activity without cytotoxicity. In the *in vivo* study, treatment with the formulated cream (Scoti-Speedwell) for 56 days significantly reduced the percentage of wrinkle area and length with 18.0% and 16.05%, respectively. Overall, *Veronica officinalis* extract containing product (Scoti-Speedwell™) can be regarded as a potent anti-wrinkle agent in human skin.

Keywords

Antioxidant, Antiwrinkle, Collagen Synthesis, *Veronica officinalis*, Scoti-Speedwell™

1. Introduction

Skin aging (whether extrinsic or intrinsic type) causes wrinkling, sagging, laxity, dyspigmentation, and telan-

---

[*]Corresponding author.

giectasia [1]. As the skin ages, the collagen (a major component of skin) and elastin in the dermis lose elasticity resulting in wrinkles. To prevent the skin from aging or wrinkles, natural phytochemical source is desirable. Plant extracts rich in phytochemicals like flavonoids, phenolic acids, tocopherols, alkaloids, monoterpenes, having antioxidant activity are being widely used for the development of anti-wrinkle topical cosmetic products [2].

Veronica officinalis belongs to the family Scrophulariaceae and is commonly called as Speedwell. The plant is herbaceous and perennial in nature and distributed mostly in Europe and western Asia. In some part of the Europe (France), the plant is used as tea substitute called "Europe tea" and is considered as a medicinal herb [3]. According to Romanian folk medicine, *Veronica officinalis* was used for kidney diseases, cough and catarrh and wound healing purposes [4]. Recently, the literature showed that the plant was rich in phytochemicals and had moderate nitric oxide scavenging activity and strong anti-inflammatory (TNF-α) activity [5]. The plant is also reported to have higher antioxidant activity [6]. In this study, our main objective was to evaluate the efficacy of plant extract and isolated compound on antioxidant, cytotoxicity and collagen synthesis activity *in vitro* and also to test the anti-wrinkle effect of formulated cream containing *Veronica officinalis* extract *in vivo*.

2. Materials and Methods

2.1. Plant Materials, Extracts Process

Dried sample of *Veronica officinalis* (whole plant) were supplied from Royal Botanical Garden Scotland, in November 2012. The plant material was air-dried at room temperature, milled, extracted with ethanol (70%) overnight, and filtered, and the process was repeated three times. The resulting ethanol extract was concentrated at reduced pressure in a rotatory evaporator at 40°C. A portion of the ethanol extract (410 g) was dissolved in distilled water, and placed in a separator funnel, and washed with n-hexane (200 mL, 15 times). The n-hexane phases were then combined and concentrated under reduced pressure. An identical process was repeated with chloroform, ethyl acetate, and butanol leaving a residual mixture of ethanol-water.

2.2. Isolation of Verbascoside Compound from *Veronica officinalis* (Speedwell)

Ethyl acetate extract (56.1 g) was fractionated by open CC using silica gel. Elution was carried out with addition of methanol to hexane-ethyl acetate mixtures in different ratios of increasing polarity until 100% methanol was reached. All fractions were analyzed by TLC. Verbascoside was obtained as the major compound by successive washes with CH_2Cl_2-MeOH (7:3) (5.02 g, 8.94% of the ethyl acetate extract). This compound was purified further by silica gel TLC using CH_2Cl_2-MeOH. The chemical structures of verbascoside was determined by comparison of spectroscopic and chromatographic data with those of authentic samples and were reported previously [7] [8].

2.3. Topical Formulation

Two percent of *Veronica officinalis* extract was mixed with a formulation containing water, Carbomer, Glycerine, Disodium EDTA (ethylene diamine tetra-acetic acid), Methylparaben, Trithanolamine, Tocopheryl acetate, Polysorbate 60, Stearyl alcohol, PEG-100 (polyethylene glycol-100) stearate, Sorbitan stearate, caprylic/capric triglyceride, Dimethicone, Mineral oil, Propylparaben, Butylene Glycol, Beeswax, and Fragrance. The placebo (control) was identical in composition, except plant extract.

2.4. Cell Culture and Cytotoxicity Determination

Fibroblast cell was purchased from the Korea cell line bank, Seoul, Korea were cultured in 96-well plates containing Dulbecco's Modified Eagle Medium (DMEM, 200 μl/well) supplemented with 10% fetal bovine serum (FBS), penicillin (100 units/ml) and streptomycin sulfate (100 μg/ml) in a humidified atmosphere of 5% CO_2. The cell viability assay of the Speedwell extract was performed with MTT (3-(4,5-dimethylthiaol-2-yl)-2-5-diphenyltetrazolium bromide) reagent following the protocol of Mosmann *et al.* [9].

2.5. Collagen Synthesis Activity in Fibroblasts

Procollagen type 1 protein synthesis test was performed according to the protocol of Tanayama *et al.* [10] with slight modification. 5×10^4 cell/well were seeded in a 24 well plate with DMEM (containing 10% FBS and 100 unit/ml penicillin-streptomycin). The plates were incubated overnight at 37°C in a humidified incubator, 5% CO_2. After incubation, the test extract or compound was added to the plate in serum free media. After incubation the plate for 24 hour at 37°C in a humidified incubator, 5% CO_2, the culture supernatant was collected after centrifuging at 13,000 rpm in 4°C for 20 min. The resultant supernatant was measured in duplicate according to the supplier's instructions (Takara, MK101). Negative control was performed with buffer and substrate but without enzyme. All assays were performed independently in duplicate.

2.6. *In Vitro* Antioxidant Activity

2.6.1. DPPH Free Radical Scavenging Assay
The antioxidant activity of extract was determined according to the method described by Bracca *et al.* [11], with slight modification. Briefly, a dilution series of ethanolic extract and isolated compound verbascoside was prepared in a 96 well plate. The reaction mixture consisted of 0.1 ml extract with 0.2 ml DPPH solution (0.15 mM in 80% methanol solution). The mixture was shaken vigorously and left to stand for 30 min at room temperature in the dark. Ascorbic acid was taken as positive control. The absorbance of the resulting solution was measured spectrophotometrically at 517 nm and the percent inhibition activity was calculated.

2.6.2. *In Vivo* Human Clinical Study (Wrinkle Area, Length Differences and Visual Score)
In vivo study was conducted in Guangzhou City, Land Proof Test Technology Co. Ltd., China. The study was a randomized, open, single-blinded, placebo-controlled, observer-blinded study which was approved by Guang-Dong light industry association institutional review committee for human testing. Twenty-one female subjects aged 45 - 65 years (without the history of serious diseases or allergic to cosmetics or pregnant women) participated in the study. The subjects' crow's feet area on both sides (right & left) were selected in which the wrinkles must not cross each other and the length of the main wrinkle must be at least 2 cm long. All subjects gave written informed consent prior to the study and evaluated for tolerance. Subjects were treated with Scoti-Speed well cream which contain 2% speedwell extract on the one side of the face (crow's feet) and with placebo (ingredients without plant extract) on the other side twice a day for 58 days. Clinical evaluations and measurements were performed on D0 (before treatment), D28 and D56. The anti-wrinkle effect of cream and placebo on wrinkled skin was evaluated by using Cutometer MPA 580 (CK Germany), Visioline VL650 (CK Germany), and SILFLO (cuDern USA).

2.7. Statistical Analysis

Statistical analyses were carried out using SPSS software (version 11.5; SPSS Inc., Chicago, IL, USA). The differences among samples were statistically evaluated via one-way analysis of variance (ANOVA) followed by Dunnett's posthoc test or Wilcoxon's test when appropriate. The level of significance was set at $p < 0.05$. Data are expressed as means ± standard errors.

3. Result

3.1. *In Vitro* Antioxidant Activity

The antioxidant efficacy of ethanolic extract of speedwell and isolated single compound verbascoside (**Figure 1**) is given in **Figure 2**. The isolated compound verbascoside showed a higher free radicle (DPPH) scavenging activity with the IC_{50} value of 36.24 ± 1.81 µg/ml. Similarly, the ethanolic extract of speedwell also showed good inhibition to DPPH radicles in dose dependent manner whose IC_{50} value was 103.50 ± 2.43 µg/ml.

3.2. Cell Viability and Collagen Synthesis Activity in Fibroblasts

The single compound verbascoside isolated from speedwell did not show significant result on Collagen synthesis activity in Fibroblasts (data not shown). However, the significantly increased in procollagen type 1 protein synthesis was observed due to the ethanolic extract of speedwell in fibroblast cell without cytotoxic effect (**Figure 3**). At a concentration of 2%, extract showed 44.6 % increase in collagen synthesis compare to the control (without extract). This activity of extract on PIP could be due to the interactions and synergistic effect of phytochemicals other than verbascoside present in the sample [12]-[14].

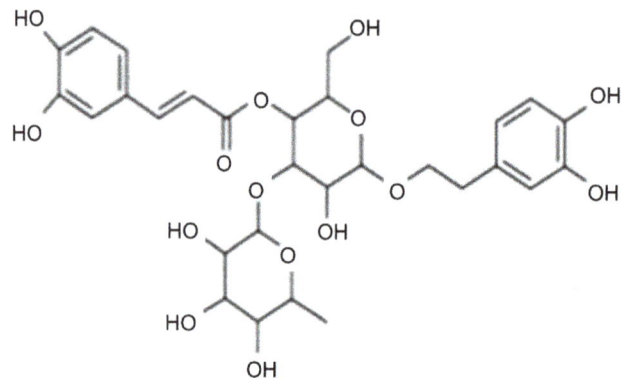

Figure 1. Verbascoside compound isolated from *Veronica officinalis.*

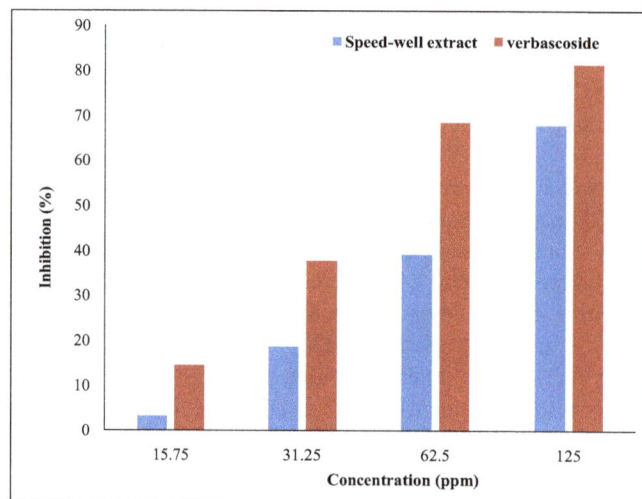

Figure 2. Antioxidant (DPPH free radical scavenging) activity in dose dependent manner exhibited by ethanolic extract of Speed-Well and the isolated compound Verbascoside.

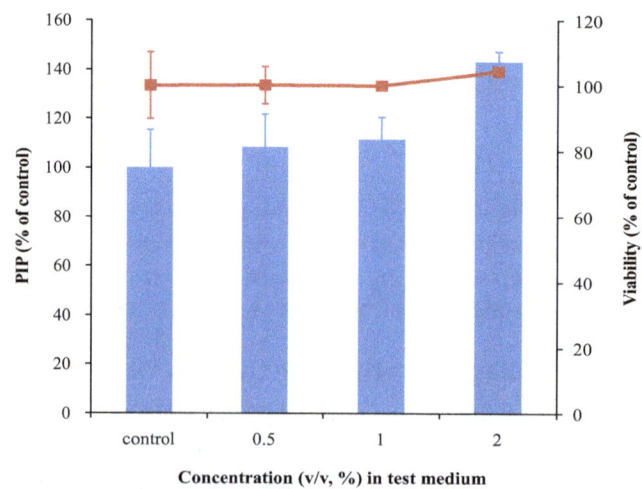

Figure 3. Pro Collagen type 1 protein synthesis test and cell viability test (MTT assay) in fibroblast cell shown by ethanolic extract of Speedwell.

3.3. Human Clinical Study

We examined the effect of topical formulated Scoti-speedwell cream on the wrinkles of crow's feet site of the eyes (**Figure 4**). The wrinkle area and length difference at the base line were analyzed to identify the differences at sample treated sites. Treatment with formulated cream for 28 days did not show any significant difference with the placebo. However, treatment for 56 days reduced significantly the percentage of wrinkle area (**Figure 5**) and wrinkle length (**Figure 6**) by 18.0% and 16.05% respectively compared with the placebo. The dermatological scores of the sides treated by the extract containing cream decreased significantly on 56 days with 66% lower than that of placebo treatment (**Figure 7**).

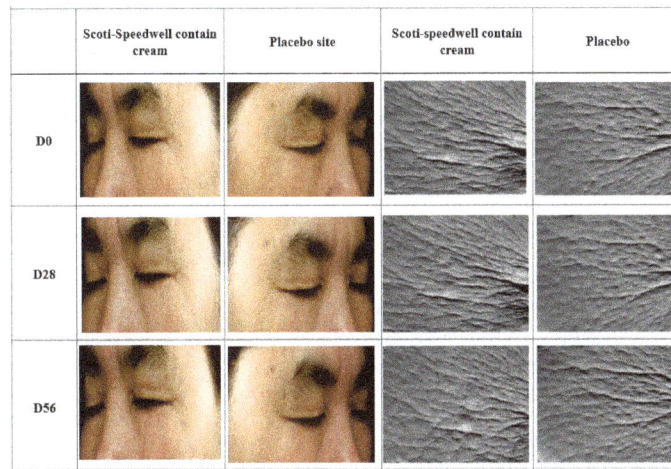

Figure 4. Photograph showing the images of wrinkles used for assessment of wrinkle area and length in the crow's feet region of the subject's eyes treated with 2% topically formulated Scoti-Speedwell extract and placebo treated for 56 days. Clinical evaluations and measurements were performed on D0 (before treatment), D28 and D56.

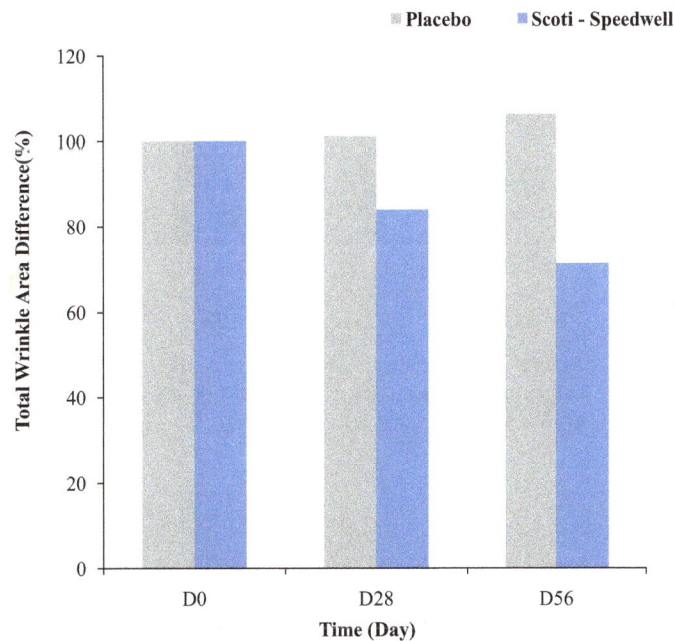

Figure 5. Differences in the wrinkle area after the treatment of topical formulated Scoti-speedwell cream or the placebo randomly on crow's feet region of eyes.

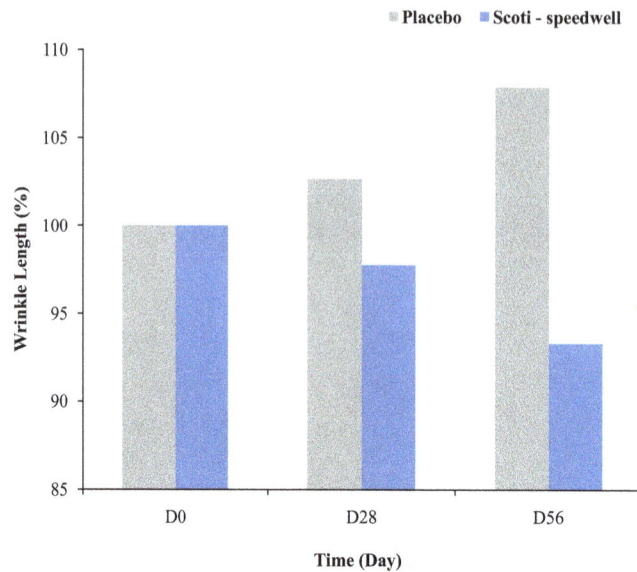

Figure 6. Differences in the wrinkle length after the treatment of topical formulated Scoti-speedwell cream or the placebo randomly on crow's feet region of eyes.

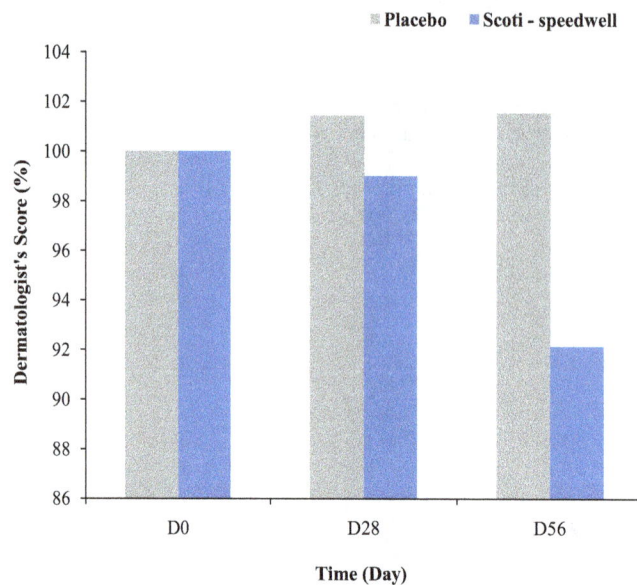

Figure 7. Differences in the visual score after the treatment of topical formulated Scoti-speedwell cream or the placebo randomly on crow's feet region of eyes.

4. Discussion

The speedwell extract showed significant anti-wrinkle activity *in vivo*. This could be due to the presence of higher radical scavenging activity of speed well extract which quenched the free radicals from the skin and thereby protected the collagen from degradation. And also, the phytochemicals present in the extract may have possible interactions with the special enzymes, mediators in the signal transduction pathway and thereby initiate the anti-wrinkle effects on skin [3]. Overall, *Veronica officinalis* extract containing product (Scoti-speedwell™) can be regarded as a potent anti-wrinkle agent in human skin.

Acknowledgements

The authors gratefully acknowledge W. Lai (MD), Z. Y. Zhong (MD), and Y. Q. Zhang (MD) of Skin Research Center of Guangzhou Land proof and Department of Dermatology, The Third Affiliated Hospital of Sun Yat-sen University, Guanhzhou, Guangdong province, China, for conducting the *in vivo* research work. This study was funded by the company Naturalsolution. Co. Ltd., South Korea.

Conflict of Interest

There are no conflicts of interest.

References

[1]   Kim, H.H., Cho, S., Lee, S., Kim, K.H., Cho, K.H., Eun, H.C. and Chung, J.H. (2006) Photoprotective and Anti-Skin-Aging Effects of Eicosapentaenoic Acid in Human Skin *in Vivo*. *Journal of Lipid Research*, **47**, 921-930. http://dx.doi.org/10.1194/jlr.M500420-JLR200

[2]   Verschooten, L., Claerhout, S., Van Laethem, A., *et al.* (2006) New Strategies of Photoprotection. *Photochemistry and Photobiology*, **82**, 1016-1023. http://dx.doi.org/10.1562/2006-04-27-IR-884.1

[3]   http://www.luontoportti.com/suomi/en/kukkakasvit/heath-speedwell

[4]   Carsten, G., Manuel, G.K., Barbara, S., Evi, S., Mathias, K., Irmgard, M., Martin, Z. and Roman, H. (2013) Traditionally Used *Veronica officinalis* Inhibits Proinflammatory Mediators via the NF-κB Signaling Pathway in a Human Lung Cell Line. *Journal of Ethnophamacology*, **145**, 118-126. http://dx.doi.org/10.1016/j.jep.2012.10.039

[5]   Vogl, S., Picker, P., Mihaly-Bison, J., Fakhrudin, N., Atanasov, A.G., Heiss, E.H., Wawrosch, C., Reznicek, G., Dirsch, V.M., Saukel, J. and Kopp, B. (2013) Ethnopharmacological *in Vitro* Studies on Austria's Folk Medicine—An Unexplored Lore *in Vitro* Anti-Inflammatory Activities of 71 Austrian Traditional Herbal Drugs. *Journal of Ethnopharmacology*, **149**, 750-771. http://dx.doi.org/10.1016/j.jep.2013.06.007

[6]   Nikolova, M. (2011) Screening of Radical Scavenging Activity and Polyphenol Content of Bulgarian Plant Species. *Pharmacognosy Research*, **3**, 256-259. http://dx.doi.org/10.4103/0974-8490.89746

[7]   Rønsted, N., Gøbel, E., Franzyk, H., Jensen, S.R. and Olsen, C.E. (2000) Chemotaxonomy of Plantago. Iridoid Glucosides and Caffeoyl Phenylethanoids Glycosides. *Phytochemistry*, **55**, 337-348. http://dx.doi.org/10.1016/S0031-9422(00)00306-X

[8]   Schilling, G., Huegel, M. and Mayer, W. (1982) Verbascoside and Isoverbascoside from *Paulownia tomentosa* Steud. *Zeitschrift für Naturforschung B*, **37**, 1633-1635. http://dx.doi.org/10.1515/znb-1982-1227

[9]   Mosmann, T. (1983) Rapid Colorimetric Assay for Cellular Growth and Survival: Application to Proliferation and Cytotoxicity Assays. *Journal of Immunological Methods*, **65**, 55-63. http://dx.doi.org/10.1016/0022-1759(83)90303-4

[10]   Tanayama, N. and Terao, T. (1992) Relationship of Serum Levels of Pro-Type I Collagen Peptide, Pro-Type III Collagen Peptide and Type IV 7S Collagen with Cervical Maturation. *Gynecologic and Obstetric Investigation*, **34**, 24-26. http://dx.doi.org/10.1159/000292719

[11]   Braca, A., Tommasi, N.D., Bari, L.D., *et al.* (2001) Antioxidant Principles from Bauhinia Terapotensis. *Journal of Natural Products*, **64**, 892-895. http://dx.doi.org/10.1021/np0100845

[12]   Wagner, H. (2006) Multitarget Therapy—The Future of Treatment for More than Just Functional Dyspepsia. *Phytomed*, **13**, 122-129. http://dx.doi.org/10.1016/j.phymed.2006.03.021

[13]   Williamson, E.M. (2001) Synergy and Other Interactions in Phytomedicine. *Phytomed*, **8**, 401-409. http://dx.doi.org/10.1078/0944-7113-00060

[14]   Tanaka, T., Okada, T., Konishi, H., *et al.* (1993) The Effect of Reactive Oxygen Species on the Biosynthesis of Collagen and Glycosaminoglycans in Cultures Human Dermal Fibroblasts. *Archives of Dermatological Research*, **285**, 352-255. http://dx.doi.org/10.1007/BF00371836

3

Relationship between Dyeing Condition and Dyeability in Hair Colouring by Using Catechinone Prepared Enzymatically or Chemically from (+)-Catechin

Takanori Matsubara, Saina Taniguchi, Shota Morimoto, Asami Yano, Aritsugu Hara, Isao Wataoka, Hiroshi Urakawa, Hidekazu Yasunaga*

Department of Biobased Materials Science, Kyoto Institute of Technology, Kyoto, Japan
Email: *yasunaga@kit.ac.jp

Abstract

Hair colouring was carried out by using catechinone prepared from (+)-catechin by enzymatic or chemical oxidation reaction. The difference of dyeability between the catechinone produced by enzymatic reaction (EC) and that produced by chemical reaction (CC) was studied changing the dyeing condition such as dye concentration, dyeing temperature, pH or the sort and concentration of salts. The colour of the hair dyed by EC or CC at 30°C is yellowish or reddish brown, respectively. The colour of the hair dyed by EC and CC is deeper at a higher dye concentration and at a higher temperature. Hair is dyed deepest by EC or CC at the solution pH = 6.04 or 5.45, respectively. The dyeability is increased by adding NaCl (≤4 M) or CaCl$_2$ (≤1 M), while it is decreased by adding AlCl$_3$. The colour fastness of the dyed hair to washing or ultraviolet light is high enough for practical use. Furthermore, it was found that colourants are obtained from tea extracts which contain catechin derivatives. Hair is dyed reddish brown by the colourants.

Keywords

Catechinone, Hair Dyestuff, Catechin, Dyeability, Tea Extract

1. Introduction

The authors have studied hair dyeing by using biobased materials (obtained from natural materials) to invent novel hair dyeing techniques, which are milder and safer for a human body and eco-friendly, in order to reduce

---
*Corresponding author.

the risks accompanying hair dyeing. This is because sensitisation symptoms, dermatitides and systemic symptoms are caused for some people by the use of the oxidation hair dyes [1]-[4]. Then it was found that a dyestuff, catechinone [5], can dye human hair yellow, orange and reddish brown, and the colour of human hair can be controlled by adding biobased materials such as natural pigments and amino acids. Catechinone is obtained from enzymatic oxidation of (+)-catechin which is contained in tea or several plants. The acute skin irritation study according to the OECD Guidelines for the testing of chemicals exhibited that catechinone does not cause skin troubles. The colour fastness to washing or daylight for the hair dyed by catechinone is high enough for practical use. The mechanisms of hair dyeing by catechinone, *i.e.* the dynamics of catechinone in the hair network, catechinone behaviours at fixation and so on, have not been clarified, because the structure of hair is extremely-complex. However, it is envisaged that the interaction between the dyestuffs and hair dye-sites can be van der Waals force, hydrogen bonding and covalent bonding.

The catechinone is also produced by chemical reaction [6] [7]. The chemical preparation of catechinone requires enough O_2 and it should be made in a basic solution for increasing the yield. The enzymatic preparation system is more specific and total reaction rate is higher than that of the chemical preparation [8]. On the other hand, the chemical preparation of catechinone has the advantages that the production condition is not so strict as compared with the enzymatic technique and the technique is economical because of without enzymes.

In the paper, the relationships between dyeing conditions such as the dye concentration of catechinone, dyeing temperature, pH or the sort and concentration of salts added and the dyeability for hair were studied comparing the enzymatically-produced catechinone (EC) with the chemically-produced one (CC). Then, the colour fastness to washing and ultraviolet (UV) light for the hair dyed by catechinone (EC and CC) was investigated. Furthermore, the authors tried to prepare hair dyestuffs from tea extracts, which contain (+)-catechin and catechin derivatives, by the chemical oxidation method, and their dyeability to hair was examined.

2. Experimental

2.1. Materials

(+)-Catechin hydrate (M_w = 290.27, Sigma) and Polyphenon® 70S (Mitsui Norin) were used without further purification. Sunphenon® ECGg, BG-3 and 90S were kindly provided from Taiyo Kagaku and the powders were used as such. The Polyphenon and Sunphenons are the extracts of green tea leaf (*Camellia sinensis*) obtained in India and Kenya and in China, respectively. They contain catechins of high concentration as shown in **Table 1** [9]. Tyrosinase from mushroom (M_w = 1.28 × 10^5 obtained by sedimentation velocity diffusion, 1.33 × 10^5 by

Table 1. Composition of catechins in tea extracts [9].

Product name	Polyphenon	Sunphenon		
	70S	EGCg	BG-3	90S
Lot No.	1008271	207051	210041	207311
	Catechins content[a]/wt%			
(+)-Catechin	2.2	0.1	2.7	1.4
(−)-Epicatechin	7.5	0.6	7.9	4.5
(−)-Gallocatechin	6.6	-	4.6	2.3
(−)-Epigallocatechin	18.2	-	16.2	3.8
(−)-Catechin gallate	0.7	-	-	0.8
(−)-Epicatechin gallate	8.9	3.9	7.4	11.9
(−)-Gallocatechin gallate	4.1	0.3	2.7	7.5
(−)-Epigallocatechin gallate	32.0	92.1	51.2	46.8
Total catechin content[a]	80.2	96.8	92.6	78.9
Total polyphenol content[b]	/[c]	≈100	90.8	92.0

(a): Measured by HPLC. The hyphen (-) indicates not detected. (b): Analysed by iron tartrate colourimetric method. (c): Not analysed.

light-scattering measurements and 1.20×10^5 by electrophoresis, Sigma) was used as received. Monoethanol amine (MEA, $M_w = 61.08$, Nacalai tesque), disodium hydrogen phosphate (Na_2HPO_4, $F_w = 141.96$, Nacalai) and sodium dihydrogen phosphate (NaH_2PO_4, $F_w = 119.98$, Nacalai) as pH regulators were used without further purification. Water was used after distillation and ethanol ($M_w = 46.07$, 99.5%, Nacalai) was used without further purification.

The human hair samples (Mathai Japan, obtained from Asians and decolourised white, length: 11 cm) were bundled by a nylon band and kept under a low humidity. Citric acid (CA, $M_w = 192.12$, Nacalai), hydrochloric acid (HCl, 35.0 - 37.0 wt%, $M_w = 36.46$, Nacalai), sodium hydroxide (NaOH, $F_w = 40.00$, Nacalai), sodium chloride (NaCl, $F_w = 58.44$, Nacalai), calcium chloride ($CaCl_2$, $F_w = 110.98$, Nacalai) and aluminium chloride hexahydrate ($AlCl_3 \cdot 6H_2O$, $F_w = 241.43$, Nacalai) were used without further purification. p-Aminophenol (PAP, $M_w = 109.13$, Katayama Chemical Industries) as an oxidation dye precursor, 5-amino-o-cresol (5AOC, $M_w = 123.16$, Tokyo Chemical Industry) as an oxidation dye coupler and ammonia solution (28 wt%, Nacalai) as a pH regulator were used without further purification. Hydrogen peroxide aqueous solution (H_2O_2, 30 wt%, $M_w = 34.01$, Santoku Chemical Industries) as an oxidising agent was diluted 5 times with distilled water. Kao Blaune Hair Manicure D13 (colour name: tea brown) was used as a commercially available acid dye, which contains orange II (C.I. 15510, C.I. Acid Orange 7), naphtol blue black (C.I. 20470, C.I. Acid Black 1), acid red (C.I. 45100, C.I. Acid Red 52) and fast acid magenta (C.I. 17200, C.I. Acid Red 33). NLES-227 (Taiko Oil Chemicals) that contains 27 wt% of sodium dodecyloxypolyoxyethylene ($n = 2$) sulphate ($C_{12}H_{25}O$ ($CH_2CH_2O)_2$ SO_3Na) was used as anionic detergent for washing hair.

2.2. Dyestuff Preparation

2.2.1. Enzymatic Oxidation Method

The dyestuff preparation was started by adding 5 ml of tyrosinase (32 kU) phosphate buffer aqueous solution (0.1 M NaH_2PO_4/Na_2HPO_4, pH = 7.0) into 495 ml of (+)-catechin (2.4 mmol) aqueous solution, which was saturated with oxygen by introducing O_2 gas ($\geq$ 99.5 vol%) for over 20 min at 30°C. The concentration of (+)-catechin in the aqueous reaction solution was 4.8 mM. The reaction was performed under O_2 atmosphere at 30°C, and 200 ml of ethanol was finally added into the reaction solution to stop the reaction. The reaction solution was filtered and the filtrate was evaporated at 50°C under below 50 hPa to obtain the powder of catechinone dye. The enzymatically-produced catechinone is abbreviated again here as EC.

2.2.2. Chemical Oxidation Method

The 100 g of (+)-catechin (0.17 $mol \cdot kg^{-1}$) solution was prepared by using MEA (0.10 $mol \cdot kg^{-1}$) water/ethanol mixed solution. The ethanol mass fraction (w_E) and the molar fraction (x_E) in the mixed solution were 0.50 and 0.28, respectively. The reaction was set off by introducing O_2 gas into the (+)-catechin solution at 100 ml min^{-1} of flow rate at 30°C. The solution was finally concentrated and then the resulting solid was ground to get catechinone dye powder. The chemically-produced catechinone is also abbreviated as CC.

2.2.3. Colourants from Commercial Tea Extracts

The colourant preparation from four kinds of tea extracts was carried out by the chemical oxidation method. Polyphenon 70S, Sunphenon EGCg, BG-3 or 90S was dissolved in MEA (0.50 $mol \cdot kg^{-1}$) water/ethanol solution ($w_E = 0.45$, $x_E = 0.25$). O_2 gas was introduced to 100 g of 5.0 wt% tea extract solution at 30°C, and then the solution was finally evaporated to obtain powder.

2.3. Hair Dyeing

The bleached white hair (0.5 g or 1.0 g) was immersed into the dye solution (50 ml or 100 ml) containing fixed amount of the colourant from (+)-catechin (EC, CC) or tea extract without or with salt (NaCl, $CaCl_2$ or $AlCl_3$), and the solutions were shaken at 100 rpm of shaking speed for 40 min at 30°C, 40°C, 50°C, 60°C or 70°C. The pH of the dyeing solution of EC or CC was adjusted by the addition of HCl and NaOH or citric acid, respectively. The dyed hair was washed with 0.27 - 0.81 wt% sodium dodecyloxypolyoxyethylene ($n = 2$) sulphate aqueous solution prepared from NLES-227 and rinsed with distilled water repeatedly at 30°C or 40°C. The hair was air-dried at room temperature.

In the oxidation dyeing, PAP (1.4 mmol), 5AOC (1.4 mmol) and ammonia (59 mmol) aqueous solution (50 g) and H_2O_2 (88 mmol) aqueous solution (50 g) were mixed, and then 0.5 g of hair was immersed into the mixed solution and it was shaken at 100 rpm at 30°C for 40 min. In the dyeing by acid dye, the viscous dye solution was applied to the bundled hair by using a comb and the hair was allowed to stand at room temperature for 20 min. The dyed hairs were washed with 300 ml of distilled water with shaking at 100 rpm and 30°C for 20 min repeatedly and were air-dried.

2.4. Measurements

The colour of hair was measured by a Konica Minolta CM-2600d spectrocolourimeter and the resulting colour was expressed in $L^*a^*b^*$ standard colourimetric system (CIE 1976). The colour measurements were made employing 10°-view angle, CIE standard illuminant D_{65} and SCI mode. All the reflection light from the sample including the regular reflection are integrated under the SCI mode. The L^* is the lightness index, and a^* and b^* are the chromaticity coordinates. The positive values of a^* indicate red and the negative values of that indicate green, and the positive values of b^* indicate yellow and the negative values indicate blue. The C^* is the chroma calculated by $C^* = \{(a^*)^2 + (b^*)^2\}^{1/2}$. The measurements of the ultraviolet-visible (UV-Vis) absorption spectra for the dyestuff aqueous solution were made by a Hitachi U-3900H spectrophotometer at 25°C. The degree of swelling of hair (q) is calculated by $q = m_s/m_d$, where m_s and m_d are the mass of the swollen and dried hair, respectively. The m_s and m_d were measured by a Mettler Toledo HG53 halogen moisture analyser at 120°C for 15 min.

The colour fastness was estimated by the colour difference, ΔE^*, for the dyed hair between before and after repeatedly washed, or the colour difference for the hair between before and after under UV irradiation. The ΔE^* is calculated by $\Delta E^* = \{(L^*_t - L^*_i)^2 + (a^*_t - a^*_i)^2 + (b^*_t - b^*_i)^2\}^{1/2}$ where L^*_t, a^*_t, b^*_t, L^*_i, a^*_i, b^*_i are L^*, a^*, b^* of treated (washed or UV irradiated) and freshly-dyed hair, respectively. In the experiments for colour fastness to washing, the dyed hair was washed with 0.27 wt% sodium dodecyloxypolyoxyethylene ($n = 2$) sulphate aqueous solution at 30°C for 20 min, rinsed twice with distilled water at 30°C for 20 min and dried by a Yamato Scientific DN400 constant temperature oven at 45°C for 1 h. The colour was measured by the spectrocolourimeter after every washing. The experiments for colour fastness to UV light for the dyed hair was made by using a Sen Lights HL100G high-pressure mercury lamp. The intensity of the light was 20.0 mW·cm^{-2} at 254 nm, 11.0 mW·cm^{-2} at 310 nm and 9.8 mW·cm^{-2} at 365 nm. The irradiation was performed for 10 h under ambient humidity. The colour was measured in the same way at each irradiation time.

3. Results and Discussion

3.1. Dyeability of EC and CC

Catechinone is prepared by both of the enzymatic oxidation in aqueous solution and the chemical oxidation in water/ethanol solution. The amount of the formed dye by the chemical method is over 20 times higher than that by enzymatic method, for the higher concentration of (+)-catechin in the water/ethanol reaction solution. However, the yield of catechinone by enzymatic preparation is 1.4 times higher than that by chemical preparation. The UV-Vis absorption spectra of EC and CC aqueous solution are approximately same but parts of the spectrum, especially at short wavelength (UV region), are little different. Both of the dyestuffs consist of catechinone (4-(3,4-dihydro-3α,5,7-trihydroxy-2H-1-benzopy-ran-2α-yl) 1,2-benzoquinone) chiefly and contain by-products [5]. The by-products are dimers, trimers and multimers, of which oxidised parts and their degrees are various. The results indicate that the EC and CC consist chiefly of catechinone and they may be different in the species and composition of the small amounts of by-products. The enzymatic oxidation reaction is specific and its rate is higher. Meanwhile, the chemical one proceeds longer under basic condition although the rate is lower than that of the enzymatic one [6] [8].

Figure 1 shows the photographs of undyed and dyed hair with EC or CC solution. The hair is coloured by both the catechinones, and the colour of EC-dyed-hair is more yellowish and vivid, while that of CC-dyed-hair is reddish brown and deeper.

The hair samples differ a little in the dyeability depending on the production lot, because the samples are human hair and, strictly speaking, no two are ever the same. Two kinds of hair differing in the lot, of which dyeability was slightly different, were used for the experiments. One was hair sample used for EC and another was for CC. Therefore, attention was focused on the tendency of the change in values of colour depending upon dyeing condition for each sample dyed by EC or CC rather than the absolute values.

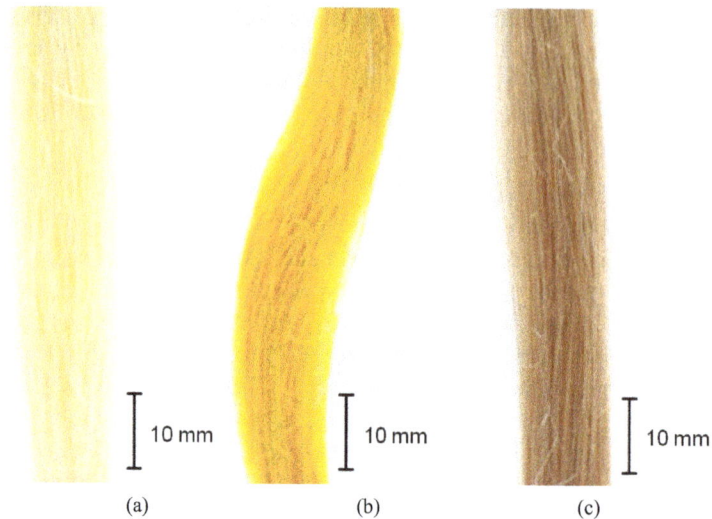

Figure 1. Photographs of the part of undyed hair (a), and hair dyed with catechinone produced by enzymatic method (EC; (b)) and chemical method (CC, (c)). The dye concentration was 1.0 wt%.

The measured colour data expressed in chromaticity coordinates and in chroma-lightness index as a function of the dye concentration (c_D) are shown in **Figure 2**. The colour of the hair dyed by EC becomes more yellowish and reddish, and the a^* and b^* increase with c_D. On the other hand, the colour obtained by CC becomes more dull, and the a^* and b^* decrease gradually with c_D. The colour of the hair dyed by both catechinones is deeper at higher c_D and the L^* decreases with c_D. The change in the colour with c_D becomes gradual for 0.60 wt% and over of EC or 1.0 wt% and over of CC. The results show that the dyeability and the tendency of the variation in the colour with the dye concentration for CC are different from those for EC. The catechinone obtained by enzymatic method consists of mainly 4-(3,4-dihydro-3α,5,7-trihydroxy-2H-1-benzopyran-2α-yl) and by-products [5]. Then the results indicate the difference in the dyestuff composition for EC and CC. In fact, the enzymatic oxidation reaction is specific, whereas the chemical one is not so specific and the preparation time is longer [6].

3.2. Effect of Dyeing Temperature

The heating effect on the dyeability of hair by catechinone was investigated in order to shorten the dyeing time. The colour of hair dyed by EC and CC at 30°C - 70°C for 40 min was measured.

The colour of hair dyed by 0.60 wt% and over of EC is about the same, and the same for 1.0 wt% and over of CC. Therefore, 0.6 wt% of EC and 1.0 wt% of CC were adopted in the temperature effect experiments taking into account also the little different dyeability of each hair sample as described above.

The results obtained by observation with the naked eye show that the colour of hair dyed by both of the EC and CC becomes deeper with an increase in the dyeing temperature. It was found that the dyeability for hair by using both of the EC and CC solution increases with increasing temperature, and the dyeing time required decreases. **Figure 3** shows the L^*, a^* and b^* for the hair dyed by EC or CC for 40 min as a function of the dyeing temperature (T). The data values obtained at 30°C differ a little from the values shown in **Figure 2**. This was caused by the variation of the dyeability of hair samples.

The L^* for the EC- and CC-dyed hair decreases with T. The a^* slightly increases with T up to 50°C and it decreases over 50°C for EC-dyed hair. The changing behaviour of a^* for CC-dyed hair is similar to that for EC-dyed one though the magnitude of the change at lower temperatures is larger than that at higher temperature. The b^* for EC- and CC-dyed hair decreases monotonously with T. It can be said that dyeability for hair by both of the EC and CC solution increases with increasing temperature up to 70°C.

The higher temperature is favourable for accelerating the dyestuff molecules diffusion in a diffusion medium (here this is hair) and depresses dye adsorption onto dye-sites and the fixation in general. However, the amount of catechinone dye molecules fixed on hair has not determined and dyeing process has not clarified. It can be said at least that the dyestuff molecules diffusion dominates the dyeability for the catechinone hair dyeing sys-

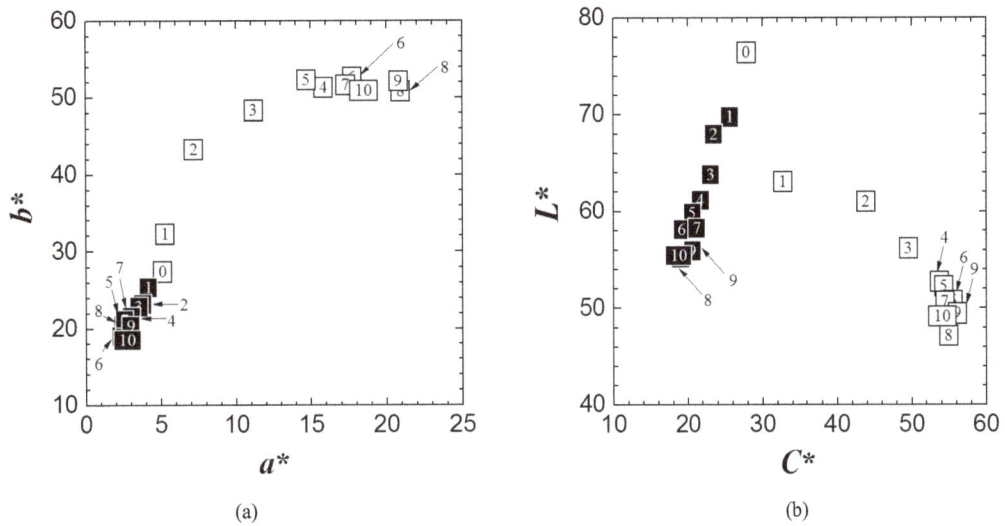

Figure 2. Chromaticity coordinates (a) and chroma-lightness index (b) relationships for hair dyed by EC at 30°C for 40 min (□) and that dyed by CC (■), and undyed one (0). The dye concentration (c_D) is 0.10 (1), 0.15 (2), 0.30 (3), 0.60 (4), 0.80 (5), 1.0 (6), 1.2 (7), 1.5 (8), 1.8 (9) or 2.0 (10) wt%. The numbers in the round brackets correspond with those in the figures.

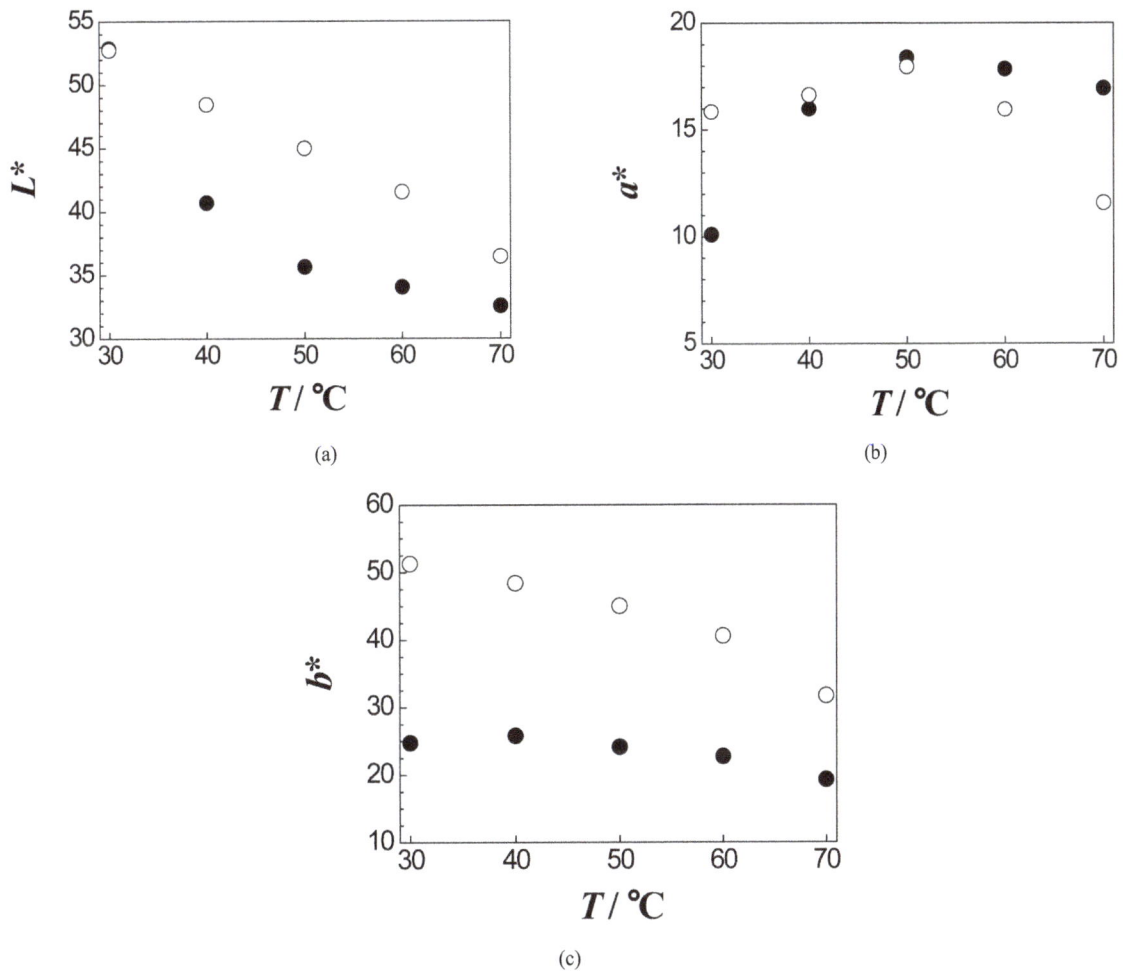

Figure 3. Dyeing temperature (*T*) dependence of the L^*(a), a^*(b) and b^*(c) for hair dyed by 0.60 wt% EC solution (○) or 1.0 wt% CC solution (●) for 40 min.

tem under the conditions. The obtained results, however, show the higher temperature is favourable for obtaining higher dyeability in a shorter time and for rapid dyeing from the practical point of view. A local heating technique, for example, may be required to realise the practical dyeing.

On the other hand, the variation of a^* for the EC and CC system is not monotonously. The colour change of dye solution during dyeing hair at higher temperature was observed. This indicates an alteration of dye molecules caused by heating. Then it was examined whether the dyestuff is altered by heating.

The results obtained from CC are presented here and **Figure 4** shows the absorption spectra of its aqueous solution. The signal intensity of the absorption spectrum increases with the rise in temperature. New signals do not appear during the development of the spectrum with temperature and the shape undergoes very little change in appearance. The temperature change in the spectra of EC is similar to that of CC. The results meant that the colourant in aqueous solution is increased by heating. The prepared catechinone dyestuff contains colourless materials such as unreacted (+)-catechin. Removing them from the dye powder and purification are difficult because the solubility and molecular weight of (+)-catechin are very close to those of catechinone. The unreacted (+)-catechin is oxidised further at higher temperature to give catechinone because of the dye solution was exposed to air during the measurement procedure and the dyeing process. The formation of coloured dimers or other coloured multimers in the solution at higher temperature may also be assumed. The formation can affect the dyeing results.

3.3. Effect of Dyeing pH

The dye solution pH is thought to be important factor for hair dyeing. Because the degree of swelling of hair and electric charge of the hair protein vary according to the pH and this may affect the dyestuff penetration into/ diffusion in hair and dyestuff fixation. Moreover, the aggregation state of dye molecules in solution may also depend upon the pH. Then the effect of the pH of dyeing solution on the dyeability of hair dyed by catechinone was investigated. The solubility of CC in each the dyeing solution of which pH is different is lower than that of EC. Then the pH-effect experiments for CC were made at higher temperature (50°C) than those for EC (30°C). The results obtained by visual observation show the colour of the hair dyed by EC is yellowish and this is almost same at pH = 1.83 - 6.04. The colour of hair dyed at pH = 6.04 by EC is deepest, and the hair is poorly dyed at pH = 8.38. Meanwhile, CC dyes hair reddish brown at pH = 4.09 - 7.48, and the colour is deepest at pH = 5.45.

Figure 5 shows the relationships between the pH and the resulting colour of hair dyed by EC or CC. The dye concentration of EC or CC was set to 0.6 or 1.0 wt% for the same reason described above. The dyeability of EC cannot be compared with that of CC in absolute terms. Here, only the tendency of each change with pH should be focused.

The L^* may take minimum and the a^* reach maximum between pH = 3 and pH = 6 for hair dyed by EC. Its b^* decreases with an increase in pH. On the other hand, the results for CC system show that L^* of the dyed hair

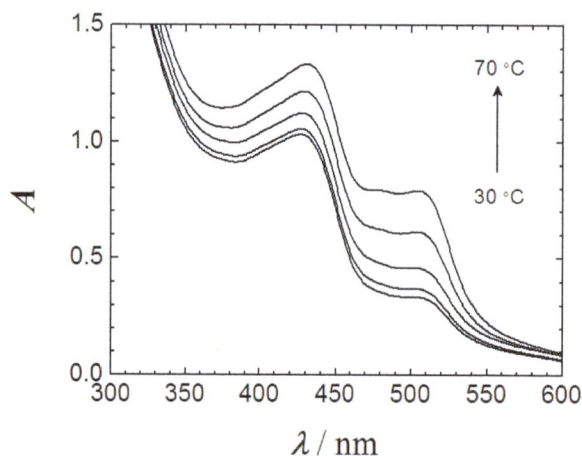

Figure 4. Absorption spectra of 0.025 wt% CC aqueous solution. The temperature of the solution was raised from 30°C to 40°C, 50°C, 60°C and 70°C with being stirred.

(a)

(b)

(c)

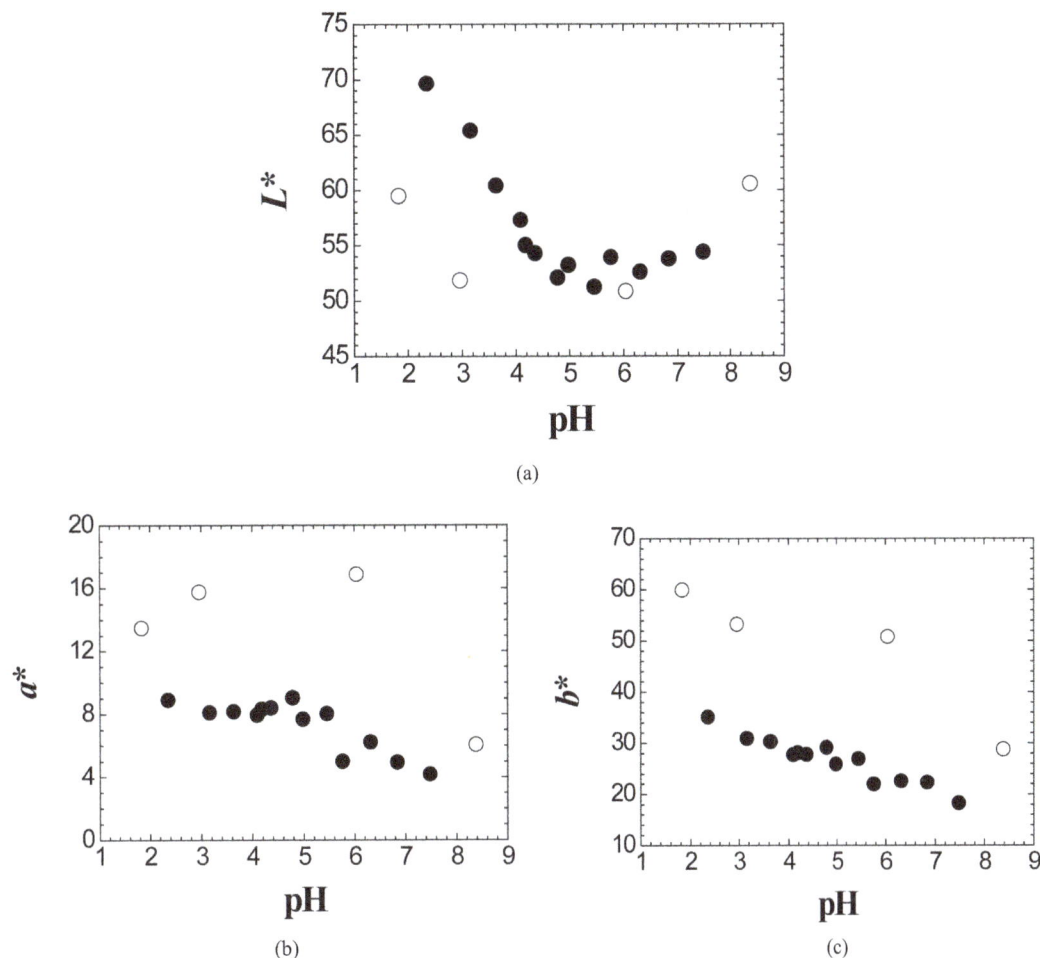

Figure 5. Relationships between pH of the dye solution and L^* (a), a^* (b) or b^* (c) for the hair dyed by 0.60 wt% EC solution at 30°C for 40 min (○) or 1.0 wt% CC solution at 50°C for 30 min (●).

decreases with increasing pH from 2.32, takes minimum at pH = 5.45 and increases slightly from pH = 5.45 and over. Its a^* decreases with increasing pH from 5.45 and b^* decreases monotonously with an increase in pH.

Subsequently, the relationship between the solution pH and the degree of swelling of hair was studied in order to clarify the mechanism of the pH effect on the dyeing. **Figure 6** shows the degree of swelling of hair (q) in CC solution against the solution pH. The q is high at pH = 3.00 - 3.20 and 6.50 - 7.10. The isoionic and isoelectric points of human hair were evaluated as 5.6 - 6.2 [10] and 3.67 [11], respectively. Therefore, the q of hair can be low approximately between pH = 3.7 and 6.2 because of the low electric interaction among hair proteins. The q takes minimum at pH $\approx$ 4 in fact as shown in **Figure 6**. The q decreases at very low and high pH and takes low values. The pH of the dyeing solution was controlled by using HCl and NaOH or citric acid, and the ionic strength for each of the solution was not adjusted. It can be thought that the decrease in the degree of swelling of hair at the very low and high pH is caused by the high ionic strength in the solution. The high ionic strength shields the electric charge repulsion among the hair protein and the hair network shrinks. The experimental results of pH-q relationship do not show clear correlation with the relationship between pH and the dyeability as seen in the Figures, although the L^* minimum appears near at the isoionic point of hair. Therefore, the pH dependence of the dyeability is not explained by the variation of q. Further investigation should be made to clarify the pH effect on the catechinone dyeability.

3.4. Effect of Added Salts

It is well known that salts play important role in dyeing of charged fibres such as wool [12]. Here, the effect of

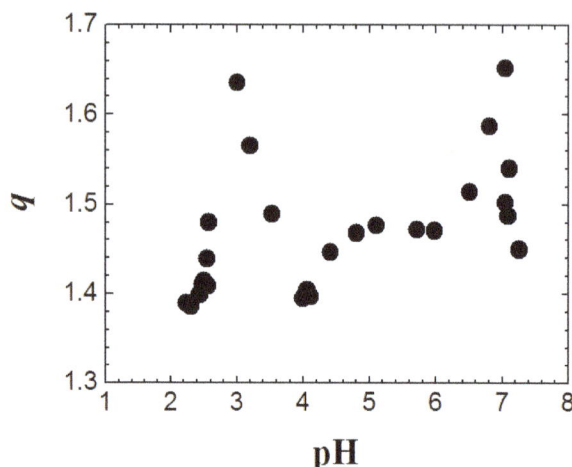

Figure 6. Relationship between solution pH and the swelling ratio of hair (q) in 1.0 wt% CC aqueous solution.

the addition of sodium chloride, calcium chloride or aluminium chloride on the dyeing by CC at 70°C and at pH = 6.7 - 7.5 was studied. The colour of the hair dyed with NaCl is deepest at c_S = 1.0 M, and it is deepest for CaCl$_2$ at c_S = 0.050 M, while it becomes paler with an increase in c_S for AlCl$_3$ in naked-eye observation. **Figure 7** shows the colour values of hair dyed with each the salt as a function of the salt concentration (c_S). The L^* of dyed hair decreases on addition of a small amount of NaCl ($c_S \leq$ 1.0 M) or CaCl$_2$ ($c_S \leq$ 0.050 M), and it increases on addition of AlCl$_3$. The a^* increases on addition of NaCl or CaCl$_2$ ($c_S \leq$ 0.5 M). The hair has negative charge as a whole in the CC solution of pH = 6.7 - 7.5 and the hydroxylphenyl groups of catechinone dissociate a little to give negative charge. The results that the addition of smaller amount of NaCl and CaCl$_2$ increases the dyeability and the addition of larger amount of salts reduces the dyeability are consistent with the negative charge state of hair and catechinone dyestuff and the shielding effect of salts. Furthermore, catechinone becomes insoluble in the solution with NaCl of $c_S \geq$ 2.0 M or with CaCl$_2$ of $c_S \geq$ 1.0 M. The shielding effect of Ca^{2+} is higher than that of Na$^+$ for the larger positive charge. The charge of Al^{3+} may be too large to promote the dyeability.

It is concluded that the addition of a small amount of NaCl or CaCl$_2$ are most effective and practical to improve the dyeability in the dyeing conditions (temperature, pH and salt addition) by comparing **Figure 3**, **Figure 5** and **Figure 7**.

3.5. Colour Fastness to Washing and UV Light

Colour fastness of hair dyed by catechinone to washing and UV light is important property for practical hair dyeing. The colour fastness of hair dyed by catechinone to washing was first examined comparing with that of hair dyed by other colourants. The colours of the hair dyed by EC, CC, an oxidation dye (PAP + 5AOC) or an acid dye are dark brownish orange, dark yellowish orange, dark reddish brown or dark reddish brown, respectively. The colour of hair dyed by each the method was not same because adjusting the colour of hair samples is not easy the important point is the comparison of the difference in the colour change.

Figure 8 shows the change in the colour difference (ΔE^*) between unwashed and washed hair dyed by each the method, as a function of number of washing (n). The ΔE^* of the hair dyed by the oxidation dye increases finally by approximately 6 with n and ΔE^* for the acid dye increases to a great extent. In contrast, the ΔE^* of the hair dyed by EC or CC at both temperatures increases by 12 - 15. However, the ΔE^* for EC and CC systems changes very slightly for $n > 6$. The change in colour is very small for visual observation. The results demonstrate that the hair dyed by EC or CC has sufficient colour fastness to washing for practical purposes.

Figure 9 shows the change in the ΔE^* between unirradiated and UV-irradiated hair dyed by each the method, as a function of UV irradiation time (t). The ΔE^* of the hair dyed by the oxidation dye or the acid dye increases with t, and it is about 6 or 9 at t = 10 h, respectively. The change in the ΔE^* of the hair dyed by EC or CC are almost as same as that of the hair dyed by the oxidation dye or the acid dye.

However, the changing behaviours of ΔE^* for [the EC and CC system] and [the oxidation and acid dyes sys-

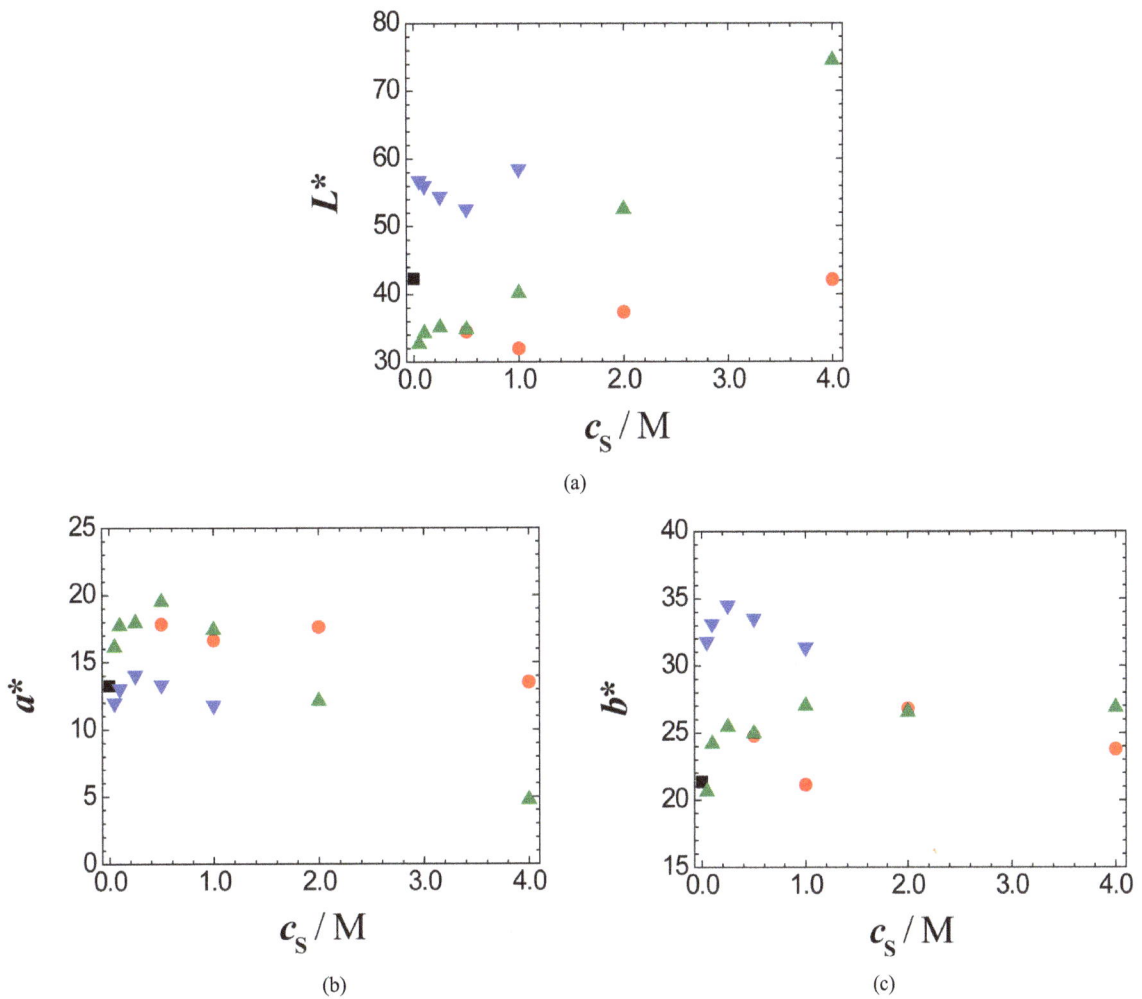

Figure 7. Change in L^* (a), a^* (b) and b^* (c) for the hair dyed by 1.0 wt% CC solution at 70˚C with NaCl (●), CaCl$_2$ (▲) or AlCl$_3$ (▼) as a function of the salt concentration (c_S). The black-closed square (■) indicates the colour values for hair dyed without salt.

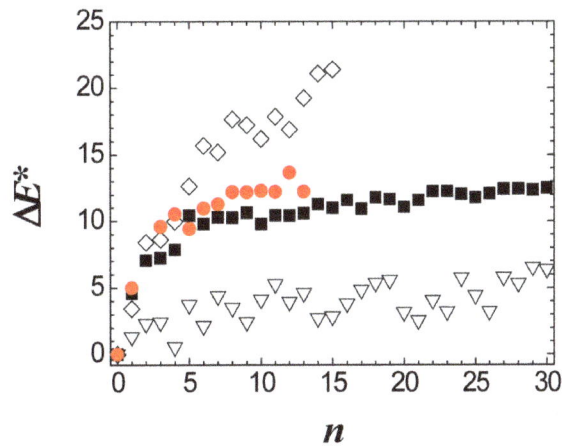

Figure 8. Change in colour difference (ΔE^*) of hair dyed by EC (■; $T = 30$˚C), CC (●; $T = 30$˚C), oxidation dye (▽; $T = 30$˚C) or acid dye (◇; room temp.) as a function of number of washing (n). The initial value at $n = 0$ means the value of the hair washed once after dyeing.

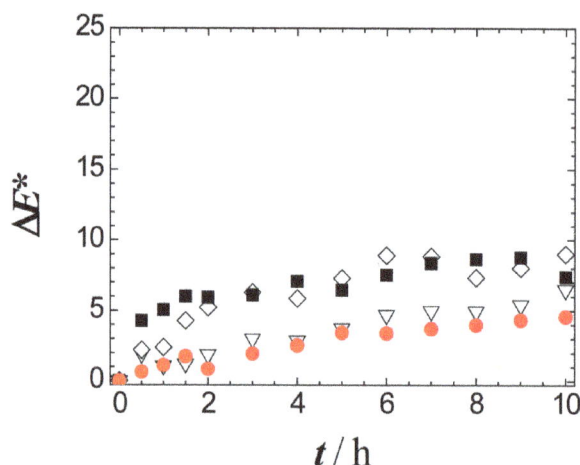

Figure 9. Change in ΔE^* of hair dyed by EC (■; $T = 30°C$), CC (●; $T = 30°C$), oxidation dye (∇; $T = 30°C$) or acid dye ($\diamond$; room temp.) as a function of UV irradiation time (t).

tem] are different. The time change in L^* of hair dyed by each the method under UV irradiation is shown in **Figure 10**. While L^* for the oxidation and acid dyes system increases monotonously with t, L^* for the EC and CC system decreases until $t = 8$ h. The results demonstrate that the hair dyed by the oxidation or acid dye only discolours by UV irradiation, whereas it dyed by EC or CC is coloured further and turns darker by the UV.

The results indicate that the hair dyed by EC or CC has enough high colour fastness to UV light. In addition, the colour fastness to visible light for the hair dyed by catechinone is also enough high [5]. Therefore, it can be said that catechinone has practical colour fastness to daily light including sunshine. Furthermore, the colour-changing into deeper for the hair dyed by EC or CC under UV irradiation is a special property of catechin. This is thought to be caused by the further progress of oxidation of (+)-catechin attaching hair with UV light.

3.6. Dyestuff Formation from Tea Extracts and Its Dyeability

It is important for the practical production of hair dyestuffs to prepare them from a massive amount of low materials. It was found that colourants are also prepared by the chemical oxidation method from four commercial tea extracts, which contain (+)-catechin and other catechin derivatives. Then, hair dyeing by using the colourants obtained from tea extracts was next examined and the high dyeing temperature (70°C) was adopted at first. The resulting colour of hair samples expressed in $L^*a^*b^*$ colourimetry, which are dyed by the obtained colourants from the tea extracts is summarised in **Table 2**. The results show that hair can be dyed by the dyestuffs obtained from tea extracts. The dyeability of them is somewhat lower than that of CC. The dyeability of the colourants prepared from Polyphenon 70S and Sunphenon BG-3 is relatively higher among them and the results imply that the dyeability depends on the composition of catechins in the tea extracts. The Polyphenon 70S and Sunphenon BG-3, which contain non-gallate catechins at a higher rate, give dyestuffs showing higher dyeability as shown in **Table 1** and **Table 2**. The non-gallate catechins such as (+)-catechin, (−)-epicatechin, (−)-gallocatechin and (−)-epigallocatechin may be profitable to obtain efficient dyestuffs. In addition, hair dyestuffs are obtained also by enzymatic oxidation of the tea extracts.

The hair dyeing by using organic compounds such as mulberry fruits, alizarin, curcumin and juglone was also tried [13]. The dyeability of the compounds is not enough high and then benzyl alcohol and 2-propernol were added to promote the dyeability. Longer dyeing time is required for mulberry fruits as 12 h at 25°C and the dyeing time is 30 min for other organic compounds. The colour fastness to washing or light for the dyed hair samples was not reported. On the other hand, guaiacol, acetosyringone, vanillic acid, syringic acid, gallic acid, homovanillyl alcohol, p-coumaric acid, vanillin, syringaldehyde, acetovanillone, ferulic acid, catechinand etc. were treated by laccase and used to dye hair [14]. Hair is dyed various colour by mixing a couple of the phenolic compounds. It takes 22 h to dye hair at 28°C. The change in colour of hair samples dyed by gallic acid + syringic acid, ferulic acid + syringic acid orcatechin + catechol was reported to be negligible up to three times of washing.

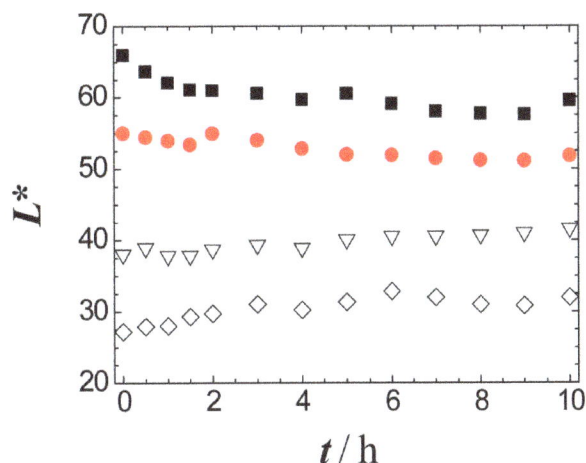

Figure 10. Change in L^* of hair dyed by EC (■; T = 30°C), CC (●; T = 30°C), oxidation dye (∇; T = 30°C) or acid dye (◇; room temp.) as a function of t.

Table 2. The colourimetric values for undyed and dyed hairs.

Sample hair dyed with	undyed	CC	dyestuffs from Polyphenon 70S	dyestuffs from Sunphenon EGCg	dyestuffs from Sunphenon BG-3	dyestuffs from Sunphenon 90S
L^*	70.8	33.3	49.2	53.4	42.7	55.7
a^*	4.47	14.5	10.7	4.54	8.77	4.01
b^*	25.8	19.3	22.7	18.8	20.0	19.3
C^*	26.2	24.1	25.1	19.3	21.9	19.7

Dyeing conditions: c_D = 1.0 wt%, T = 70°C and t = 40 min.

4. Conclusion

Catechinone is obtained from (+)-catechin by both the enzymatic and chemical oxidation method. Hair is dyed deeper red brown of the higher dye concentration, for longer dyeing time and at higher dyeing temperature. Hair is dyed darkest by EC at pH = 6.04 and by CC at pH = 5.45. A small amount of NaCl and $CaCl_2$ addition into the dye solution increases the dyeability. The colour fastness to washing and UV light for the hair dyed by catechinone is high enough for practical use. Hair dyestuff is obtained from commercially available tea extracts.

Acknowledgements

This study was financially supported partly by the Japan Society for the Promotion of Science Research Foundation Grant (No. 21500732), Japan Science and Technology Agency as Adaptable & Seamless Technology Transfer Program through Target-driven R&D (No. AS2211611E) and Kyoto Institute of Technology Venture Laboratory in VL Research Project 2012 Category I (No. I-01).

References

[1]   Corbett, J.F. (1976) Hair Dyes—Their Chemistry and Toxicology. *Cosmetics & Toiletries*, **91**, 21-28.

[2]   Bourgeois-Spinasse, J. (1981) Reactions to Hair Products. In: Orfanos, C.E., Montagna, W. and Stüttgen, G., Eds., *Hair Research: Status and Future Aspects, Proceedings of the First International Congress on Hair Research*, Hamburg, 13-16 March 1981, Springer-Verlag Berlin Heidelberg New York, 543-547. http://dx.doi.org/10.1007/978-3-642-81650-5_87

[3]   Søsted, H., Agner, T., Andersen, K.E. and Menné, T. (2002) 55 Cases of Allergic Reactions to Hair Dye: A Descriptive, Consumer Complaint-Based Study. *Contact Dermatitis*, **47**, 299-303. http://dx.doi.org/10.1034/j.1600-0536.2002.470508.x

[4]   Ishida, W., Makino, T. and Shimizu, T. (2011) Severe Hair Loss of the Scalp Due to a Hair Dye Containing Para Phenylenediamine. *ISRN Dermatology*, **2011**, 947284. http://dx.doi.org/10.5402/2011/947284

[5]   Yasunaga, H., Takahashi, A., Ito, K., Ueda, M. and Urakawa, H. (2012) Hair Dyeing by Using Catechinone Obtained from (+)-Catechin. *Journal of Cosmetics, Dermatological Sciences and Applications*, **2**, 158-163. http://dx.doi.org/10.4236/jcdsa.2012.23031

[6]   Matsubara, T., Wataoka, I., Urakawa, H. and Yasunaga, H. (2013) Effect of Reaction pH and $CuSO_4$ Addition on the Formation of Catechinone Due to Oxidation of (+)-Catechin. *International Journal of Cosmetic Science*, **35**, 362-367. http://dx.doi.org/10.1111/ics.12051

[7]   Matsubara, T., Wataoka, I., Urakawa, H. and Yasunaga, H. (2014) High-Efficient Chemical Preparation of Catechinone Hair Dyestuff by Oxidation of (+)-Catechin in Water/Ethanol Mixed Solution. *Sen'i Gakkaishi*, **70**, 19-22. http://dx.doi.org/10.2115/fiber.70.19

[8]   Yasunaga, H. (2011) Hair Dyeing Using Dyestuffs Obtained from Biobased Materials. *Proceedings of the 11th Asian Textile Conference*, Daegu, 1-4 November 2011, 85-90.

[9]   The Data Provided from Mitsui Norin Co. Ltd. and Taiyo Kagaku Co. Ltd.

[10] Freytag, H. (1964) Hautbewirkte Änderungen Der pH-Werte Wässriger Lösungen. *Journal of the Society of Cosmetic Chemists*, **15**, 265-279.

[11] Wilkerson, V.A. (1935) The Chemistry of Human Epidermis: II. The Isoelectric Points of the Stratum Corneum, Hair, and Nails as Determined by Electrophoresis. *The Journal of Biological Chemistry*, **112**, 329-335.

[12] Vickerstaff, T. (1954) The Physical Chemistry of Dyeing. 2nd Edition, Oliver and Boyd, London.

[13] Boga, C., Delpivo, C., Ballarin, B., Morigi, M., Galli, S., Micheletti, G. and Tozzi, S. (2013) Investigation on the Dyeing Power of Some Organic Natural Compounds for a Green Approach to Hair Dyeing. *Dyes and Pigments*, **97**, 9-18. http://dx.doi.org/10.1016/j.dyepig.2012.11.020

[14] Jeon, J.-R., Kim, E.-J., Murugesan, K., Park, H.-K., Kim, Y.-M., Kwon, J.-H., Kim, W.-G., Lee, J.-Y. and Chang, Y.-S. (2013) Laccase-Catalysed Polymeric Dye Synthesis from plant-Derived Phenols for Potential Application in Hair Dyeing: Enzymatic Colourations Driven by Homo- or Hetero-Polymer Synthesis. *Microbial Biotechnology*, **3**, 324-335. http://dx.doi.org/10.1111/j.1751-7915.2009.00153.x

Dead Sea Minerals-Induced Positive Stress as an Innovative Resource for Skincare Actives

Meital Portugal-Cohen[1,2*], Maria F. Dominguez[3], Miriam Oron[1,2], Robert Holtz[4], Ze'evi Ma'or[1,2]

[1]Ahava-Dead Sea Laboratories, Lod, Israel
[2]Dead Sea and Arava Science Center, The Laboratory for Skin Biochemistry and Biotechnology, Ein Gedi, Israel
[3]Lonza-Personal Care, South Plainfield, USA
[4]BioInnovation Laboratories Inc., Lakewood, USA
Email: [*]meital.p@ahava.com

Abstract

Objective: Exposure to certain stresses in small doses might lead to a protective effect by improving resistance to other stressors. Dead Sea (DS) minerals can be a relevant source to induce positive stress due to their high salinity and unique mineral combination. This concept could be further optimized using advanced unique cell biotechnology. The purpose of this study was to elucidate the innovative concept of DS minerals (water extract and black mud) supplementation in small amount to *Pichia pastoris* yeast growth media as a positive stress by testing the capability of accepted fermentation compounds to affect the appearance of skin. Methods: Skin equivalents were topically applied with different *Pichia pastoris* fermentations (Metabiotics™). Skin elasticity biomarkers were tested, since loss of elasticity and suppleness is a natural skin aging process leading to deeper wrinkles and loss of firmness. A preliminary screening at the gene level using DNA microarray was performed and subsequently, the following proteins were detected using ELISA or immunoblotting assays: elastin, fibulin-1, lysyl oxidase (LOX), metalloproteinase 3 (MMP-3), E-cadherin, claudin 4, tight junction protein (TJP)-1 and TJP-2. UVB irradiation was selected as a stressor. Results: Fermentation compounds generated in the presence of small doses of DS minerals affected the expression of various elasticity-related genes in skin. Moreover, they significantly attenuated the abnormal UVB-induced alterations, the proteins elastin, fibulin-1, LOX, MMP-3, E-cadherin and TJP-2. Conclusions: The observations clearly demonstrate that when DS Metabiotics™ compounds are topically applied, significant alterations in several biomarkers that contribute to skin elasticity occur. Thus, these novel compounds have the potential to serve as skincare actives.

---

[*]Corresponding author.

Keywords

Skin Elasticity Biomarkers, Skin Aging, Active Ingredients, Dead Sea Minerals, Positive Stress

1. Introduction

1.1. Positive Stress and Hormesis

Stressors, both endogenous and exogenous, are encountered constantly through an organism's life cycle. As a first line of defense against external insults, skin frequently works to protect itself and to effectively shield the internal tissues against threats such as, UV irradiation, free radicals attack and exposure to environmental agents. Over time, damage to the skin occurs, which leads to drastic changes in skin's integrity and to the activation of aging processes. Researchers from various scientific disciplines such as toxicology, medicine and cosmetology have studied the effects of skin exposure to various chemicals stressors at different concentrations at the tissue, organ and whole organism level [1]. Major advances have been made in screening and evaluation processes which help to determine more accurately the damaging effects of substance exposure (chemicals or other stressors) on skin health [2]. Following dose-response work, the phenomenon of "hormesis" was proposed, in which a damaging substance surprisingly elicited a positive effect when used in small concentrations [1]. Extensive research has been carried out exploring hormetic effects of a wide range of substances, ranging from antioxidants, to biological intermediates etc. [2].

1.2. Dead Sea Environment as a Positive Stressor

The Dead Sea (DS), although famous worldwide for its healing properties, is a stressful living environment: DS water and mud with their almost saturated natural salinity prevents organisms, such as fish and aquatic plants, from living in these conditions. At the same time, in spite of their living restrictions, it is known that DS water and mud can be therapeutic for different skin and arthritis disorders in moderate doses of exposure [3].

DS water, as compared to seawater, contains a tenfold concentration and an unusual composition of various cations; mainly magnesium, sodium, calcium, potassium and strontium. These metal cations are balanced with halogen anions mainly chlorides and bromides [4]. DS black mud, which contains antibacterial and hyperemic properties, is rich in minerals similarly to DS water [5]. The therapeutic properties of DS water and mud have been thoroughly investigated and published. Clinical studies demonstrate that DS water and mud contribute to a significant improvement in patients' symptoms of skin disorders, mainly psoriasis, atopic dermatitis, seborrheic dermatitis and vitiligo [6]-[8].

Recently, it has been demonstrated that photo-damage protective effects occur in human skin organ culture following exposure to DS water extract or DS mud at certain doses [9]-[12].

Due to its extreme and unusual conditions, it is well-known that the DS area contains unique flora and botanicals which have adaptogenic characteristics [4] [12]. This allows an organism to pre-adapt itself in a manner that contributes to its survival against various endogenous stressors (aging and different pathological processes) and exogenous stressors (extreme conditions such as radiation, temperature, dryness, etc.). Secondary metabolites consist of enzymes, vitamins, and various natural components are presented in the extract and can contribute to protection against various stressors [13]. Thus, here DS-induced stress has a positive effect by producing secondary metabolites enabling better coping with harsh environmental conditions. Indeed, DS region-originated botanical extracts, such as palm date (*Phoenix dactilifera*) extracts, *Dunaliella salina* green algae extract and Jujube (zyziphus) extracts, were reported to have beneficial skin healing effects.

1.3. Metabiotics™ Technique Using DS Minerals as a Positive Stress for *Pichia pastoris* Yeast Growth

DS water's and DS mud's potency to induce positive stress was assumed due to their high salinity, unique mineral combination and well established therapeutic effects. Based on hormesis concepts, we investigated how their positive stress could be further optimized using advanced unique cell biotechnology, Metabiotics™ (international patent application is WO2010/011885 A1). In this respect, DS water extract and DS mud were provided as nutrients in small doses for the yeast *Pichia pastoris* (*P. pastoris*), which utilized and completely metabolized them as positive stress supplement by fermentation. Hence, this fermentation product might have biological effects on skin and serve as a potent skincare active. In this work, DS minerals supplementation as a positive stress to *P. pastoris* was examined by testing the effect of fermentation extracts on 3D human skin equivalents.

2. Materials and Methods

2.1. DS Water Extract and DS Mud Supplementation to *Pichia pastoris* (*P. pastoris*)

2.1.1. Materials

P. pastoris was obtained from ATCC (# 60372) and maintained on yeast-peptone-dextrose (YPD) agar plates. The culture is grown in shaker flasks containing YPD liquid media. The fermentation media is Yeast Nitrogen-Base (YNB) growth media supplemented with glycerol, containing 2.7% H_3PO_4, 0.09% $CaSO_4$, 1.8% K_2SO_4, 1.5% $MgSO_4$, 0.41% KOH, 4% glycerol (Sigma St. Louis, MO), 1% and 2% sterile Dead Sea water extract (Osmoter™), 1% and 2% sterile Dead Sea Mud (Ahava-Dead Sea Laboratories, Inc., Israel). Antifoam sigma-emulsion B was used at onset of fermentation only (Sigma, St. Louis, MO).

2.1.2. Fermentation

P. pastoris cultures maintained on YPD agar plates were grown in YPD liquid media at 30°C, 250 rpm, for 24 hours, until Optical Density (OD) reaches 2.0 at 600 nm. Scale up into 2L bioreactor (2L New Brunswick Scientific, Edison NJ) using Yeast Nitrogen-Base (YNB) growth media and supplemented with glycerol and 1.0% sterile DS Mud after 24 hours post-inoculation with *P. pastoris*. The pH was kept constant at 5.0 ± 0.5 with 2 M NH_4OH. The dissolved oxygen (DO) levels were maintained at 30% saturation by regulating the agitation between 100 and 600 rpm. The air flow into the vessel was maintained at 1VVM, throughout the process. The fermentation continued until OD reaches 2.5 at 600 nm, approximately 50 hours post inoculation. At this time the fermentation was considered complete and the batch was harvested and processed.

2.2. Skin Tissue Preparation

Upon arrival, the tissues were stored at 4°C until used. For use, the tissues were removed from the agarose-shipping tray and placed into a 6-well plate containing 2 ml of assay medium and incubated at $37°C \pm 2°C$ and $5\% \pm 1\%$ CO_2 overnight.

2.3. Treatment of the Tissues

After the initial overnight incubation, the tissues were treated topically with the test materials or phosphate buffered saline (PBS) for untreated controls for 24 hours. At the end of this incubation period the test material was rinsed from the tissues using PBS and then selected tissues were exposed to 225 mJ/cm^2 UVB. Immediately after the UVB exposure the test material or PBS was reapplied to the tissues and the tissues were incubated further for 48 hours. Two sets of tissues were prepared and treated for this study. At the end of this second incubation period, the tissues were washed again and the first set of tissues was used to assess changes in viability (MTT assay), the second set was used for immunoblotting assays. Media from the second set of tissues was used for the ELISA assays and the lysyl oxidase activity assay.

2.4. Skin Viability by MTT Assay

After the final wash the tissue culture media was replaced with 2 ml of tissue culture media supplemented with 1 mg/ml MTT and the tissues were incubated for 3 hr at $37°C + 2°C$ and $5\% \pm 1\%$ CO_2. After the incubation with the MTT solution the tissues were rinsed and placed into wells containing 4 ml of isopropyl alcohol to extract the purple formazin crystals. The extraction was allowed to continue overnight, after which 200 μl of the isopropyl extracts was transferred to a 96-well plate and the plate was read at 540 nm using isopropyl alcohol as a blank.

2.5. DNA Micro-Array for Gene Expression

Total RNA was isolated using Ambion RNAqueous Kit. mRNA amplification was performed by Ambion MessageAmp aRNA kit which included first and second strand cDNA synthesis, cDNA purification and *in-vitro* transcription to synthesize aRNA and aRNA purification. aRNA was labeled with fluorescent dyes using PerkinElmer ASAP RNA Labeling Kit and concentrated by Molecular Probes Ribogreen Assay.

To purify the labeled aRNA, a Millipore Microcon YM-30 filter column was inserted into a collection tube and filled with 400 µl of TE buffer. The Cy3 and Cy5 probes were combined and then added to the Microcon filter and thoroughly mixed with the TE buffer. The filter was centrifuged at 12,000 RPM for 8 minutes and the flow through was discarded. The column was then washed twice with 400 µl of TE buffer, discarding the flow though after each centrifugation (12,000 RPM for 8 minutes). After the final wash the filter column was inverted, placed into a new collection tube and centrifuged at 12,000 RPM for 2 minutes to collect the probe.

Microarray Hybridization and Washing was performed by Agilent Technologies Microarrays. The microarrays were then scanned with an Axon GenePix 4100A Scanner with the scanning resolution set to 5 µm and analyzed with GenePix Pro software. During the initial scan the PMT gains for the scanner were adjusted such that the Cy5/Cy3 image count ratios were between 0.95 and 1.05.

2.6. Determination of Elastin Level by Competitive ELISA

Soluble α-elastin was dissolved in 0.1 M sodium carbonate at a concentration of 1.25 µg/ml. 150 µl of this solution was then applied to the wells of a 96-well Maxisorp Nunc plate and the plate was incubated overnight at 4°C. On the following day the wells were saturated with PBS containing 0.25% bovine serum albomine (BSA) and 0.05% Tween 20. The plate was then incubated with this blocking solution for 1 hour at 37°C and then washed two times with PBS containing 0.05% Tween 20.

An anti-elastin antibody solution was prepared (the antibody was diluted 1:100 in PBS containing 0.25% BSA and 0.05% Tween 20) and 20 µl of the solution was added to the tube. The tubes were then incubated overnight at 4°C ± 2°C. On the following day, 150 µl was transferred from each tube to the 96-well elastin ELISA plate, and the plate was incubated for 1 hr at room temperature. The plate was then washed 3 times with PBS containing 0.05% Tween 20. After washing, 200 µl of a solution containing a peroxidase linked secondary antibody diluted in PBS containing 0.25% BSA and 0.05% Tween 20 was added, and the plate was incubated for 1 hr at room temperature. After washing the plate three times as described above, 200 µl of a substrate solution was added and the plate was incubated for 10 to 30 minutes in the dark at room temperature. After this final incubation the plate was read at 460 nm using a plate reader.

2.7. Lysyl Oxidase Activity Assay (Abcam Lysyl Oxidase Activity Assay Kit, Red Fluorescence)

For this assay, 50 µl of each cell culture media was added to the wells of a 96-well plate, followed by the addition of 50 µl of reaction mix (fluorescent substrate and horse radish peroxidase, mixed in lysyl oxidase assay buffer). The plate was then incubated at 37°C for 30 minutes. At the end of the incubation period the plate was read using a fluorometer with an excitation wavelength of 540 nm and an emission wavelength of 590 nm. Enzyme activity was measured in relative fluorescence units.

2.8. Quantification of MMP-3 and Fibulin-1 Levels by ELISA Procedure

2.8.1. Tissue Preparation for ELISA

The ELISA plates were prepared by diluting the appropriate capture antibody in PBS. Next, 100 µl of the diluted capture antibody was added to the wells of a 96-well ELISA plate and the plate was incubated overnight at room temperature. On the following day the plate was washed three times with 300 µl wash buffer (0.05% Tween 20 in PBS) and then blocked by adding 300 µl of blocking buffer (1% BSA in PBS) to each well. The plate was incubated with the blocking buffer for at least one hour. After the incubation the blocking buffer was removed and the plate was washed three times as described above.

2.8.2. MMP-3 Levels by ELISA Procedure

After sample incubation the plate was washed three times as described above. Once the last wash was removed, 100 µl of a biotin conjugated detection antibody was added. After incubating the plate for two hours at room temperature the plate was washed again as described above. 100 µl of HRP-streptavidin was then added to each well and the plate was incubated for 20 minutes at room temperature. Once the last wash was removed, 100 μl of substrate solution (hydrogen peroxide + tetramethylbenzidine as a chromagen) was added to each well. Once a sufficient level of color development had occurred, 50 μl of stop solution (2 N sulfuric acid) was added to each well and the plate was read at 460 nm using a Packard Spectra Count plate reader.

2.8.3. Fibulin-1 ELISA Procedure

A series of standards were prepared and 100 μl of each of these standards was dispensed into two wells (duplicates) in the appropriate 96-well plate. Subsequently, 100 μl of each sample was added to additional wells and the plate was incubated for two hours at 37°C. After the incubation the plate was aspirated but not washed, and then 100 μl of a biotin conjugated detection antibody was added. After incubating the plate for one hour at 37°C the plate was washed three times with wash buffer. 100 μl of HRP-streptavidin was then added to each well and the plate was incubated for one hour at 37°C. Once the last wash was removed, 100 μl of substrate solution (hydrogen peroxide + tetramethylbenzidine as a chromagen) was added to each well. Once a sufficient level of color development had occurred, 50 μl of stop solution (2 N sulfuric acid) was added to each well and the plate was read at 460 nm using a Packard Spectra Count plate reader.

2.9. Quantification of E-Cadherin, ZO-1, ZO-2 by Immunoblotting

2.9.1. Tissue Preparation for Immunoblotting

At the end of the treatment period the tissues were homogenized in 500 μl of CelLytic MT Cell Lysis Reagent supplemented with protease inhibitors. The homogenates were then centrifuged at 13,500 RPM (4°C) for 10 min and the supernatant was retained. Prior to use, the protein concentration was determined using a BCA protein assay.

2.9.2. Bicinchoninic Acid (BCA) Protein Assay

Fifty volumes of Reagent A (BCA solution) was combined with 1 volume of Reagent B (4% (w/v) $CuSO_4$-5 H_2O) in a 15-ml centrifuge tube. Two hundred microliters of this combined reagent was then be dispensed into a 96-well plate. Next, 10 μl of each of the standards or sample was added to respective wells (standards were made using 2 mg/ml bovine serum albumin dissolved in PBS, and a series of 50% dilutions were made). The plate was then covered and incubated it at 37°C ± 2°C for 30 ± 5 min and then read at 540 nm using a microplate reader.

2.9.3. Immunoblotting

A membrane was equilibrated in PBS and assembled into a Bio-Dot microfiltration apparatus. After assembly, 200 μl of PBS was added to each well used in the Bio-Dot and the vacuum was applied to ensure that there was adequate flow through all of the wells. Next, each sample (approximately 10 μg) was assigned a well in the apparatus and was applied to the appropriate well. The samples were filtered under low vacuum. PBS was added to wells not assigned a sample to ensure that the membrane did not dry out during the procedure. At the end of the blotting procedure an additional 200 μl of PBS was applied and filtered through each well. The membrane was then removed from the Bio-Dot apparatus, washed in PBS for 5 - 10 minutes and then placed into blocking solution (PBS, 1% BSA) and allowed to incubate for at least 1 hour at room temperature on a rocking platform.

After blocking, the membrane was transferred to 20 ml of PBST (PBS with 0.1% Tween-20) and 0.5% BSA with an appropriate dilution of detection antibody and allowed to incubate overnight at 4°C on a rocking platform. After this incubation the membrane was washed 3 times (1× for 15 minutes and 2× for 5 minutes) in PBST. The secondary antibody (conjugated with a fluorophore) was then incubated with the membrane in 15 ml of PBST with 0.5% BSA for 1 hour at room temperature and then washed 3 times with PBS (1× for 15 minutes, 2× for 5 minutes). After the final wash, the membrane was placed into a BioRad Molecular Imager FX and scanned using an excitation laser and emission filter combination appropriate for the fluorophore. Images produced by the scanner were then analyzed using ImageJ image analysis software.

2.10. Data Analysis

Values are expressed as mean ± standard deviation. Differences between average values were tested for significance using the Student t-test and considered significant for $p \leq 0.05$. Each experiment included four repetitions.

3. Results

P. pastoris fermentation with DS water extract or DS mud was completed successfully. Thus, the fermentation extracts were utilized for a further analysis by application to skin equivalents.

Skin equivalents were topically treated with 2% of different Metabiotics™ preparations: *P. pastoris* ferment as a vehicle, DS water extract (Osmoter™) ferment, DS mud ferment and DS mud ferment at 1:1 ratio. For analyzing skin viability, MTT mitochondrial activity assay was used. Skin viability was not changed following topical application of all tested preparations (**Figure 1**). Thus, all preparations were further analyzed for different proteins playing an important role in skin elasticity, as loss of elasticity and suppleness is a natural skin aging process leading to deeper wrinkles and loss of firmness [14]. These proteins were selected based on a previous micro-array gene analysis on skin equivalents showing that Metabiotics™ preparations may alter gene expression-related to extracellular matrix (ECM) formation and cell to cell adhesion.

Table 1 describes several elasticity-related genes following the different treatments.

Elasticity-related protein expression or activity was detected following topical application with the different DS ferments. Skin elasticity is impaired as a result of aging or photo-damage and elasticity proteins can be expressed abnormally due to UVB irradiation. Hence, ECM proteins and adhesion dermal-epidermal junction proteins were tested with and without UVB irradiation.

Elastin, fibulin-1, lysyl oxidase (LOX) and metalloproteinase 3 (MMP-3) play an important role in ECM structure. Elastin level significantly increased by 75% following skin UVB irradiation (**Figure 2**). This increase was eliminated by pre-treatment with most of the different DS ferments. Elastin level was the most similar to the basal level (control, non-irradiated) following application of DS mud ferment. Pre-treatment with a mixture of DS water extract and DS mud led to a decrease of elastin levels, below the original non-irradiated baseline levels. In non-irradiated skin samples, elastin levels were significantly elevated by 34% following application of DS mud ferment.

Fibulin-1 is a secreted glycoprotein that is found in association with extracellular matrix structures including elastin-containing fibers. Fibulin-1 levels significantly increased following UVB irradiation more than two-fold (**Figure 3**). Pre-treatment with DS mud and DS water extract ferments attenuated this elevation.

Lysyl oxidase (LOX) is an extracellular enzyme that catalyzes the oxidation of lysine residues in collagen and elastin precursors resulting in cross-linking of collagen and elastin. This function is essential for stabilization of collagen fibrils and for the integrity and elasticity of mature elastin in skin. LOX activity significantly increased following UVB irradiation by 46%. Among the treatments, only *P. pastoris* ferment demonstrated a significant increase in LOX activity by 58% in non-irradiated skin. All three DS ferments significantly abolished UVB-induced LOX activity (**Figure 4**).

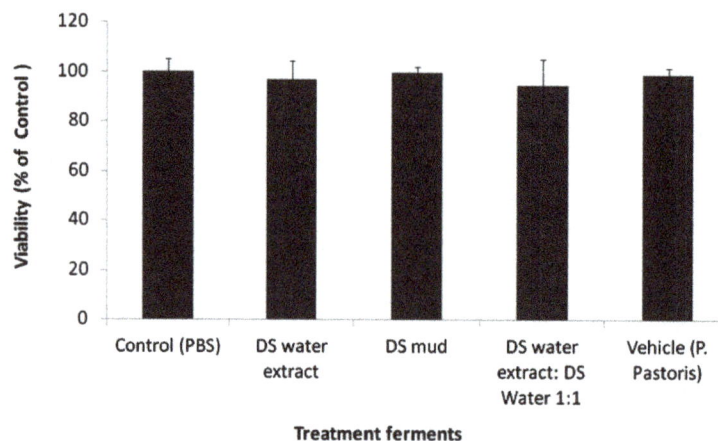

Figure 1. Skin viability following treatment with different *P. pastoris* ferments. MatTek full thickness skin tissues were treated with different *P. pastoris* ferments for 72 hr and their viability was tested by MTT assay as described in the methods section. Data are presented as mean ± SD.

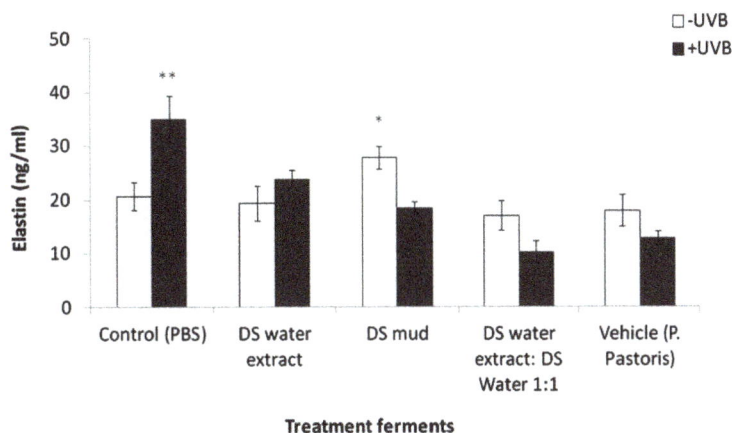

Figure 2. Skin elastin levels following treatment with different *P. pastoris* ferments. MatTek full thickness skin tissues were treated with different *P. pastoris* ferments for 24 hr and UVB irradiated at 225 mJ/cm^2 after the removal of preparations. Immediately after the UVB exposure the test materials were reapplied to the tissues and the tissues were incubated for 48 hours. Elastin levels were tested by ELISA as described in the methods section. Data are presented as mean ± SD. $^{**}p < 0.01$ irradiated vs. non-irradiated-control; $^{*}p < 0.05$ DS mud ferment vs. control-non-irradiated, irradiated vs. non-irradiated-DS water extract:DS mud ferment 1:1.

Table 1. Selected elasticity-related genes expression following different *P. pastoris* fermentation preparations.

Gene name	Gene expression vs. control (PBS)			
	2% *P. pastoris* ferment	2% DS water extract ferment	2% DS mud ferment	1% DS water extract ferment + 1% DS mud ferment
Elastin	NC	NC	NC	+
Fibulin-1	NC	+	+	+
Lysyl oxidase	NC	NC	NC	+
MMP-3	-	-	-	-
E-cadherin	NC	+	+	+
Claudin-4	NC	+	+	+
TJ protein 1	+	NC	+	+
TJ protein 2	NC	NC	NC	+

*Ratio of median: +: >1.3 significant up-regulation; −: <0.7 significant down-regulation; NC = no change.

MMP-3 is an enzyme involved in the breakdown of extracellular matrix and is known to increase following irradiation. MMP-3 levels were significantly increased by 11% following irradiation in the control group. This elevation was eliminated following topical application of the different ferments. In non-irradiated samples, a significant increase of MMP-3 by 12% was observed following application of DS water extract ferment (**Figure 5**).

E-cadherin, Claudin 4, TJP-1 and TJP-2 play a significant role in dermal epidermal junction structure.

E-cadherin is a calcium dependent protein and is important in cell adhesion, forming adherent junctions to bind cells within tissues together. E-cadherin levels declined by 34% following irradiation. Pre-treatment with DS water extract ferment and a mixture of DS water and mud ferments attenuated this reduction. In non-irradiated samples, treatment with DS mud ferment significantly decreased E-cadherin levels by 30% (**Figure 6**).

Claudin 4 is an integral membrane protein, which is an important component of the cell junctions, which form the paracellular barrier. With regard to Claudin 4 expression, neither treatment with the ferments nor the

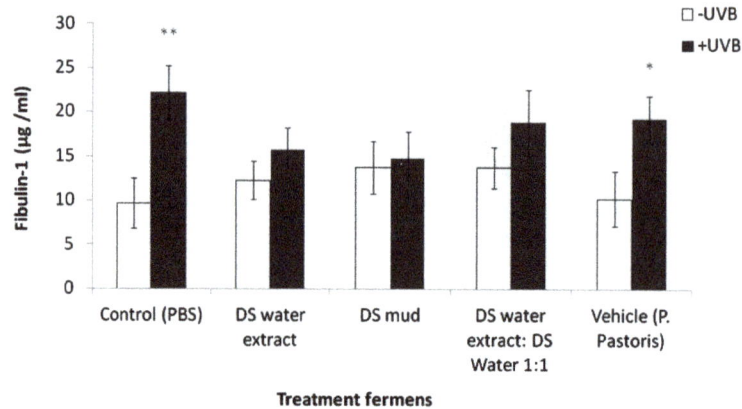

Figure 3. Skin fibulin-1 levels following treatment with different *P. pastoris* ferments. MatTek full thickness skin tissues were treated with different *P. pastoris* ferments for 24 hr and UVB irradiated at 225 mJ/cm^2 after the removal of preparations. Immediately after the UVB exposure the test materials were reapplied to the tissues and the tissues were incubated for 48 hours. Fibulin-1 levels were tested by ELISA. Data are presented as mean ± SD. $^{**}p < 0.01$ irradiated vs. non-irradiated-control; $^{*}p < 0.05$ irradiated vs. non-irradiated-vehicle.

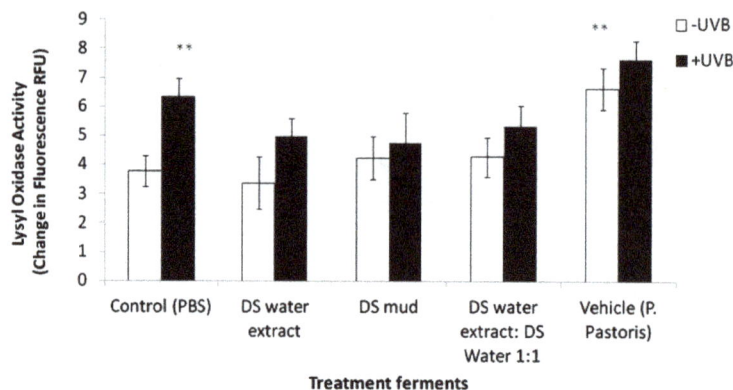

Figure 4. Skin lysyl oxidase (LOX) activity following treatment with different *P. pastoris* ferments. MatTek full thickness skin tissues were treated with different *P. pastoris* ferments for 24 hr and UVB irradiated at 225 mJ/cm^2 after the removal of preparations. Immediately after the UVB exposure the test materials were reapplied to the tissues and the tissues were incubated for 48 hours. LOX activity was tested by Lysyl Oxidase Activity Assay Kit (ABCAM) as described in the methods section. Data are presented as mean ± SD. $^{**}p < 0.01$ irradiated vs. non-irradiated-control; vehicle vs. control-non-irradiated.

combined UVB exposure and ferments were observed to have an impact. Claudin 4 expression was not observed to be significantly different with any of the treatments (**Figure 7**).

TJP-1, 2 are involved in signal transduction at cell-cell junctions, anchoring strands of the cytoskeleton and are located on the peripheral membrane.

TJP-1 levels significantly increased by 47% following UVB irradiation. All ferment treatments reduced this elevation. In non-irradiated skin, vehicle ferment significantly increased TJP-1 levels by 24% compared to control (**Figure 8**).

Contrary to TJP-1, TJP-2 levels significantly decreased by 35% following UVB irradiation. Only pre-treatment with DS water + DS mud ferment attenuated this decrease. In non-irradiated skin TJP-2 decreased by 24% following application of vehicle ferment (**Figure 9**).

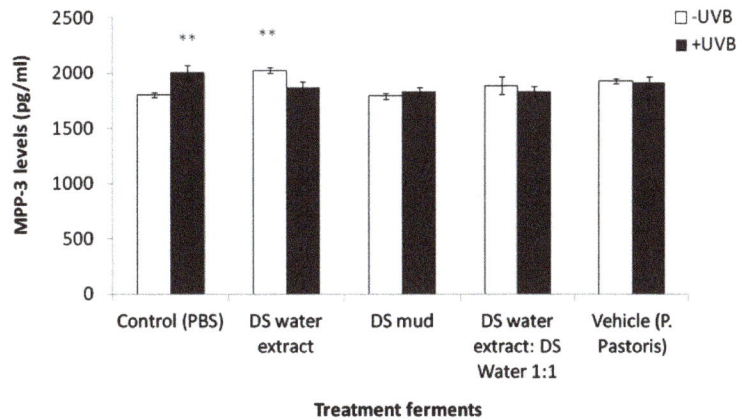

Figure 5. Skin matrix metalloproteinase 3 (MMP-3) levels following treatment with different *P. pastoris* ferments. MatTek full thickness skin tissues were treated with different *P. pastoris* ferments for 24 hr and UVB irradiated at 225 mJ/cm^2 after the removal of preparations. Immediately after the UVB exposure the test materials were reapplied to the tissues and the tissues were incubated for 48 hours. MMP-3 levels were tested by ELISA as described in the methods section. Data are presented as mean ± SD. $^{**}p < 0.01$ irradiated vs. non-irradiated-control; DS water extract ferment vs. control-non-irradiated.

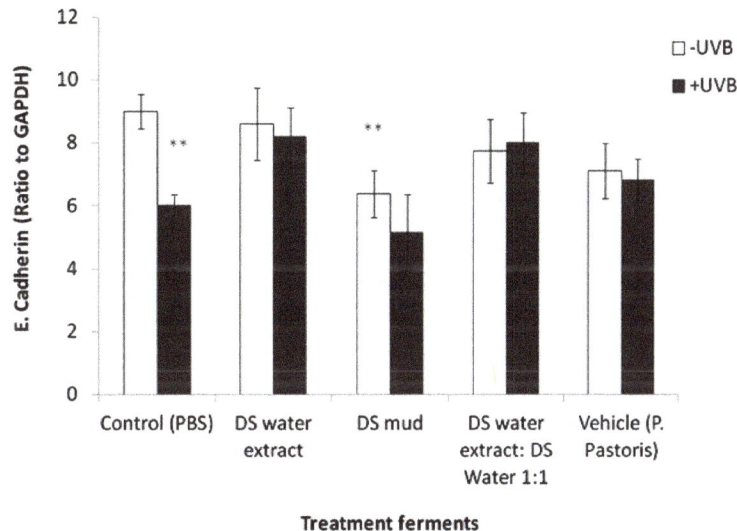

Figure 6. Skin E-cadherin levels following treatment with different *P. pastoris* ferments. MatTek full thickness skin tissues were treated with different *P. pastoris* ferments for 24 hr and UVB irradiated at 225 mJ/cm^2 after the removal of preparations. Immediately after the UVB exposure the test materials were reapplied to the tissues and the tissues were incubated for 48 hours. E-cadherin levels were tested using immunoblotting as described in the methods section. Data are presented as mean ± SD. $^{**}p < 0.01$ irradiated vs. non-irradiated-control; DS mud ferment vs. control-non-irradiated.

4. Discussion

Different mechanisms to cope with stressors have evolved in organisms. Interestingly, exposure to certain stresses in small doses might lead to protective effects by improving resistance to other exogenous and endogenous stressors. Thus, positive stress can be beneficial for well-functioning and survival of cells and organisms.

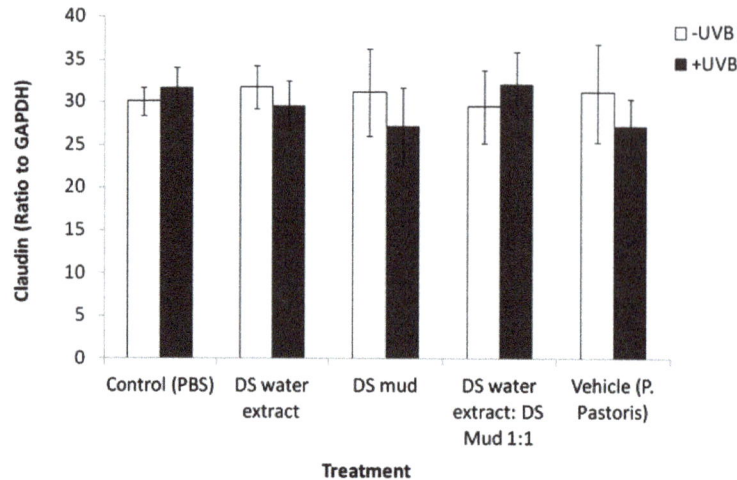

Figure 7. Skin claudin 4 levels following treatment with different *P. pastoris* ferments. MatTek full thickness skin tissues were treated with different *P. pastoris* ferments for 24 hr and UVB irradiated at 225 mJ/cm^2 after the removal of preparations. Immediately after the UVB exposure the test materials were reapplied to the tissues and the tissues were incubated for 48 hours. Claudin 4 levels were tested using immunoblotting as described in the methods section. Data are presented as mean ± SD.

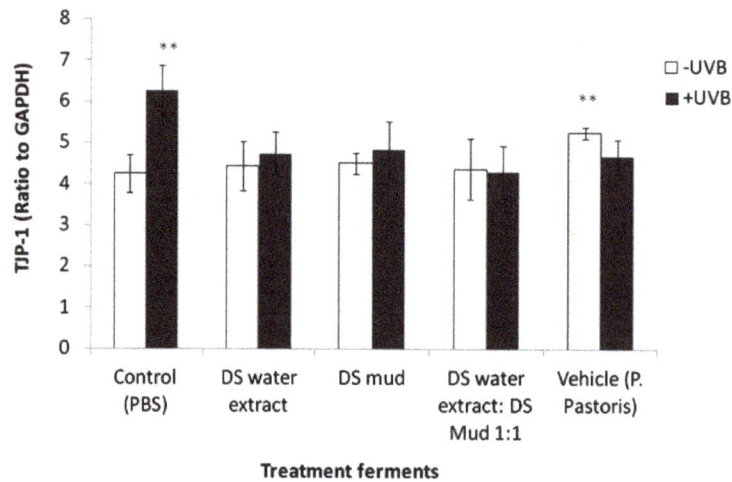

Figure 8. Skin tight junction protein 1 (TJP-1) levels following treatment with different *P. pastoris* ferments. MatTek full thickness skin tissues were treated with different *P. pastoris* ferments for 24 hr and UVB irradiated at 225 mJ/cm^2 after the removal of preparations. Immediately after the UVB exposure the test materials were reapplied to the tissues and the tissues were incubated for 48 hours. TJP-1 levels were tested using immunoblotting as described in the methods section. Data are presented as mean ± SD. $^{**}p < 0.01$ irradiated vs. non-irradiated-control; vehicle vs. control-non-irradiated.

This study elucidated the effect of positive stress metabolites, derived from the yeast *P. pastoris* fermentation on human skin equivalents. This was performed by adding DS water extract and DS mud in small doses as nutrients supplements. *P. pastoris* was used as the microorganism mainly because its long history of exploitation in the pharmaceutical industry recognized as safe by the FDA, and only recently being explored for personal care applications.

In this study, the innovative concept of DS minerals supplementation as a positive stress to *P. pastoris* was investigated by testing the capability of yeast fermentation compounds to elicit beneficial effects on human skin

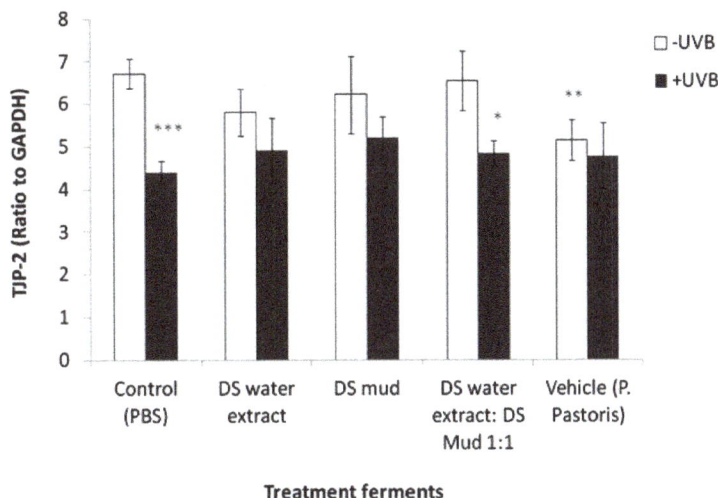

Figure 9. Skin tight junction protein 2 (TJP-2) levels following treatment with different *P. pastoris* ferments. MatTek full thickness skin tissues were treated with different *P. pastoris* ferments for 24 hr and UVB irradiated at 225 mJ/cm^2 after the removal of preparations. Immediately after the UVB exposure the test materials were reapplied to the tissues and the tissues were incubated for 48 hours. TJP-2 levels were tested using immunoblotting as described in the methods section. Data are presented as mean ± SD. $^{***}p < 0.001$ irradiated vs. non-irradiated-control; $^{**}p < 0.01$ vehicle vs. control-non-irradiated; $^{*}p < 0.05$ irradiated vs. non-irradiated-DS water extract: DS mud 1:1.

using 3D human skin equivalents. The purpose was to test whether these compounds could serve as potent skincare actives. The main focus was on their effect on skin elasticity. Skin elasticity is crucial for skin appearance and supports lifting, firming and tightening and its properties can be reflected by different proteins related to extracellular matrix (ECM) and to dermal epidermal junctions (DEJ).

The observations clearly show that topical applications with fermentation compounds derived from *P. pastoris* exposed to DS minerals as a positive stress, have significant effects on the expression or activity of proteins related to skin elasticity. The major fermentation compounds' impact is on UVB-irradiated skin, where it can be seen that damage UVB-related proteins alteration effects can be attenuated.

Chronic exposure to UV solar radiation is usually the main environmental insult to human skin. Since UV exposure leads to skin photo-damage and consequently to skin aging, it has been selected as a stressor in this study.

Various protein biomarkers related to skin elasticity were tested in UVB-irradiated and non-irradiated skin equivalent samples following treatment with different *P. pastoris* ferments derived from exposure to DS water or mud.

From the results, it can be seen that skin exposure to UVB irradiation significantly led to the induction of different proteins related to ECM: elastin, fibulin-1 and LOX activity.

Elastin is one of the important components of elastic fibers in skin's ECM. Solar UV exposure leads to connective tissue damage that includes accumulation of abnormal elastic fibers. Studies show that UVB irradiation stimulates synthesis of elastin in human skin and experimental animals [15] [16] as well as of tropoelastin, a monomer precursor of elastin increased in human reconstituted skin [17].

Elastic fibers formation is catalyzed by LOX enzyme, which is crucial for the initiation of elastin formation by covalent cross-linking of tropoelastin monomers into elastin polymers. Therefore, it is expected that elastin formation will be associated with LOX activity.

Another protein which contributes to the elastic properties of connective tissue fibers and is involved with the process of fibrogenesis is the elastic fiber component Fibulin-1 [18].

The link among elastin, LOX and fibulin-1 in this study is emphasized due to their elevation following UVB irradiation, suggesting abnormal elastosis. However, pre-treatment with the different *P. pastoris* ferments has a photo-protective effect via eliminating or diminishing these 3 biomarkers UVB-induced elevation.

Among all tested ferments, DS water extract ferment and DS mud ferment were the only ferments which significantly attenuated all three biomarkers that were induced following irradiation (**Figures 2-4**).

The mixture of DS water extract ferment and DS mud ferment reduced UVB-induced elastin and UVB-induced LOX, whilst the vehicle reduced only UVB-induced elastin. One proposed mode of action for reducing elevation of UVB-induced elastic fiber by DS elements-derived ferments can be via elastin cross-linking mechanism.

In non-irradiated skin only DS mud ferment significantly increased elastin level. However, this elevation was not accompanied by LOX activity elevation or fibulin level elevation. Here pre-treatment with DS mud ferment possesses a selective impact on elastin level, which differs between irradiated skin and non-irradiated skin. Thus, there is a possibility that the moderate increase in elastin level due to DS mud ferment application might occur due to another mechanism and may even have a positive effect on non-irradiated skin as no stress. This can be further elucidated by protein localization and structure.

Proteins of the matrix metalloproteinase (MMP) family are involved in the breakdown of ECM and during tissue remodeling in normal physiological processes as well as in pathological conditions. Exposure to UVB irradiation leads to inflammatory process affecting also on MMPs induction and might disrupt the balance towards abnormal ECM breakdown [19]. Among MMPs family MMP-3 can activate MMP-1, MMP-7 and MMP-9 and therefore plays an important role in mediation of ECM degradation. In this study MMP-3 activity significantly increased as expected. All ferments reduced this UVB-induced activity (**Figure 5**). This result supports the protective effect against UVB-induced ECM degradation. MMP-3 degrades collagen, but also proteoglycans, fibronectin, laminin and elastin [20]. It has been demonstrated that in irradiated skin there is a strong link between enhancement in MMP-3 activity and collagen degradation [21]. The fact that not only elastin, but also other ECM protein serve as a target for MMP-3 can explain the elevation in elastin following irradiation despite the increase in MMP-3 activity. Moreover, it was reported that among MMP family members MMP-12 is the most active MMP against elastin [22]. This also explains that UVB irradiation may contribute to the accumulation of elastotic material and prevents the normal formation of elastic fibers in human skin and that different Metabiotics™ preparations can diminish this effect.

E-cadherin is the main cadherin in the human epidermis and controls epidermal adherent junctions. It is the major adhesion mediator between epidermal melanocytes and keratinocytes [23] [24]. Loss of E-cadherin appears to lead to malignant processes resulting in skin cancers such as melanoma and basal cell carcinoma [25] [26]. It has been shown previously that UVB irradiation induced the cleavage of E-cadherin in HaCaT cells [26]. In this study, UVB irradiation also led to a significant decrease in E-cadherin levels, suggesting damage to epidermal junctions (**Figure 6**). Application of DS water extract ferment and a mixture of DS water extract ferment and DS mud ferment prevented the decrease of E-cadherin following irradiation and hence, may provide a protection against this phenomenon. However, pre-treatment with DS mud ferment did not attenuate UVB-induced E-cadherin decrease, and led to a slight decrease in E-cadherin basal level and hence, might have a negative effect on this protein. Nevertheless, it is possible that in other concentrations this effect will be significantly reduced.

Tight junction proteins have been shown to be involved in barrier function of the skin by organizing the intracellular junctions. UVB irradiation is known to result in functional deterioration of tight junctions [27]. Tight junctions protein 1 (TJP-1) and tight junction protein 2 (TJP-2) expression was indeed altered following irradiation. TJP-1 level was elevated after irradiation, probably due an abnormal accumulation. Moreover, it has been shown that the location of TJP-1 alters after exposure to UVB [28]. All fermentation compounds prevented the UVB-induced over-expression of TJP-1 thus, might provide protection. TJP-2 level however, declined following irradiation pointing other damage mechanism to this protein by UVB and a complex damage to the TPs network. This decrease was not fully recovered by pre-treatment with fermentation compounds.

5. Conclusion

In conclusion, in this study, we managed to implement the positive stress concept by adding small amounts of Dead Sea minerals to the growth medium of the yeast *P. pastoris* and testing the generated fermentation compounds on human skin equivalents. The observations demonstrate that when these compounds are topically applied in a low concentration *in-vivo* (2%) similarly to those of skincare actives, significant alterations in several proteins contributing to skin elasticity occur. Since a disruption in skin elasticity is a main phenomenon in aged or photo-damaged skin, these compounds are potent to serve as skincare actives. It is important to note that the *in-vivo* implications of an increase or decrease in a particular protein level are not always fully understood. However, these alterations provide a good basis for further elucidation of the altered protein localization and their structure as well as for *in-vivo* tests.

References

[1] Mattson, M.P. (2008) Hormesis Defined. *Ageing Research Reviews*, **7**, 1-7. http://dx.doi.org/10.1016/j.arr.2007.08.007

[2] Mattson, M.P. and Cheng, A. (2006) Neurohormetic Phytochemicals: Low-Dose Toxins That Induce Adaptive Neuronal Stress Responses. *Trends in Neurosciences*, **29**, 632-639. http://dx.doi.org/10.1016/j.tins.2006.09.001

[3] Sukenik, S., Buskila, D., Neumann, L., Kleiner-Baumgarten, A., Zimlichman, S. and Horowitz, J. (1990) Sulphur Bath and Mud Pack Treatment for Rheumatoid Arthritis at the Dead Sea Area. *Annals of the Rheumatic Diseases*, **49**, 99-102. http://dx.doi.org/10.1136/ard.49.2.99

[4] Moses, S.W., David, M., Goldhammer, E., Tal, A. and Sukenik, S. (2006) The Dead Sea, a Unique Natural Health Resort. *Israel Medical Association Journal*, **8**, 483-488.

[5] Ma'or, Z., Henis, Y., Alon, Y., Orlov, E., Sorensen, K.B. and Oren, A. (2006) Antimicrobial Properties of Dead Sea Black Mineral Mud. *International Journal of Dermatology*, **45**, 504-511. http://dx.doi.org/10.1111/j.1365-4632.2005.02621.x

[6] Even-Paz, Z. and Efron, D. (1996) The Dead Sea as a Spa Health Resort. *Israel Journal of Medical Sciences*, **32**, S4-S8.

[7] Hodak, E., Gottlieb, A.B., Segal, T., Politi, Y., Maron, L., Sulkes, J. and David, M. (2003) Climatotherapy at the Dead Sea Is a Remittive Therapy for Psoriasis: Combined Effects on Epidermal and Immunologic Activation. *Journal of the American Academy of Dermatology*, **49**, 451-457. http://dx.doi.org/10.1067/S0190-9622(03)00916-2

[8] Proksch, E., Nissen, H.P., Bremgartner, M. and Urquhart, C. (2005) Bathing in a Magnesium-Rich Dead Sea Salt Solution Improves Skin Barrier Function, Enhances Skin Hydration, and Reduces Inflammation in Atopic Dry Skin. *International Journal of Dermatology*, **44**, 151-157. http://dx.doi.org/10.1111/j.1365-4632.2005.02079.x

[9] Portugal-Cohen, M., Afriat-Staloff, I., Soroka, Y., Frusic-Zlotkin, M., Schlippe, G., Voss, W. and Ma'or, Z. (2014) Protective Effects of a Novel Preparation Consists of Concentrated Dead Sea Water and Natural Plants Extracts against Skin Photo-Damage. *Journal of Cosmetics, Dermatological Sciences and Applications*, **4**, 7-15. http://dx.doi.org/10.4236/jcdsa.2014.41002

[10] Portugal-Cohen, M., Soroka, Y., Ma'or, Z., Oron, M., Zioni, T., Bregegere, F.M., Neuman, R., Kohen, R. and Milner, Y. (2009) Protective Effects of a Cream Containing Dead Sea Minerals against UVB-Induced Stress in Human Skin. *Experimental Dermatology*, **18**, 781-788. http://dx.doi.org/10.1111/j.1600-0625.2009.00865.x

[11] Soroka, Y., Ma'or, Z., Leshem, Y., Verochovsky, L., Neuman, R., Bregegere, F.M. and Milner, Y. (2008) Aged Keratinocyte Phenotyping: Morphology, Biochemical Markers and Effects of Dead Sea Minerals. *Experimental Gerontology*, **43**, 947-957. http://dx.doi.org/10.1016/j.exger.2008.08.003

[12] Wineman, E., Portugal-Cohen, M., Soroka, Y., Cohen, D., Schlippe, G., Voss, W., Brenner, S., Milner, Y., Hai, N. and Ma'or, Z. (2012) Photo-Damage Protective Effect of Two Facial Products, Containing a Unique Complex of Dead Sea Minerals and Himalayan Actives. *Journal of Cosmetic Dermatology*, **11**, 183-192. http://dx.doi.org/10.1111/j.1473-2165.2012.00625.x

[13] Molnar, K. and Farkas, E. (2010) Current Results on Biological Activities of Lichen Secondary Metabolites: A Review. *Zeitschrift für Naturforschung C*, **65**, 157-173. http://dx.doi.org/10.1515/znc-2010-3-401

[14] Takema, Y., Yorimoto, Y., Kawai, M. and Imokawa, G. (1994) Age-Related Changes in the Elastic Properties and Thickness of Human Facial Skin. *British Journal of Dermatology*, **131**, 641-648. http://dx.doi.org/10.1111/j.1365-2133.1994.tb04975.x

[15] Schwartz, E., Feinberg, E., Lebwohl, M., Mariani, T.J. and Boyd, C.D. (1995) Ultraviolet Radiation Increases Tropoelastin Accumulation by a Post-Transcriptional Mechanism in Dermal Fibroblasts. *Journal of Investigative Dermatology*, **105**, 65-69. http://dx.doi.org/10.1111/1523-1747.ep12312576

[16] Starcher, B., Pierce, R. and Hinek, A. (1999) UVB Irradiation Stimulates Deposition of New Elastic Fibers by Modified Epithelial Cells Surrounding the Hair Follicles and Sebaceous Glands in Mice. *Journal of Investigative Dermatology*, **112**, 450-455. http://dx.doi.org/10.1046/j.1523-1747.1999.00553.x

[17] Seo, J.Y., Lee, S.H., Youn, C.S., Choi, H.R., Rhie, G.E., Cho, K.H., Kim, K.H., Park, K.C., Eun, H.C. and Chung, J.H. (2001) Ultraviolet Radiation Increases Tropoelastin mRNA Expression in the Epidermis of Human Skin *in Vivo*. *Journal of Investigative Dermatology*, **116**, 915-919. http://dx.doi.org/10.1046/j.1523-1747.2001.01358.x

[18] Roark, E.F., Keene, D.R., Haudenschild, C.C., Godyna, S., Little, C.D. and Argraves, W.S. (1995) The Association of Human Fibulin-1 with Elastic Fibers: An Immunohistological, Ultrastructural, and RNA Study. *Journal of Histochemi-*

stry & Cytochemistry, **43**, 401-411. http://dx.doi.org/10.1177/43.4.7534784

[19] Cox, T.R. and Erler, J.T. (2011) Remodeling and Homeostasis of the Extracellular Matrix: Implications for Fibrotic Diseases and Cancer. *Disease Models & Mechanisms*, **4**, 165-178. http://dx.doi.org/10.1242/dmm.004077

[20] Quan, T., Qin, Z., Xia, W., Shao, Y., Voorhees, J.J. and Fisher, G.J. (2009) Matrix-Degrading Metalloproteinases in Photoaging. *Journal of Investigative Dermatology Symposium Proceedings*, **14**, 20-24. http://dx.doi.org/10.1038/jidsymp.2009.8

[21] Rittie, L. and Fisher, G.J. (2002) UV-Light-Induced Signal Cascades and Skin Aging. *Ageing Research Reviews*, **1**, 705-720. http://dx.doi.org/10.1016/S1568-1637(02)00024-7

[22] Chen, Z., Seo, J.Y., Kim, Y.K., Lee, S.R., Kim, K.H., Cho, K.H., Eun, H.C. and Chung, J.H. (2005) Heat Modulation of Tropoelastin, Fibrillin-1, and Matrix Metalloproteinase-12 in Human Skin *in Vivo*. *Journal of Investigative Dermatology*, **124**, 70-78. http://dx.doi.org/10.1111/j.0022-202X.2004.23550.x

[23] Furukawa, F., Fujii, K., Horiguchi, Y., Matsuyoshi, N., Fujita, M., Toda, K., Imamura, S., Wakita, H., Shirahama, S. and Takigawa, M. (1997) Roles of E- and P-Cadherin in the Human Skin. *Microscopy Research and Technique*, **38**, 343-352. http://dx.doi.org/10.1002/(SICI)1097-0029(19970815)38:4<343::AID-JEMT2>3.0.CO;2-K

[24] Gruss, C. and Herlyn, M. (2001) Role of Cadherins and Matrixins in Melanoma. *Current Opinion in Oncology*, **13**, 117-123. http://dx.doi.org/10.1097/00001622-200103000-00006

[25] Fuller, L.C., Allen, M.H., Montesu, M., Barker, J.N. and Macdonald, D.M. (1996) Expression of E-Cadherin in Human Epidermal Non-Melanoma Cutaneous Tumours. *British Journal of Dermatology*, **134**, 28-32. http://dx.doi.org/10.1111/j.1365-2133.1996.tb07835.x

[26] Hung, C.F., Chiang, H.S., Lo, H.M., Jian, J.S. and Wu, W.B. (2006) E-Cadherin and Its Downstream Catenins Are Proteolytically Cleaved in Human HaCaT Keratinocytes Exposed to UVB. *Experimental Dermatology*, **15**, 315-321. http://dx.doi.org/10.1111/j.0906-6705.2006.00411.x

[27] Yuki, T., Hachiya, A., Kusaka, A., Sriwiriyanont, P., Visscher, M.O., Morita, K., Muto, M., Miyachi, Y., Sugiyama, Y. and Inoue, S. (2011) Characterization of Tight Junctions and Their Disruption by UVB in Human Epidermis and Cultured Keratinocytes. *Journal of Investigative Dermatology*, **131**, 744-752. http://dx.doi.org/10.1038/jid.2010.385

[28] Yamamoto, T., Kurasawa, M., Hattori, T., Maeda, T., Nakano, H. and Sasaki, H. (2008) Relationship between Expression of Tight Junction-Related Molecules and Perturbed Epidermal Barrier Function in UVB-Irradiated Hairless Mice. *Archives of Dermatological Research*, **300**, 61-68. http://dx.doi.org/10.1007/s00403-007-0817-y

5

Melasma, Melasma-Like Lichen Planus Actinicus, and Butterfly Lichen Planus Actinicus Build up One Spectrum (Clinico-Histopathological Study)

Khalifa E. Sharquie[1,2]*, Adil A. Noaimi[1,2], Maha A. Al-Shukri[3]

[1]Department of Dermatology, College of Medicine, University of Baghdad, Baghdad, Iraq
[2]Arab Board for Dermatology and Venereology, Baghdad Teaching Hospital, Medical City, Baghdad, Iraq
[3]Department of Dermatology, Baghdad Teaching Hospital, Medical City, Baghdad, Iraq
Email: *ksharquie@ymail.com, adilnoaimi@yahoo.com, dr.mahaameer2012@gmail.com

Abstract

Background: Facial melanosis is a major pigmentery problem seen in the daily clinical practice. Melasma and lichen planus actinicus are among these common causes. Still some facial melanosis that had features of melasma and butterfly lichen planus actinicus but could not be classified to either of them. Objective: To evaluate melasma, lichen planus actinicus and cases that could not be classified into one or either of them using clinical picture, Wood's lump examination, and histopathological assessment. Patients and Methods: This is a case descriptive, comparative, clinical and histopathologicasl study carried out in Department of Dermatology, Baghdad Teaching Hospital, Baghdad, Iraq during the period from December 2012-May 2014. Forty patients with facial hyperpigmentation were included in this study. Twelve (30%) were males and 28 (70%) were females with female to male ratio: 2.3:1. Mean age ± SD of studied patients was 37.07 ± 9.63 years. History, physical examination, Wood's lump examination and photographic pictures were done for all patients. Punch biopsy was taken from each patient, and processed and stained with Hematoxylin-Eosin (HE) and Fontana-Masson (FM) for histological evaluations. Results: These diseases were classified into: melasma with 11 patients, female to male ratio: 4.5:1 with mean age ± SD was 33.64 ± 6.516 years, melasma-like lichen planus actinicus with 21 patients, female to male ratio: 2.5:1,mean age ± SD: 39 ± 8.349 years, butterfly lichen planus actinicus with 8 patients, female to male ratio: 1:1, mean age ± SD: 36.75 ± 15.088 years. This classification depends on the following findings: some of these results could be more frequent and intense in one than others; they were the diseases of young age group, that had more tendency to affect females than males, sun light exposure and outdoor activities were the main etiological factors, but these factors were more triggering in lichen planus actinicus followed by melasma-like lichen planus actinicus and to less-

---

*Corresponding author.

er extent in melasma. The skin types were mostly III, the location and distribution of pigmentation were almost similar, Wood's lamp findings were similar although was not conclusive. The histopathological findings especially the level of melanin deposition and inflammatory infiltrate were comparable but the melanin deposition was more intense in butterfly lichen planus and melasma-like lichen planus actinicus and to lesser extent in melasma. Conclusion: From the epidemiological, clinical and histopathological findings of the present work, we can suggest a conclusion that melasma, butterfly lichen planus actinicus, and melasma-like lichen planus actinicus were inflammatory skin diseases that build up one spectrum where melasma at one pole and lichen planus actinicus at the other pole and melasma-like lichen planus actinicus at the middle. The young age group, during their active reproductive life, will have these diseases in relation to sun light exposure with seasonal variations.

Keywords

Melasam, Butterfly Lichen Planus Actinicus, Melasma-Like Lichen Planus Actinicus, Spectrum

1. Introduction

Facial melanosis is a major cosmetic problem among people especially in people with dark complexion and we can categorise the commonest causes of facial melanosis as follows [1]-[3].

Melasma is representing 61%, frictional melanosis 12%, postinflamatory hyperpigmentation 9.5%, butterfly lichen planus actinicus (LPA) 8%, acanthosis nigricans 7.5%, nevus of Ota 1%, phytophotodermatitis 0.5%, gazelle eye like facial melanosis 0.5% [4].

Facial melanosis could be defined as increase in the melanin stores either in the epidermis or dermis or both as a result of increase in the number or function of melanocytes as seen in inflammatory conditions like melasma and lichen planus [5].

Although melasma and butterfly lichen planus actinicus are considered distinctive clinical entities but they share many epidemiological, clinical and histopathological features as both diseases are common in the dark skin colored peoples and especially seen in countries of Middle East [6]-[8]. Sun exposure is the main etiological triggering factors in both conditions plus other additional factors and both diseases are seen in outdoor activities with seasonal variations [6]-[9]. They are diseases of young age people with more tendency to affect females with positive family history [10] [11]. The location and distribution on the face are similar and both share the same melanin depositions in the epidermis and dermis [12]-[14].

There are some cases that are seen commonly in clinical practice share features of both melasma and butterfly lichen planus actinicus and often could not classify to either of them. Hence we think that there is a spectrum of diseases where melasma at one pole and butterfly lichen planus actinicus (LPA) at the end of the other pole and some cases lie at the middle of spectrum that have features of both diseases and deserve the name melasma-like lichen planus actinicus (MLPA).

Accordingly, the present work is arranged to support the spectrum hypothesis of these pigmentery diseases.

2. Patients and Methods

A *case* descriptive, comparative, clinical and histopathological study carried out in the Department of Dermatology and Venereology-Baghdad Teaching Hospital, Baghdad, Iraq during the period from December 2012 to May 2014.

Forty patients with facial melanosisthat had mainly butterfly distribution were enrolled in this study.

Inclusion Criteria: Patients clinically presented with facial melanosis with butterfly distribution, with no history of treatment for at least 6 months.

Exclusion Criteria: Pregnant and lactating females, patients with chronic illness like: liver, kidney, heart, blood dyscrasia, connective tissue diseases, photodermatosis, and any endocrine disease that interfere with skin pigmentation. Patients receiving drugs that involved with skin pigmentation especially female on hormonal therapy including oral contraceptive pills and immune suppressed patients. Also, patients with fascial melanosis that refused biopsy were not included in this study.

History was taken from each patient stressing on the followings: age, gender, onset and duration of facial melanosis, activity of the disease, history of remissions and relapses, history of seasonal variations, marital status, frictional or rubbing habits, use of cosmetics, family history of same condition, history of outdoor working, sun exposure, sunscreen applications and drug history, drug allergy, bleeding tendency, history of keloid formation after trauma or surgery. For female patients also asked about pre menstrual flare up, history of pregnancy and use of oral contraceptive pills.

All patients were photographed at first visit at fix distance with natural light source using a digital SONY16.1 MEGA PIXEL camera, The need for photos was explained to the patients. The nature and aim of this study were explained for each patient. Formal consent was taken from them before taking the biopsy, after full explanation about the nature of the disease and the study. The ethical approval was given by the Scientific Council of Dermatology & Venereology-Iraqi Board for Medical Specializations.

All patients were examined under natural sun light for following features: distribution of rash, type of rash whether macular or papular, colour of rash, types of pigmentation either superficial so called stuck on appearance or dermal. Site of involvement, other sites of involvement apart of face were also assessed.

Wood's lamp examination done for all patients and was used to evaluate the level of melanin deposition in the skin whether epidermal, dermal or in combination.

Punch biopsy was be taken from lesional skin of the face for all forty patients using sterilized reusable stainless punch biopsy as 3 mm punch biopsy instrument. Each biopsy specimen was processed and stained with Hematoxylin-Eosin (HE), Fontana-Masson (FM) for histological evaluations. To evaluate the intensity of melanophages in the dermis, the following score was invented using 40 high power field on Fontana stain;

Nil: No melanophage.

Few: (1 - 5) from one to five melanophages.

Frequent: (6 - 15) from six to fifteen melanophages.

High number: (16<) sixteen and above melanophages.

Patients were categorized into following groups depending on history and clinical pictures:

1—Typical melasma 11 patients, with brown and dark brown pigemented butterfly patches associated with histopathological features of melasma (increase epidermal melanosis, basal melanosis, dermal melanophages).

2—Typical LPA butterfly type 8 patients, with gray brown pigmented butterfly like configuration patches associated with histopathological features of LPA (orthokeratosis, hypergranulosis, irregular acanthosis, vacuolar alteration of the basal layer, and a band like dermal melanosis.

3—An overlap cases 21 patients with facial melanosis that had melasma-like distribution but the pigmentation was mainly brown, dark brown, red brown, and gray brown in color and hands could be involved and couldn't be categorized clinically as LPA or melasma. Also, the histopathological picture was more in favor LPA.

Data were statistically described in term range, mean, stander deviation (±SD), and frequencies (number of cases) and relative frequencies (percentages). Comparison between different groups in the present study was done using Chi square test. Fisher's Exact Test was used when one of the cells in the table has zero value. A probability value (P value) less than 0.005 was considered significant. All statistical calculations were done using computer statistical programs SPSS ver.20 (Statistical Package for the Social Science; SPSS Inc. Chicago, IL, USA).

3. Results

Forty patients with facial hyperpigmentation were included in this study, twelve (30%) were males and 28 (70%) were females with female to male ratio (2.3:1).The mean age ± SD of studied patients was 37.07 ± 9.63 years. Patients were categorized into following groups depending on history and clinical pictures:

1—Typical melasma 11 patients.

2—Typical LPA butterfly type 8 patients.

3—Melasma-like lichen planus actinicus (MLPA) 21 patients with facial melanosis that had melasma-like distribution but the pigmentation was mainly brown, dark brown, red brown, and gray brown in color and hands could be involved and couldn't be categorized clinically as LPA or melasma. Also, the histopathological picture was more in favor LPA.

3.1. Melasma

Clinical study: All 11 patients were of skin type III, with female to male ratio (4.5:1), the mean age ± SD was 33.64 ± 6.516 years. One (9.1%) patient had pruritus. Color of the lesions were brown in all patients. Three (27.3%) patients were outdoor workers with sun exposure at mid-day for more than 3 hours, 4 (36.4%) patients had positive family history for the same problem. In addition 4 (36.4%) patients had positive family history of LP. Morphological forms of skin lesions were observed as macular/patch with stuck on like appearance in all patients. Also, patients had butterfly distribution. Three (27.3%) patients had a seasonal exacerbation of their skin lesions during summer and spring especially at April and August. Wood's light examination showed that 7 (63.6%) patients had epidermal lesions, 3 (27.3%) dermal and one (9.1%) mixed (**Figure 1(a)**).

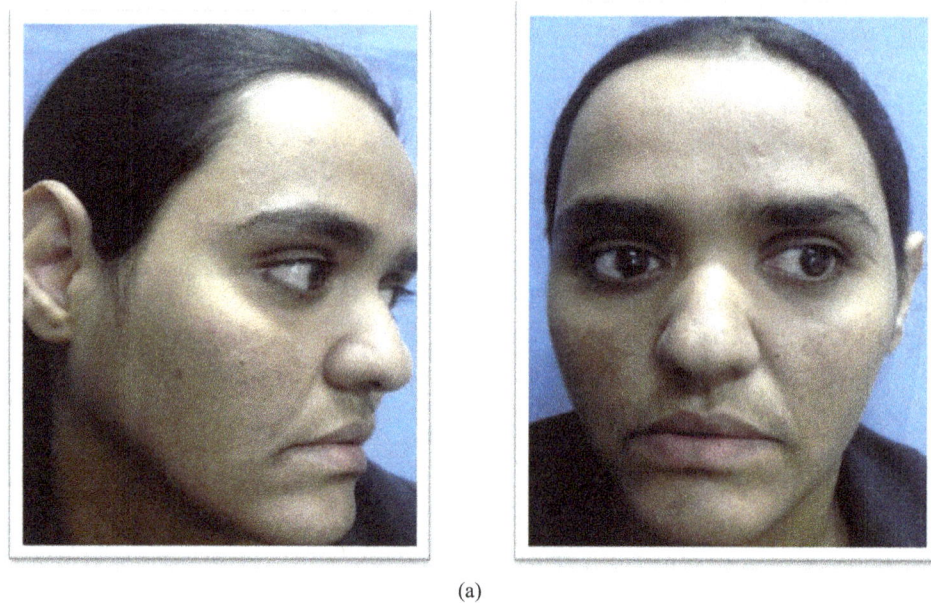

(a)

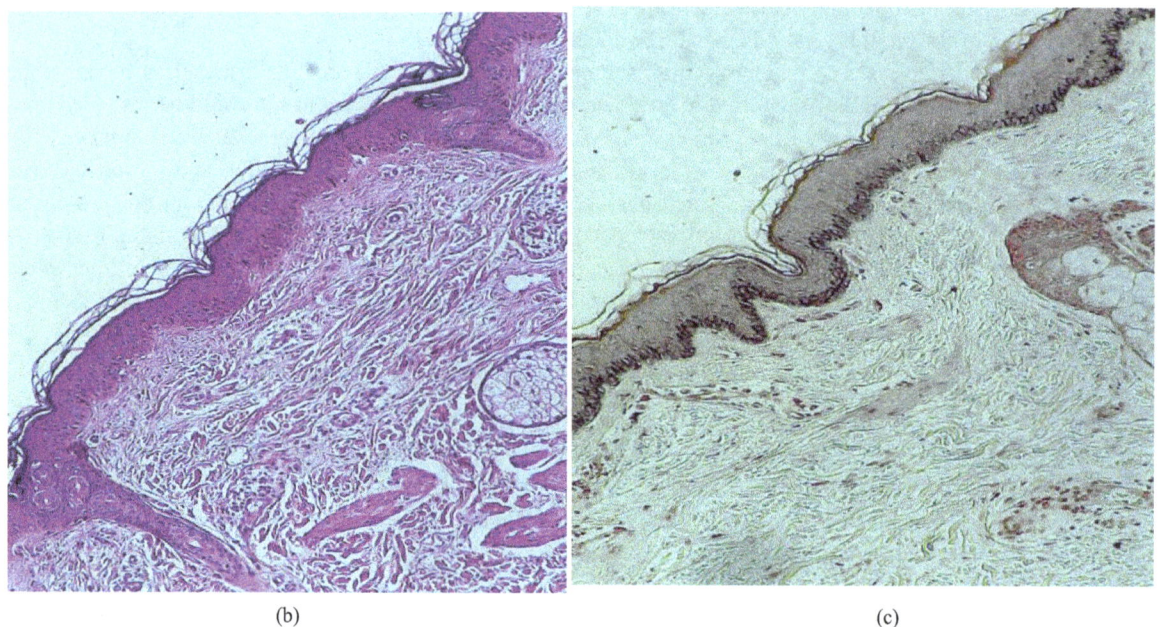

(b)   (c)

Figure 1. (a) Twenty eight years old female with typical picture of butterfly melasma; (b) H & E stain ×10; (c) Fontana Stain ×10. (b) (c) Histopathological pictures of melasma showing basal melanosis with few dermal melanophages with sparse perivascular lymphocytic infiltrate.

H & E Stain: All patients with melasma had normal epidermis. Basal liquefaction were not present in all patients while basal melanosis were present in 10 (90.9%) patients. Ten (90.9%) patients had sparse superficial perivascular lymphocytic infiltrate and one (9.1%) had no infiltrate. Five (45.45%) patients had no melanophages in the dermis, 5 (45.45%) had few and one (9.1%) had frequent melanophages (**Figure 1(b)**).

Fontana Stain: Basal melanosis were presented in 10 (90.9%) patients, dermal melanophages seen in five (45.5%) as few dermal melanophages and 5 (45.5%) patients had frequent melanophages (**Figure 1(c)**).

Wood's light examination was statistically different from histopathology in identifying depth of pigment in melasma (P value= 0.032).

3.2. Lichen Planus Actinicus

Clinical study: Six (75%) out of 8 patients had skin type III while 2 (25%) skin type IV, with female to male ratio (1:1) The mean age ± SD was 36.75 ± 15.088 years. All patients (100%) had pruritus. One (12.5%) patient had lesion with brown color, one (12.5%) gray brown and 6 (75%) red brown skin lesions. Seven (87.5%) patients were outdoor workers. One (12.5%) patient had positive family history of LPA while 2 (25%) patients had positive family history of melasma. Six (75%) patients had macular/patch lesions and 2 (25%) had maculopapular form. Six (75%) patients had butterfly-like lesions while 2 (25%) had mask like distribution of lesion. All patients had seasonal exacerbation. Wood's light examination showed that 2 (25%) patients had epidermal lesions, 4 (50%) dermal and 2 (25%) mixed (**Figure 2(a)**).

H & E Stain: Five (62.5%) patients had thin epidermis while 3 (37.5%) had acanthosis with hypergranulosis. Focal basal liquefaction was seen in 2 (25%) patients and were diffuse in 4 (50%) patients. Basal melanosis present in 4 (50%) patients. Three (37.5) had sparse infiltrate and 5 (62.5%) had band like infiltrate. Four (50%) patients had few melanophages and 4 (50%) had frequent melanophages (**Figure 2(b)**).

Fontana Stain: Basal melanosis were presented in 4 (50%) patients. Three (37.5) patients had sparse infiltrate and 5 (62.5%) had band like infiltrate. Four (50%) patients had frequent melanophages while 4 (50%) had high numbers of melanophages (**Figure 2(c)**).

Wood's light examination was statistically not different from histopathology in identifying depth of pigment in LPA (P value= 0.264).

3.3. Melasma-Like LPA

Clinical study: Fifteen (71.4%) out of 21 patients had skin type III, while 3 (14.3%) had skin type II and other 3 (14.3%) had skin type IV, with female to male ratio (2.5:1), the mean age ± SD was 39 ± 8.349 years. Seventeen (81%) patients had pruritus. The skin lesions were gray brown 10 (47.6%), brown in 6 (28.6%) patients, red brown in 3 (14.3%), and dark brown in 2 (9.5%) patients. Twelve (57.1%) patients were outdoor workers. Five (23.8%) patients had positive family history of LPA while 8 (38.1%) patients had positive family history of melasma. Sixteen (76.2%) patients had macular/patch lesions and 5 (23.8%) had maculopapular form. Nine (42.95) patients had butterfly distribution, 6 (28.6%) on forehead, 4 (19%) had butterfly plus lesions on dorsa of hand and forearm and 2 (9.5%) had mask like distributions plus lesions on dorsa of hand and forearm. Seventeen (81%) patients had seasonal exacerbation. Wood's light examination showed that 6 (28.6%) patients had epidermal lesions, 13 (61.9%) dermal and 2 (9.5%) mixed (**Figure 3(a)**).

H & E Stain: Thirteen (61.9%)patients had thin epidermis, 7 (33.3%) patients had normal epidermis, and one (4.8%) acanthosis. Four (19%) patients had focal and 5 (23.8%) had diffuse basal liquefaction. Basal melanosis was present in 16 (76.2%) patients. Twelve (57.1%) patients had sparse lymphocytic infiltrate and 9 (42.9%) had band infiltrate. Eight (38.1%) patients had few melanophages and 13 (61.9%) had frequent melanophages (**Figure 3(b)**).

Fontana stain: Basal melanosis was seen in 16 (76.2%) patients. Twelve (57.1%) patients had sparse infiltrate and 9 (42.9%) had band infiltrate. Three (14.3%) patients had few melanophages, while 5 (23.8%) had frequent melanophages and 13 (61.9%) had high score of melanophages (**Figure 3(c)**).

Wood's light examination was statistically different from histopathology in identifying depth of pigment in MLPA (P value = 0.001).

Comparison between the three group of facial melanosis many common things were noticed in the clinical findings and histopathological pictures including H & E and Fontana stains (**Tables 1-4** and **Figure 4**).

Table 1. Most common clinical findings between the 3 groups.

Demographic data	Melasma	LPA	MLPA
Gender (♂:♀ratio)	1:4.5	1:1	1:2.5
Skin type III	100%	75%	71.4%
Skin color	**Brown** (100%)	**Gray Brown** (75%)	**Gray Brown** (47.6%)
Pruritus	(9.1%)	(100%)	(81%)
Outdoor	(27.3%)	(87.5%)	(57.1%)
Family history of same condition	(36.4%)	(12.5%)	(23.8. %)
Family history of other condition	36.4%	(25.0%)	(38.1%)
Type of lesion (Macular)	(90.9%)	(75%)	(76.2%)
Distribution of lesion (Butterfly)	100%	87.5%	42.9%
Seasonal exacerbation	(27.3%)	(100%)	(81%)

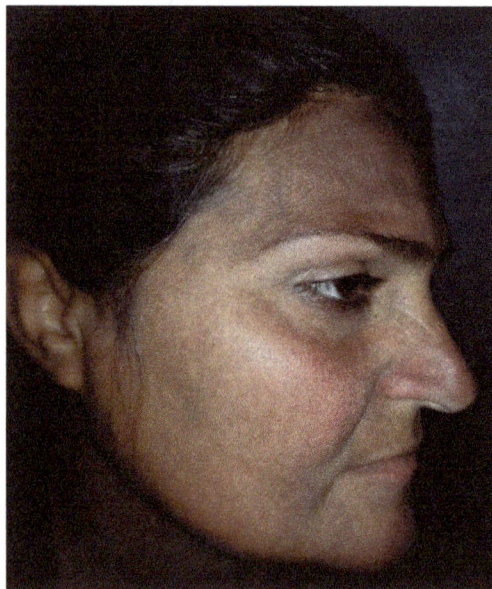 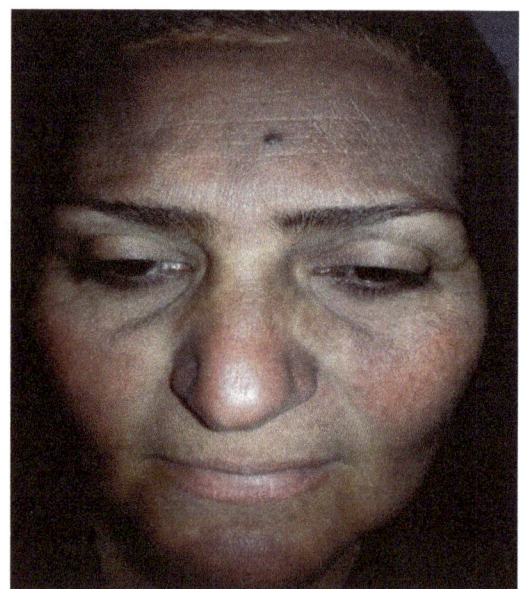

(a)

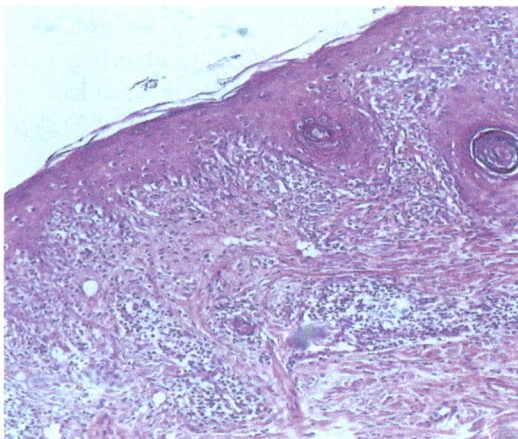 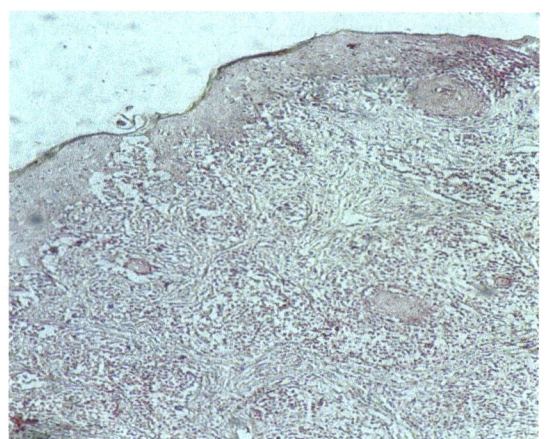

(b)   (c)

Figure 2. (a) Thirty eight years old female with melasma mask like lichen planus actinicus; (b) HE Stain ×10; (c) Fontana Stain ×10; (b) (c) Histopathological pictures showing acanthosis, basal liquefaction with marked perivascular infiltrate admixed with many melanophages.

Table 2. The most common histopathological (H & E stain) findings between the 3 groups.

Histopathology by H & E stain	Melasma %	LPA %	MLPA %
Epidermal changes	0%	(62.5%)	(61.9%)
Basal liquefaction	0%	(50.0%)	(23.8%)
Basal melanosis	(90.9%)	(50.0%)	(76.2%)
Dermal cell infiltrates	(90.9%)	(100. %)	(100%)
Intensity of melanophages	(45.45%)	(100%)	(100%)
Level of pigmentation	Mixed (54.5%)	Mixed (50%)	Mixed (71.4%)

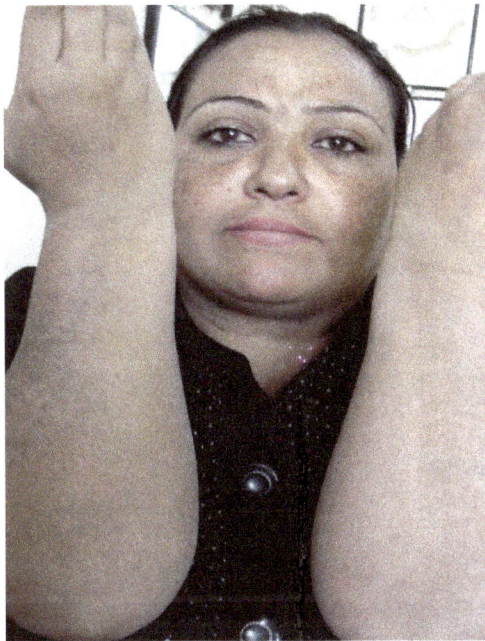
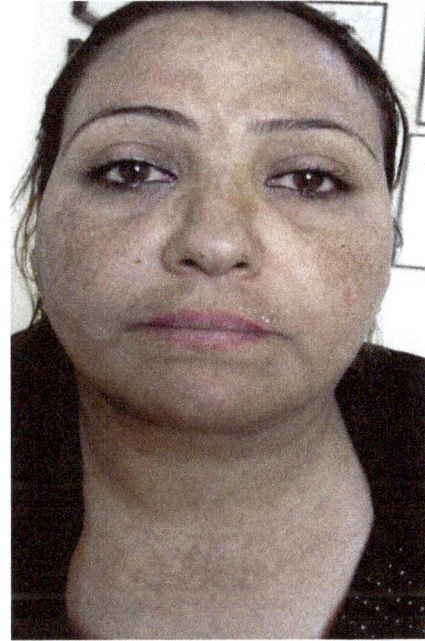

(a)

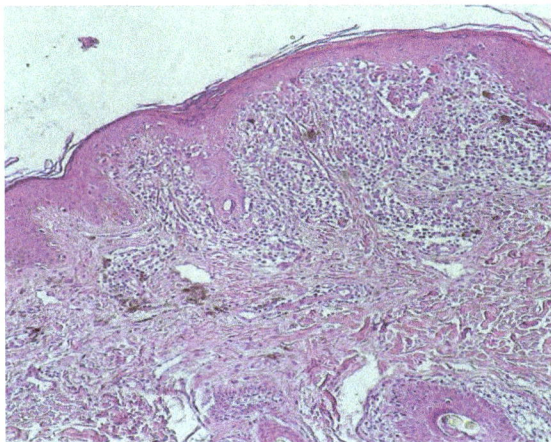
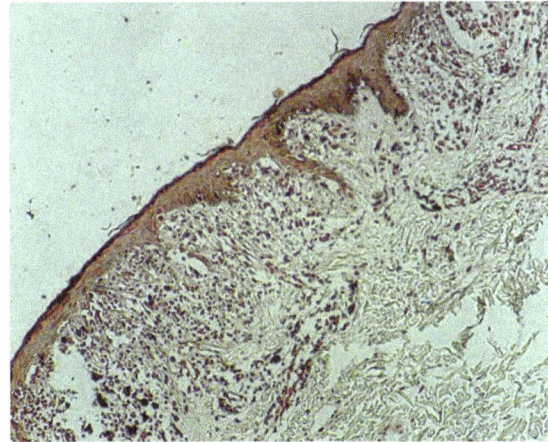

(b)	(c)

Figure 3. (a) Thirty four years old female showing butterfly melasma-like lichen planus actinicus with involvement of dorsa of both hands and V-area of chest; (b) H & E Stain ×10; (c) Fontana Stain ×10; (b) (c) Histopathological pictures showing features of melasma-like lichen planus actinicus like hypergranulosis, acanthosis, basal liquefacation, band infiltrate of lymphocyte with high number of melanophages.

Table 3. The most common histopathological findings between the 3 groups using Fontana stain.

Histopathology by Fontana stain	Melasma %	LPA %	MLPA %
Basal melanosis	90.9%	50.0%	76.2%
Melanophages	(45.45%)	(100%)	(100%)
Level of pigmentation	Mixed (90.9%)	Mixed (50%)	Mixed (63.6%)

Table 4. Comparison between Woods's light and histopathological findings regarding the level of pigmentation in patients in all groups.

Depth of pigmentation		Melasma		LPA		MLPA		P-value
		N	%	N	%	N	%	
Wood's light	Epidermal	7	63.6%	2	25.0%	6	28.6%	
	Dermal	3	27.3%	4	50.0%	13	61.9%	0.217
	Mixed	1	9.1%	2	25.0%	2	9.5%	
Histopathology H&E stain	Epidermal	5	45.5%	0	0.0%	0	0.0%	
	Dermal	0	0.0%	4	50.0%	6	28.6%	0.001
	Mixed	6	54.5%	4	50.0%	15	71.4%	

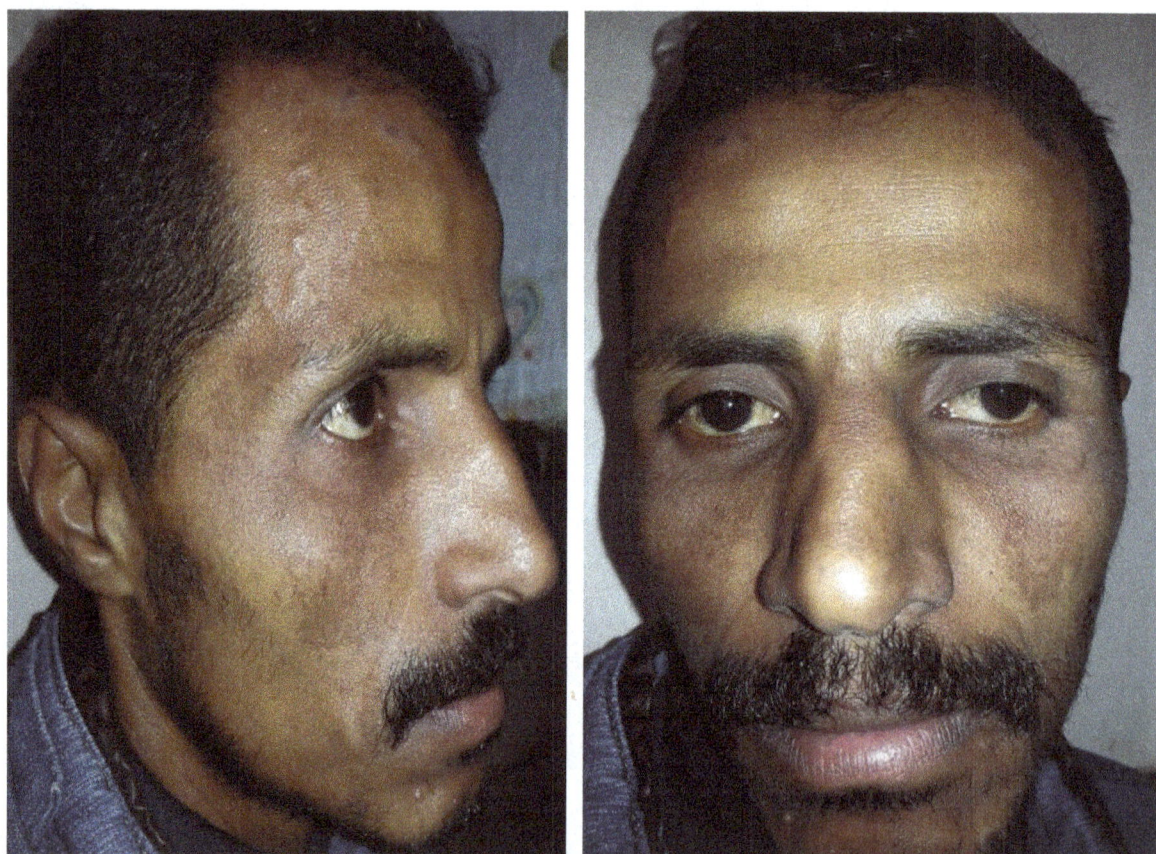

Figure 4. (a) Thiry six years old male showing clinical feature of annular LPA on the forehead with melasma features on both cheecks.

4. Discussion

Facial melanoses are group of facial pigmentation where there is increase of skin melanin whether epidermal or dermal and these disorders are major health problems in Iraqi population [6] [10]. Melasma and facial LPA constitute the main causes of facial melanosis where the sun light is the main etiological factor involved in their etiopathogenesis [4].

During our daily clinical practice, we see cases that are similar to melasma but there is clinical and histopathological difference. In addition we see cases where they have melasma in winter time but change to LPA in summer time. These observations encouraged us to conduct the present work where three group of diseases are classified: classical melasma, classical facial LPA butterfly type, and cases where couldn't categorized into melasma or LPA were evaluated by clinical and HP studies so called MLPA.

The present study showed many similarities between these three diseases and from these similarities we can draw spectrum where melasma at one end and LPA in other end while MLPA is in the middle (**Figure 5**).

Age is comparable as these diseases affect young age group in their active reproductive life, such as melasma: mean age ± SD was (33.64 ± 6.516), LPA mean age ± SD (36.75 ± 15.088) while MLPA had mean age ± SD (39 ± 8.349). Females are mainly affected in melasma (female to male ratio 4.5:1) and in MLPA (female to male ratio 2.5:1), while in LPA gender was equal. Family history was positive for the same disease in all three groups as in melasma (36.4%), in MLPA (23.8%), and LPA (12.5%).Outdoor activity was more frequent in LPA 87.5% and MLPA 57.1%, while in melasma 27.3%. The rash was macular in melasma (100%) but in MLPA was macular in 76.2% and papular in 23.8% of cases while in LPA was macular in75% and papular in 25% of patients. Itching might occur in all three diseases but in different frequency such as in melasma (9.1%), MLPA (81%), and in LPA (100%).

In the three groups of these diseases, there are two sharing etiological factors mainly they are a disease of active reproductive life and sharing sun light exposure with outdoor activities. Somebody might raise question: what are the role of sex hormones especially during pregnancy in the etiopathogenesis of melasma. It is difficult to answer this question but we can speculate that sex hormones mainly estrogen and progesterone might act as cofactors like by sensitising the skin to sun light action in females patient and even in males.

In the present study, families were seen where one sister had melasma while the other sister had LPA or MLPA. Also, patient with melasma had positive family history of LPA (36.4%), while MLPA patients had positive family history of melasma (38.1), and LPA patients had positive family history of melasma (25%). Seasonal variation was noticed in all three diseases where there was a seasonal exacerbation in summer time but mainly in

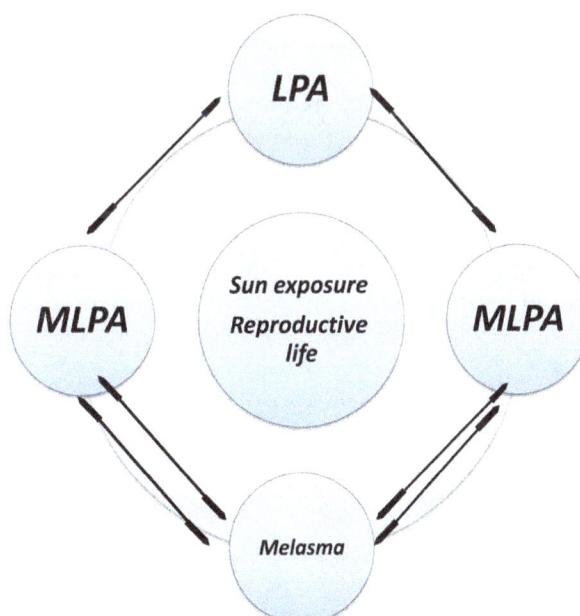

Figure 5. Showing the spectrum and the overlap between melasma, MLPA, butterfly LPA.

April and September and decline in winter time as in melasma showed exacerbation in (27.3%), in MLPA (81%), and in LPA was (100%). Some patients with LPA or MLPA might change into ordinary melasma in winter time and change into LPA in summer time while some cases of melasma might change into into LPA or MLPLA in summer time.

Skin types were found almost similar as skin type III in melasma was (100%), while in MLPA (71.4%), and in LPA (75%). The color of the rash is variable but in general was brown in melasma (100%), gray brown in MLPA (47.6%), and red brown in LPA (75%).

Distribution of rash was similar in these three groups usually sharing butterfly distribution like in melasma (100%), in MLPA (42.9%), and in LPA (75%), even could be mask type in LPA (25%), MLPA (9.5%). Extra facial rash were noticed on the hand, forearm, and V area of the chest in MLPA (28.5%) and some cases of LPA.

Wood's lump examination was variable but usually in melasma showed epidermal pigmentation in (63.6%), while in MLPA was dermal pigmentation in (61.9), and in LPA was dermal melanosis in (50%). But there was major controversy between Wood's lump examination and histopathological examination as seen in **Table 4**. Accordingly Wood's lump examination is not a good predictive test to asses depth of melanin deposition in skin.

By histopatholgial evaluation using HE stain, lymphocytic infiltrate was mild in melasma, moderate in MLPA, and severe in LPA. Basal liquefaction was nil in melasma, while present in LPA ((75%) and in MLPA was (42.9%). In addition basal melanosis was positive in all three groups. While dermal melanophages by HE stain were seen in melasma 45.5%, MLPA (100%), and in LPA (100%). But in all groups, Fontana stain showed great discrepancy with HE stain as melanophages few by HE stain while was frequent or high by Fontana stain, but in general there were few in melasma frequent in MLPA and high in number in LPA. When the results of three groups were compared with each other, we can draw a diagram as seen in **Figure 5** showing the overlap of these three groups with each other that could change to another group according to season and severity of sun light exposure.

5. Conclusions

✓ Melasma, LPA, and MLPA are important causes for facial melanosis and they affect mainly female patients in the same age group mostly during reproductive age with a similar skin type which is type III. Also they have the same distribution of rash mainly facial butter fly.

✓ These three diseases are sharing the history of sun exposure, and seasonal exacerbation in summer time which give a clue for the same etiological factors.

✓ Positive family history was seen in all three diseases for the same diseases and also positive family history for each other.

✓ All these three diseases are inflammatory in nature as seen by histopathological study in a form of superficial perivasculer lymphocytic infiltrate with basal melanosis and dermal pigmentations as dermal melanophages were seen in all these groups.

✓ Wood's lump examinations are not dependable test to assess the depth of pigmentations whether epidermal or dermal in all groups.

✓ From clinical and histopathological findings of the present work, we can give a debatable conclusion that melasma, LPA, and MLPA could form a spectrum of diseases as melasma at one end of spectrum and butterfly LPA at the other end while MLPA lie at the middle of spectrum.

Disclosure

This study was an independent study and not funded by any drug companies.

References

[1]   Anstey, A.V. (2010) Disorders of Skin Colour. Rook's Textbook of Dermatology. 8th Edition, Wiley-Blackwell Publishing Company, Singapore, 2923-2982.

[2]   Chang, M.W. (2012) Disorders of Hyperpigmentation. *Dermatology Jean L Bolognia*, 3rd Edition, Elsever Saundres, 1052-1053.

[3]   Pandya, A.G. and Guevara, I.L. (2000) Disorders of Hyperpigmentation. *Dermatologic Clinics*, **18**, 91-98.

http://dx.doi.org/10.1016/S0733-8635(05)70150-9

[4] Sharquie, K.E. and Noaimi, A.A. (2014) Gazelle Eye Like Facial Melanosis (Clinico-Histopathological Study). *Journal of Pigmentary Disorders*, **2**, 111.

[5] Sharquie, K.E., Noaimi, A.A. and Al-Ogaily, S.M. (2015) Acanthosis Nigricans as a Cause of Facial Melanosis (Clinical and Histopathological Study). *IOSR Journal of Dental and Medical Science*, in Press.

[6] Mohammad, K.I. (1989) Melasma in Iraq. Clinical and Epidemiological Study. A Diploma Dissertation in Dermatology and Venereology, College of Medicine, University of Baghdad, Baghdad.

[7] Sharquie, K.E. and Dhahir, S.A. (2000) Melasma in Iraqi Women, a Clinical, Histopathological and Histochemical Study. *Journal of Pan-Arab League of Dermatologists*, **3**, 111-117.

[8] Tetsuo, S. and Yoko, K. (2012) Lichen Planus and Lichenoid Dermatoses. In: Bolognia, J.L., Jorizzo, J.L. and Schaffer, J.V., Eds., *Dermatology Jean L Bolognia*, 3rd Edition, Elsever Saundres, 183-195.

[9] Al-Waiz, M.M. (1999) Lichen Planus among IRAQI Patients a Clinico-Epidemiological Study. *Iraqi Journal Community Medicine*, **12**, 63-66.

[10] Al-Waiz, M.M. (1999) Treatment of Lichen Planus Actinicus by PUVA Therapy. *Iraqi Journal Community Medicine*, **12**, 55-57.

[11] Lattif, E.A. (1991) Lichen Planus Actinicus among Iraqi Patients. A Diploma Dissertation in Dermatology & Venereology, College of Medicine, University of Baghdad, Baghdad.

[12] Kang, W.H., Yoon, K.H., Lee, E.S., Kim, J., Lee, K.B., Yim, H., Sohn, S. and Im, S. (2002) Melasma: Histopathological Characteristics in 56 Korean Patients. *British Journal of Dermatology*, **146**, 228-237. http://dx.doi.org/10.1046/j.0007-0963.2001.04556.x

[13] Salman, M.S., Kibbi, A.G. and Shukrallah, Z. (1989) Actinic Lichen Planus. Aclinicopathologic Study of 16 Patients. *Journal of American Academy Dermatology*, **20**, 226-231. http://dx.doi.org/10.1016/S0190-9622(89)70026-8

[14] Parihar, A., Sharma, S., Bhattacharya, S.N. and Singh, U.R. (2014) A Clinicopathological Study of Cutaneous Lichen Planus. *Journal of the Saudi Society of Dermatology & Dermatologic Surgery*, **12**, 1.

6

Strategic Trial to Find Aging Face Print

Khalifa E. Sharquie[1]*, Sabeeh A. Al-Mashhadani[1], Ali Thamer Hameed[2]

[1]Department of Dermatology, College of Medicine, University of Baghdad, Iraqi and Arabic Board of Dermatology, Baghdad, Iraq
[2]Department of Dermatology and Venereology, Baghdad Teaching Hospital, Medical City, Baghdad, Iraq
Email: *ksharquie@ymail.com

Abstract

Background: Wrinkling of face is a common feature of aging and each individual could have his own feature of disease. Objective: To categorize the wrinkles of each individual in order to find the characteristic picture of each individual aiming to find so called a print of aging. Patients and Methods: An observational study was done on 1011 cases their ages more than 30 years. 679 subjects (67.2%) were males and 332 (32.8%) were females. Their ages ranged between 30 - 86 years. Cases attended Department of Dermatology/Baghdad Teaching Hospital, Baghdad, Iraq in period from April 2012 to April 2013. The distribution and the types of wrinkling were mapped in all individuals. Regional variations including forehead, glabellae, periorbital, nasolabial, perioral and sides of the face were well studied. Results: Forehead horizontal pattern was presented in 860 (85%) subjects, forehead vertical pattern in 84 (8.3%), glabella horizontal pattern in 705 (69.7%) and glabella vertical in 698 (69%). Periorbital pattern was presented in 885 (87.5%) subjects and nasolabial angle in 540 (53.4%). Glabella vertical and horizontal patters were significantly more in males than females. Also, the males were significantly more affected by periorbital and nasolabial folds. Conclusion: Each individual or group of individual has characteristic morphological pattern of wrinkling that starts early in life and becomes mature often with time and this pattern might deserve the name of a print.

Keywords

Wrinkles, Mapping, Aging Face, Nasolabial Angle

1. Introduction

Facial aesthetics begin with the marriage of hard and soft tissue integration; however, it is the changing balance

---

*Corresponding author.

of these elements that is the hallmark of the aging process [1]. The major forces responsible for facial aging include: gravity, soft tissue maturation, skeletal remodeling, muscular facial activity, and solar changes. Clearly, a person's age often is judged on the appearance of his or her skin. Although much has been written on cutaneous gerontology, it is really the balance of skeletal structure, soft tissue, and skin that is responsible for the appearance of cutaneous senescence [1] [2].

Wrinkles or facial lines may be divided into: coarse, medium and fine. Wrinkles are the most clinically apparent changes in the aging skin. Both intrinsically aged skin and extrinsically aged skin show wrinkling. As the skin ages, a redundancy of tissue develops as the collagen and elastin fibers in the dermis weaken and the subcutaneous fat atrophies. The muscular attachment to the skin remains during the aging process with excess skin overlying the facial muscles buckling, resulting in wrinkling [3] [4].

Human skin, like all organs, undergoes chronological aging. In addition, unlike other organs, skin is in direct contact with the environment and therefore undergoes aging as a consequence of environmental damage. The primary environmental factor that causes human skin aging is UV irradiation from the sun [5] [6]. Wrinkling of face is a common feature of aging and each individual could have his own characteristic picture of disease. This work is conducted to categorize the wrinkles of each individual in order to find the characteristic picture of each individual aiming to find so called a print of aging.

2. Patients and Methods

This is an observational study that had been carried out in Department of Dermatology-Baghdad Teaching Hospital, Baghdad, Iraq from April 2011 through April 2013. It included (1011) patients with their ages more than 30 years.

Each subject's face wrinkles were examined closely while the subject was sitting with facial muscles relaxed in a well-illuminated room. The forehead, glabella, periorbital, nasolabial, side of the face and perioral areas were examined closely.

Wrinkles of glabella and forehead were described as horizontal or vertical. The number of wrinkles from each was calculated and categorized as either one, two or more. Vertical wrinkles on glabella were divided into one vertical line, Triangular shape, palm-tree shape and Mercedes shape.

In this study, Modified Fitzpatrick Wrinkle Scale (MFWS) for the assessment of nasolabial folds were used (**Figure 1**). Wrinkle depth is based on physical measurement by Digital Vernier Caliper and mechanical pencil. The depth of the wrinkle was measured by mechanical pencil, then the length of emerging micro carbon from mechanical pencil was measured by Digital Vernier Caliper (**Figure 2**).

Color photographs for each patient were performed. Frontal, right and left views were taken using Sony-digital, high sensitivity, 16.1 megapixel camera with fixed illumination and distance. These photos to be evaluated

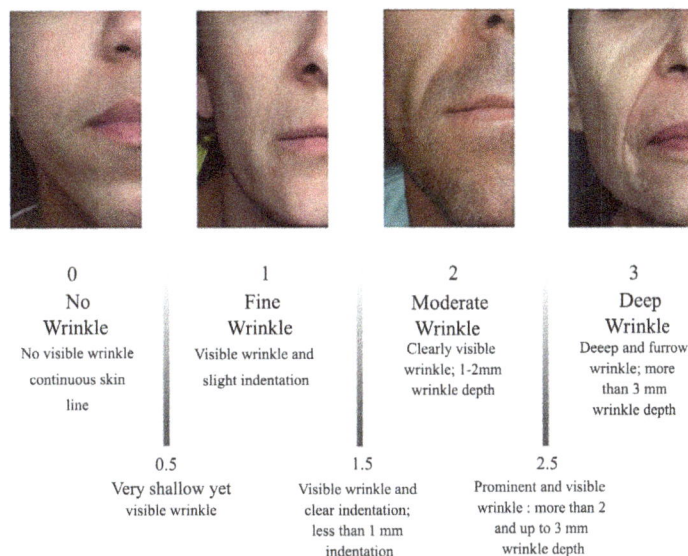

0	1	2	3
No Wrinkle	Fine Wrinkle	Moderate Wrinkle	Deep Wrinkle
No visible wrinkle continuous skin line	Visible wrinkle and slight indentation	Clearly visible wrinkle; 1-2mm wrinkle depth	Deeep and furrow wrinkle; more than 3 mm wrinkle depth

0.5	1.5	2.5
Very shallow yet visible wrinkle	Visible wrinkle and clear indentation; less than 1 mm indentation	Prominent and visible wrinkle : more than 2 and up to 3 mm wrinkle depth

Figure 1. Reference photographs of the four main classes for MFWS.

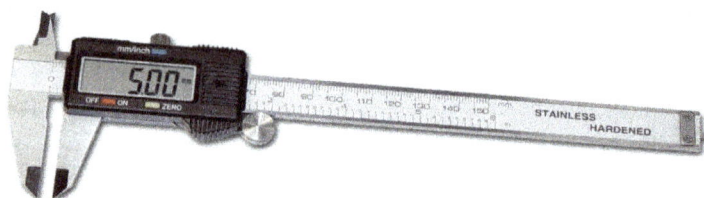

Figure 2. The Digital Vernier Caliper.

within each individual and to be compared with other cases in order to assess the morphology of wrinkle and other signs of face aging (sagging).

Formal consent was taken from each patient after full explanation about nature of present study and the goal of the present work. Also ethical approval was taken from the Scientific Council of Dermatology and Venereology-Iraqi Board for Medical Specializations.

Data were statistically described in terms of range, mean, standard deviation ($\pm$SD), median, mode and frequencies (number of cases) and relative frequencies (percentages). Comparison between different groups in the present study was done using Chi square (X^2) test. A probability value (P value) less than 0.05 was considered significant. All statistical calculations were done using SPSS ver.20 (Statistical Package for the Social Science; SPSS Inc. Chicago, IL, USA).

3. Results

One thousand and eleven subjects were recruited in this study. Their age range from 30 - 86 years and mean $\pm$ SD age was 51.47 $\pm$ 17.32 years. Most subjects (284; 28.2%) were above 69 years, 679 subjects (67.2%) were males and 332 (32.8%) were females with male to female ratio equal to 2:1.

This study showed that glabella was affected by vertical and horizontal wrinkles. Vertical patterns were one line in 270 (26.7%) subjects, triangular shape 265 (26.2%), palm-tree shape 121 (12%) and Mercedes shape in 42 (4.2%) subjects. Horizontal patterns were one horizontal line in 482 (47.7%), two lines in 205 (20.3%) and more than two lines in 18 (1.8%) subjects.

Forehead was also affected by vertical and horizontal lines. One vertical line was presented in 36 (3.6%) subjects, two lines 24 (2.4%) and more than two lines in 24 (2.4%). One horizontal line was presented in 180 (17.8%) subjects, two lines 300 (29.7%) and more than two lines in 380 (37.6%) (**Table 1**, **Figure 3** and **Figure 4**).

Nasolabial folds were mildly affected 1n 174 (17.2%), moderately affected 336 (33.2%) and severely affected in 447 (44.2%) subjects. More than 835 (82.6%) of subjects had Crow's foot pattern in peri-orbital area while 50 (4.9%) had Arboriform pattern. Perioral area was affected in 673 (66.6%) of subjects and not affected in 338 (33.4%) of subjects.

Glabella vertical and horizontal patters were significantly more in males than females (p value < 0.0001 and < 0.023 respectively) as well as forehead horizontal and vertical lines (p value < 0.0001 for both). Most affected males had glabellar T shape (28.4%), one glabellar horizontal line (48.5%) and more than two forehead horizontal lines (39.9%). (**Table 2**)

Also the males were significantly more affected by periorbital and nasolabial folds (p value < 0.0001 for both). Most of them had crow's feet pattern (46.1%) and severely affected nasolabial folds (35.8%). There was significant difference between male and female regarding perioral involvement (p value 0.043) (**Table 2**).

4. Discussion

Aging is a normal natural process that affects every human being. There are many exacerbating factors that provoke the natural process like sun light exposure, smoking and plus others [1] [7]. This aging process affects every structure of the face including epidermis, dermis, fatty layer, underlying muscles and bones [1] [8] but these structures are not affected in equal amount and in parallel way as some individual might have the aging

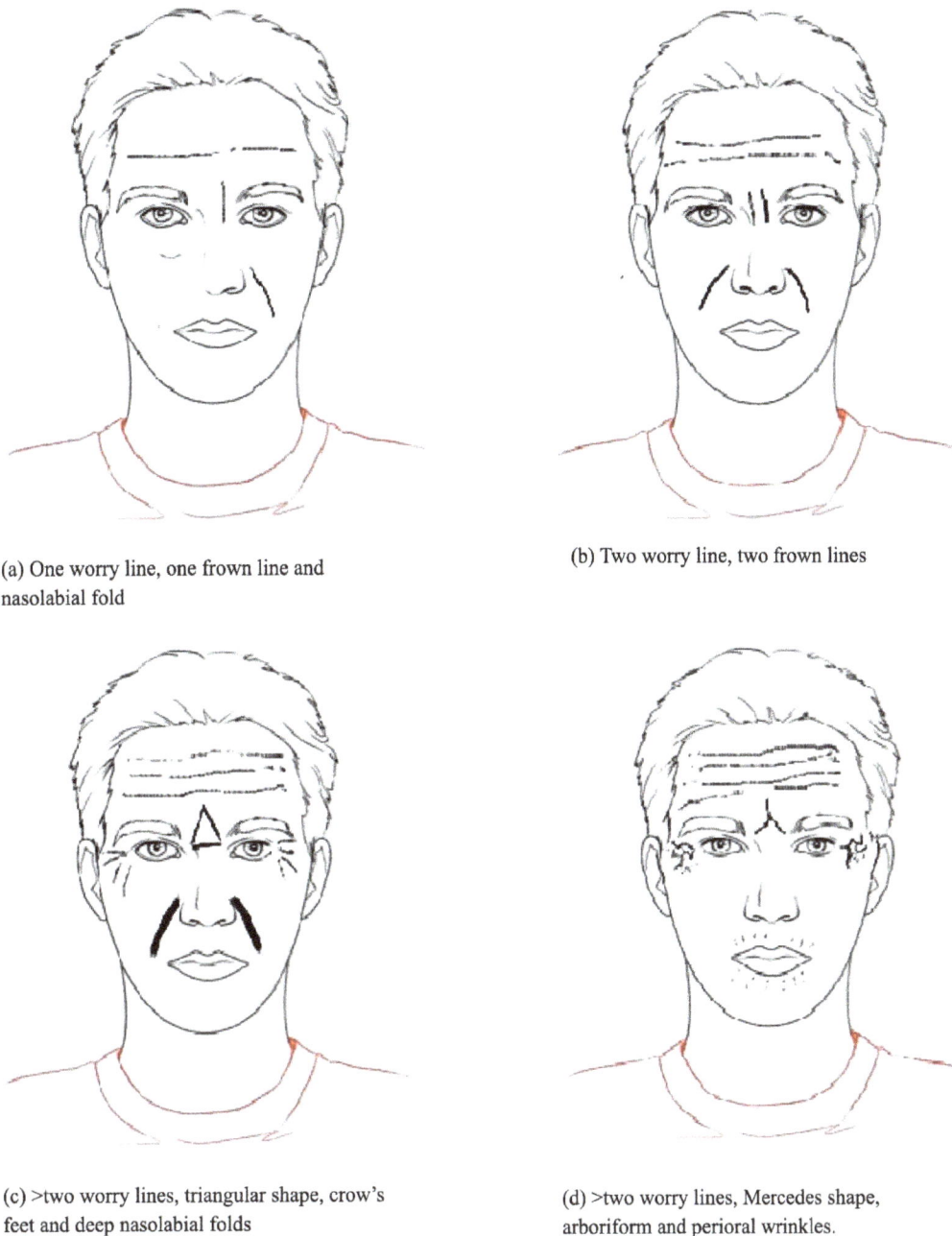

(a) One worry line, one frown line and nasolabial fold

(b) Two worry line, two frown lines

(c) >two worry lines, triangular shape, crow's feet and deep nasolabial folds

(d) >two worry lines, Mercedes shape, arboriform and perioral wrinkles.

Figure 3. Schematic draws of horizontal wrinkle patterns.

process affecting mainly the epidermis and dermis and appear as wrinkling [9] while other might have involvement of fatty layer, fatty lobules of the face that end with sagging of skin rather than wrinkling [10]. While in some people all structures might be affected including the bone and might appear as mom mated individual. [11].

Wrinkling is an important feature and marker of aging that could be also variable among people. The wrinkling could be fine or coarse and could affect one region more than the other [4] [12]. So according to regional variation, each individual might have his own wrinkles giving him or her characteristic morphological picture that could simulate a print. These patterns of wrinkling unfortunately are not well studied in the medical literature although the aging process is a very well-studied and evaluated. Hence, the present work is to best of our knowledge is the first study that dealt with morphology of the wrinkles rather than with descriptive terms of the cause of the wrinkles. The previous literatures described wrinkles depending entirely on the action of facial muscles that produced the wrinkles. The present study described morphological criteria for evaluation of wrinkles particularly upper half of the face.

In present study, we noticed many patterns of wrinkling in each region of face which are not described in details in the previous literatures. The previous studies mentioned the worry lines as forehead wrinkles while our study found many patterns. In forehead, the wrinkles can be classified according to orientation of lines to vertical and horizontal lines. Vertical and horizontal lines were one line, two lines and more than two lines.

Also, previous literatures noted frown lines on glabella, while this study revealed many wrinkle's pattern. In glabella, the wrinkle patterns can be divided to vertical, horizontal lines or both. Vertical patterns were classified according to line patterns to one line, triangular shape, palm-tree shape and Mercedes shape. Horizontal patterns were classified into one line, two lines and more than two lines.

This study showed same patterns which were mentioned in previous literatures like crow's foot which was found in peri-orbital areas and nasolabial fold grades which might be not affected at all, mildly affected, moderately af-

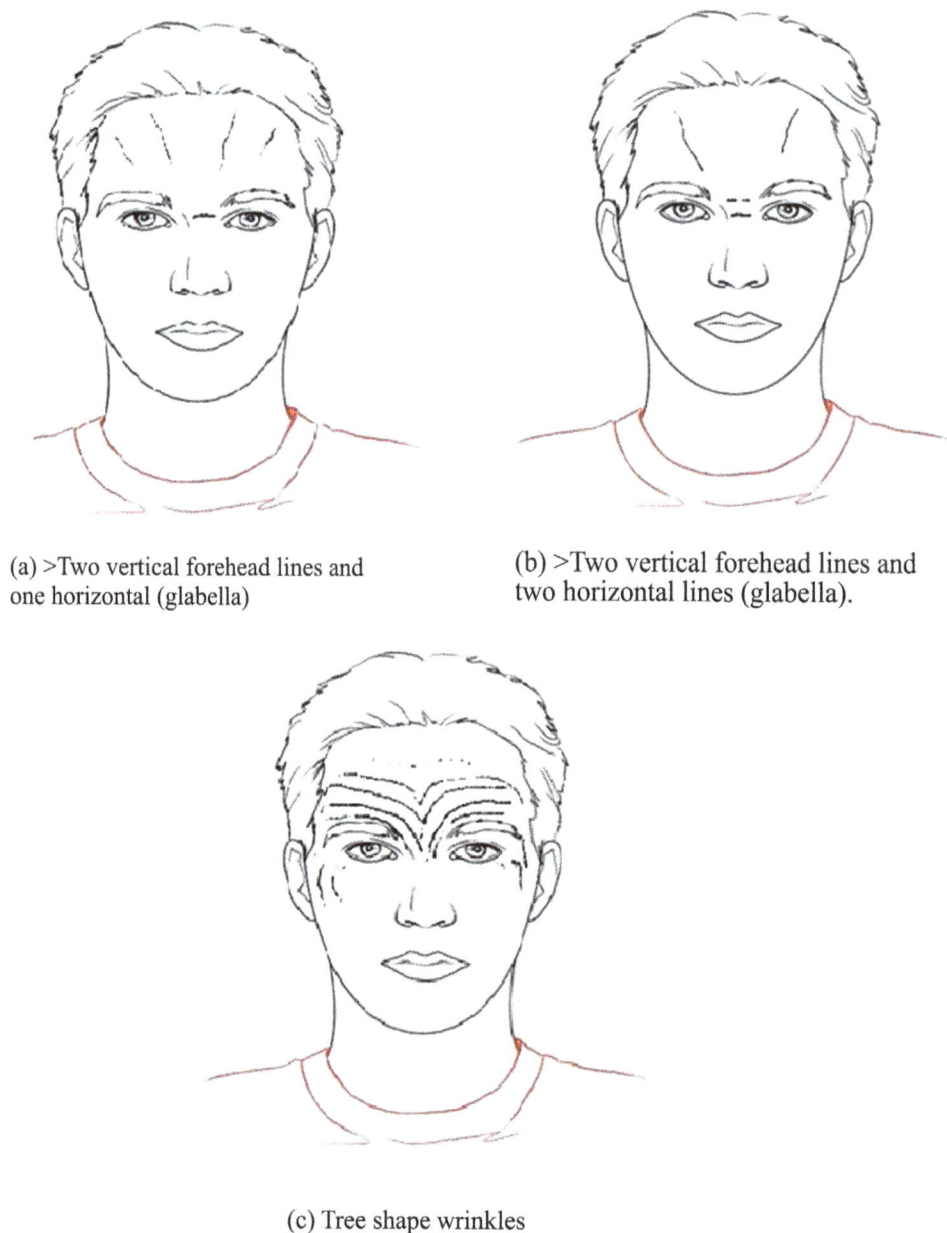

(a) >Two vertical forehead lines and one horizontal (glabella)

(b) >Two vertical forehead lines and two horizontal lines (glabella).

(c) Tree shape wrinkles

Figure 4. Schematic draws of vertical wrinkle patterns.

Table 1. Frequency of observed wrinkles according to site.

		N (1011)	(%)
Glabella vertical patterns	• Absent	313	31.0
	• One line (frown line)	270	26.7
	• Triangular shape	265	26.2
	• Palm-Tree shape	121	12.0
	• Mercedes shape	42	4.2
	Total	1011	100.0
Glabella horizontal patterns	• Not affected	306	30.3
	• One line	482	47.7
	• Two lines	205	20.3
	• > two lines	18	1.8
	Total	1011	100.0
Forehead vertical patterns	• Not affected	927	91.7
	• One line	36	3.6
	• Two lines	24	2.4
	• >two lines	24	2.4
	Total	1011	100.0
Forehead horizontal patterns	• Not affected	151	14.9
	• One line (worry line)	180	17.8
	• Two lines (worry lines)	300	29.7
	• >two lines (worry lines)	380	37.6
	Total	1011	100.0
Nasolabial	• Not present	54	5.3
	• Mildly affected	174	17.2
	• Moderate	336	33.2
	• Sever affected	447	44.2
	Total	1011	100.0
Periorbital	• Absent	126	12.5
	• Crow's feet	835	82.6
	• Arboriform	50	4.9
	Total	1011	100.0
Perioral area	• Not affected	673	66.6
	• Affected	338	33.4
	Total	1011	100.0

fected or severely affected [13].

Men showed increased forehead and glabellar wrinkles compared with women. In contrast, gender-dependent differences were found in perioral wrinkles as women were affected more than men significantly. Other facial

Table 2. Frequency of observed wrinkles according to gender.

		Male N (%)	Female N (%)	Total N (%)	P value
Glabella vertical pattern	• One line	198 (28.4%)	72 (10.3%)	270 (38.7)	**0.0001**
	• Triangular shape	162 (23.2%)	103(14.8%)	265 (38.0)	
	• Tree shape	96 (13.8%)	25(3.6%)	121 (17.3)	
	• Mercedes shape	24 (3.4%)	18 (2.6%)	42(6.0)	
	Total	480 (68.8%)	218 (31.2%)	698 (100%)	
Horizontal line	• 1 line	342 (48.5%)	140 (19.9%)	482 (68.4%)	**0.023**
	• 2 lines	151 (21.4%)	54 (7.7%)	205 (29.1%)	
	• >2 lines	18 (2.6%)	0 (0)	18 (2.6%)	
	Total	511 (72.5%)	194 (27.5%)	705 (100%)	
Forehead horizontal pattern	• 1 line	108 (12.6%)	72 (8.4%)	180 (20.9%)	**0.0001**
	• 2 lines	222 (25.8%)	78 (9.1%)	300 (34.9%)	
	• >2 lines	343 (39.9%)	37 (4.3%)	380 (44.2%)	
	Total	673 (78.3%)	187 (21.7%)	860 (100%)	
Forehead vertical pattern	• 1 line	24 (28.6%)	12 (14.3%)	36 (42.9%)	**0.0001**
	• 2 lines	24 (28.6%)	0 (0.0%)	24 (28.6%)	
	• >2 lines	24 (28.6%)	0 (0.0%)	24 (28.6%)	
	Total	72 (85.7%)	12 (14.3%)	84 (100.0%)	
Periorbital	• Crows foot	601 (67.9%)	234 (26.5%)	835 (94.4%)	**0.0001**
	• Arboriform	42 (4.7%)	8 (0.9%)	50 (5.6%)	
	Total	643 (72.7%)	242 (27.3%)	885 (100%)	
Nasolabial	• Mildly affected	96 (10.0%)	78 (8.2%)	174 (18.2%)	**0.0001**
	• Moderate	210 (21.9%)	126 (13.2%)	336 (35.1%)	
	• Severe	343 (35.8%)	104 (10.9%)	447 (46.7%)	
	Total	649 (67.8%)	308 (32.2%)	957 (100.0%)	
Perioral	• Affected	108 (32%)	230 (68%)	338 (100%)	**0.043**

wrinkles were greater in men than in women in like periorbital, side of the face and nasolabial folds [13]-[15]. All these results were agreed with Tsukahara *et al.* except for perioral wrinkles in which wrinkles in women were equal to those in men [15].

The study agreed with Emma *et al.* [14] that all of the following could be contributing factors to the presence of more and deeper perioral wrinkles in women:

• Women's perioral skin contains fewer sweat glands and sebaceous glands which could influence the natural filling of the skin.
• Women's perioral skin contains fewer blood vessels and, therefore, is less vascularized compared to men, which could accelerate the development of wrinkles.
• In women, the closer attachment of the muscular fibers surrounding the orifice of the mouth to the dermis may cause an inward traction, thereby creating deeper wrinkles. In conclusion each individual or groups of individual has characteristic morphological pattern that might deserve the name of a print.

Disclosure

This study is an independent study and not funded by any of drug company.

References

[1]   Rabe, J.H., Mamelak, A.J., McElgunn, P.J., Morison, W.L. and Sauder, D.N. (2006) Photoaging: Mechanisms and Repair. *Journal of the American Academy of Dermatology*, **55**, 1-19. http://dx.doi.org/10.1016/j.jaad.2005.05.010

[2]   Hiatt, J.L. and Gartner, L.P. (2009) Textbook of Head & Neck Anatomy. 4th Edition, Lippincott Williams and Wilkins, Philadelphia, 31-39.

[3]   Fisher, G.J., Kang, S. and Varani, J. (2002) Mechanisms of Photoaging and Chronological Skin Aging. *Archives Dermatology*, **138**, 1462-1470. http://dx.doi.org/10.1001/archderm.138.11.1462

[4]   Prystowsky, J.H. and Siegel, D.M. (1999) Anatomy of Facial Lines and Wrinkles. In: Blitzer, A., Binder, W.J., Bayed, J.B. and Carruthers, A., Eds., *Management of Facial Lines and Wrinkles*, 2nd Edition, Lippincott Williams and Wilkins Publication, Philadelphia, 1-3.

[5]   Ghersetich, I., Troiano, M., De Giorgi, V. and Lotti, T. (2007) Receptors in Skin Ageing and Antiageing Agents. *Dermatologic Clinics*, **25**, 655-662. http://dx.doi.org/10.1016/j.det.2007.06.018

[6]   Sharquie, K.E., Al-Rawi, J.R. and Al-Amily, B.D. (2004) Aging Changes around Auricles. *Iraqi Journal of Community Medicine*, **17**, 224-229.

[7]   Scharffetter-Kochanek, K., Brenneisen, P. and Wenk, J. (2000) Photoaging of the Skin: From Phenotype to Mechanisms. *Experimental Gerontology*, **35**, 307-316. http://dx.doi.org/10.1016/s0531-5565(00)00098-x

[8]   Bhawan, J., Andersen, W. and Lee, J. (1995) Photoaging versus Intrinsic Aging: A Morphologic Assessment of Facial Skin. *Journal of Cutaneous Pathology*, **22**, 154. http://dx.doi.org/10.1111/j.1600-0560.1995.tb01399.x

[9]   Nguyen, H.T., Isaacowitz, D.M. and Rubin, P.A. (2009) Age and Fatigue-Related Markers of Human Faces: An Eye-Tracking Study. *Ophthalmology*, **116**, 355-360. http://dx.doi.org/10.1016/j.ophtha.2008.10.007

[10]   Marquardt, S.R. and Stephen, R. (2002) Marquardt on the Golden Decagon and Human Facial Beauty. Interview by Dr. Gottlieb. *Journal of Clinical Orthodontics*, **36**, 339-347.

[11]   Oldenburg, M., Kuechmeister, B., Ohnemus, U., Baur, X. and Moll, I. (2013) Extrinsic Skin Ageing Symptoms in Seafarers Subject to High Work-Related Exposure to UV Radiation. *European Journal of Dermatology*, **12**, 112-114.

[12]   Boissieux, L., Kiss, G., Thalmann, N.M. and Kalra, P. (2000) Simulation of Skin Aging and Wrinkles with Cosmetics Insight. *Eurographics* 2000, 15-27. http://dx.doi.org/10.1007/978-3-7091-6344-3_2

[13]   Shoshani, D., Markovitz, E., Onstrey, S.J.M. and Narins, D.J. (2008) Measurement Tool for Nasolabial Wrinkle Severity Assessment. *Dermatologic Surgery*, **34**, 85-91.

[14]   Paes, E.C., Teepen, H.J.L.J.M., Koop, W.A. and Kon, M. (2009) Perioral Wrinkles: Histologic Differences between Men and Women. *Aesthetic Surgery Journal November*, **29**, 467-472. http://dx.doi.org/10.1016/j.asj.2009.08.018

[15]   Tsukahara, K., Hotta, M., Osanai, O., Kawada, H., Kitahara, T. and Takema, Y. (2013) Gender-Dependent Differences in Degree of Facial Wrinkles. *Skin Research and Technology*, **19**, 65-71. http://dx.doi.org/10.1111/j.1600-0846.2011.00609.x

7

In Vitro and *in Vivo* Anti-Inflammatory Effect of a Biotechnologically Modified Borage Seed Extract: Evidence for Lipid Pro-Resolving Mediators' Implication in the Enhancement of Psoriatic and Atopic Dermatitis Lesions

Gérald Chene[1], Vincent Baillif[1], Emeline Van Goethem[1], Jean-Eric Branka[2], Toni Ionescu[3], Géraldine Robert[3], Luc Lefeuvre[3*]

[1]Ambiotis SAS, Cana Biotech 2, Toulouse, France
[2]EPHYSCIENCE, Nantes, France
[3]Laboratoires Dermatologiques d'Uriage, Siège Social, Courbevoie, France
Email: *luc.lefeuvre@uriage.com

Abstract

Aim: Resolvins, maresins and lipoxins are lipid mediators issued from essential polyunsaturated fatty acids which are the first anti-inflammatory and pro-resolving signals identified during the resolution phase of inflammation. As borage oil and/or borage seed extracts have shown beneficial action in treatment of atopic dermatitis or eczema in human and canine, we have modified a borage oil component by using biotechnology in order to get a compound structurally related to a polyunsaturated fatty acid, and we have studied its ability to reduce inflammation mediators production through the generation of resolvins, maresins and/or lipoxins. Additionally, we have demonstrated the potent anti-inflammatory effect of this new compound which consists in borage seed oil aminopropanediol amides, through an *in vivo* study concerning subjects suffering from psoriasis or atopic dermatitis. Study Design/Methods: For the *in vitro* study, inflammation was induced in co-cultures of human dendritic cells and normal keratinocytes by the addition of PMA and the calcium ionophore A23187. Ability of our borage seed oil aminopropanediol amides to increase resolvin D2, maresin 1 and lipoxins A4 and B4 synthesis was then measured. Pro-inflammatory cytokines (IL-1β, IL-6, IL-8) and PGE2 productions were also quantified. For the *in vivo* study, 36 subjects suffering from psoriasis or atopic dermatitis have used twice a day during 30 days, a formulation containing borage seed oil aminopropanediol amides. Before the beginning of the study and after 30 days' treatment, the severity of psoriasis and of atopic dermatitis was evaluated by using the PGA and the SCORAD scoring scales, respectively. Results: Borage seed oil aminopropanediol amides were able to significantly increase the resolvin D2, maresin 1 and lipoxins A4 and B4 synthesis. Concomitantly, they were also able to significantly inhibit the production of IL-1β, IL-6, IL-8 and PGE2 induced by the PMA and the calcium ionophore A23187 in the *in vitro* co-culture model used. Introduced in formulation, borage seed oil aminopropanediol amides significantly reduced the clinical manifestations of psoriasis and atopic dermatitis. Conclusion: Our *in vitro* and *in vivo* study clearly showed the anti-inflammatory activity of borage seed oil aminopropanediol amides and emphasized the putative role of pro-resolving lipid mediators in the treatment of atopic dermatitis, psoriasis or other inflammation-induced skin diseases.

Keywords

Human Skin, Biotechnologically Modified Borage Extract, Interleukins, Inflammation, Psoriasis, Atopic Dermatitis, Resolvins, Maresins, Lipoxins

1. Introduction

Resolvins, protectins, maresins and lipoxins are lipid mediators issued from essential polyunsaturated fatty acids (PUFAs) which are the first anti-inflammatory and pro-resolving signals identified during the resolution phase of inflammation (for a review, see [1]). Resolvins derived from both eicosapentaenoic (EPA) and docosahexaenoic acid (DHA), lipoxins (AA metabolites), protectins and maresins (DHA metabolites), all participate to reduce inflammation and were all able to inhibit pro-inflammatory cytokines production in various situations such as obesity [2], asthma [3], chronic airway inflammation diseases [4], cigarette smoke-induced lung inflammation [5] and pulmonary inflammation in general [6], synovial inflammation [7], chronic disorders of the colon and colon cancer [8].

In these conditions, the use of these lipid mediators, or of products able to induce their production, seems to be of a great therapeutic value in the management of human skin inflammatory disorders.

Interestingly, fish or borage oil for example, which contains significant quantities of PUFAs like eicosapentaenoic acid (EPA) and docosahexaenoic acid (DHA), has showed potent anti-inflammatory effects in animal [9] and human skin suffering from atopic dermatitis [10]-[13], eczema [14] [15], or psoriasis [16]. Dietary supplementation with borage oil even showed significant efficacy in increasing hydration of human elderly skin [17].

According to various scientific works, generation of lipid pro-resolving mediators from PUFAs contained in fish and borage oils, is the most likely explanation for these anti-inflammatory and curative effects (for a review, see [18]).

Nevertheless, in a very surprising way, nor resolvins, protectins, maresins or lipoxins, nor products able to induce their production, were already tested for their ability to enhance atopic dermatitis or other inflammatory skin diseases after a topical application on the human cutaneous tissue.

Taking advantage of the possibility to use biotechnological process to create a borage oil derivative structurally related to a polyunsaturated fatty acid, we have created borage seed oil aminopropanediol amides (BSOAA) and we have studied their anti-inflammatory effects in an *in vitro* model of human dendritic cells and normal keratinocytes co-cultures. In this first part of the study, the ability of our biotechnological product to induce the lipid pro-resolving mediators' production, and to reduce the pro-inflammatory cytokines and the PGE2 production, was evaluated.

In the second part of this study, we have evaluated the *in vivo* capacity of our borage seed oil aminopropanediol amides to enhance psoriatic and atopic dermatitis lesions of patients suffering from these diseases.

2. Materials and Methods

2.1. Reagents and Materials

Macrophage-SFM and Alamar Blue were purchased from Life Technologies (Saint Aubin, France). Keratinocytes growth medium (KGM-2) and Normal Human Epidermal Keratinocyte (NHEK) were purchased from Promocell (Heidelberg, Germany). GM-CSF and IL-4 were purchased from Peprotech (Neuilly-Sur-Seine, France). PMA and A23187 were purchased from Sigma-Aldrich (Saint Quentin Fallavier, France). PUFA, DHA and EPA, came from Larodan (Solna, Suède). All plastics for cell culture were produced by Falcon and purchased from D. Dutscher (Brumath, France). Turbocapture mRNA kit for mRNA was purchased from Qiagen (Courtaboeuf, France). Maxima First Strand cDNA Synthesis kit was purchased from Thermo Fisher Scientific (Illkirch, France). The kit used for cytokines multiplex analysis came from Merck Millipore (Saint-Quentin en Yvelines, France). For PCR, SsoFast EvaGreen super mix were purchased from BioRad (Marnes la coquette, France). Oasis HLB 96 wells solid phase extraction were purchased from Waters (Saint Quentin en Yvelines, France).

2.2. Dendritic Cells and Normal Human Epidermal Keratinocytes Co-Culture

Dendritic cells (DCs) were differentiated from human peripheral blood mononuclear cells (PBMCs). PBMCs were obtained from healthy blood donor buffy coats by a standard Ficoll-Hypaque gradient method. Monocytes were isolated from PBMCs by adherence to plastic for 2 hours in serum-free medium (SFM) optimized for macrophage culture, at 37°C in a humidified atmosphere containing 5% CO_2. Monocytes were then incubated for 7 days with GM-CSF (10 ng/ml) and IL-4 (10 ng/mL) to be differenciated in dendritic cells. In parallel of dendritic cells differenciation, Normal Human Epidermal Keratinocytes (NHEK) were set in culture. At the end of diferenciation step, NHEK were seeded in inserts and were placed with dendritic cells to recreate a skin compartment.

Compounds tested were mixed with the DC/NHEK co-culture 24 hours prior to the inflammatory stimulation with PMA (50 nM) and A23187 (1 μM).

2.3. Test of Viability

Borage seed oil aminopropanediol amides were evaluated on monocyte viability. For that PBMCs were seeded in 96-wells plate at the density of 3.125×10^6 cells/cm^2 for 2 hours. After subsequent washes with PBS, borage seed oil aminopropanediol amides were introduced at 0.005% (v/v) in culture medium for 24 hours. During the last 6 hours, Alamar Blue was introduced in the cell culture and conversion of resazurin to the fluorescent molecule, resorufin, was measured as an indicator of cell death. Measurement was done thanks to the spectrofluorimeter Tecan Infinite F500.

2.4. Specialized-Proresolving Mediators Quantification

The extraction protocol and LC/MS/MS analysis were performed by Ambiotis SAS (France) as described in Le Faouder et al., J. Chrom. B., 2013 adapted from Ambiotis Standard Operating Procedure. Briefly, samples were extracted using oasis HLB 96 wells solid phase extraction (Waters). LC-MS/MS analysis was performed on UHPLC system (Agilent LC1290 Infinity) coupled to Agilent 6460 triple quadrupole MS (Agilent Technologies) equipped with electro-spray ionization operating in negative mode. Reverse-phase UHPLC was performed using ZorBAX SB-C18 column (2.1 mm × 50 mm × 1.8 μm) (Agilent Technologies). We thank Pr Charles Serhan for PD1 standard.

2.5. Genes Expression

mRNAs of DCs were extracted by using specific extraction system, Turbocapture mRNA (Qiagen). Then a reverse transcription was made to obtain cDNA (Fermentas). cDNA have been used in the Applied Biosystems 7500 Fast Real Time PCR system with the SsoFast EvaGreen Supermix (BioRad) and specific primer of gene interest.

2.6. Cytokine Quantification

Cell supernatant was collected after 24 hours of stimulation and analyzed thanks to Millipore kit for expression of IFN-g, IL-1b, IL-2, IL-4, IL-6, IL-8, IL-10, IL-13 and TSLP in accordance with manufacturer instruction.

2.7. *In Vivo* Study

2 groups of 18 subjects (one group suffering from psoriasis, one group suffering from atopic dermatitis), male and female, aged from 3.5 months to 63.1 years, were included in this study. All the subjects have used twice a day, a cosmetic formulation (see below) containing our borage seed oil aminopropanediol amides. Before and after a 30 days' treatment, 5 dermatologists have scored psoriasis severity by using the Physician Global Assessment (PGA) [19] and severity of atopic dermatitis by using the standardized quotation of the SCORAD [20]. Dermatologists also determined for each group, the SRRC Index score (evaluating scaling roughness, redness and cracks) (for a review, see [21]).

Additionally, before and after a 30 days' treatment, volunteers have answered to an auto-evaluation questionnaire regarding the efficacy of the product. Sensations of itching, tightness and discomfort were then evaluated; the Infant's Dermatitis Quality of Life Index [22] and the Dermatology Life Quality Index [23] were also determined.

2.8. Cosmetic Formulation Composition

AQUA (WATER)-URIAGE THERMAL SPRING WATER-BUTYROSPERMUM PARKII (SHEA BUTTER)-CETEARYL ISONONANOATE-ISODECYL NEOPENTANOATE-BUTYLENE GLYCOL–GLYCERIN-HYDROGENATED POLYDECENE-DIMETHICONE-SQUALANE-STEARETH-2-STEARETH-21-CETYL ALCOHOL-PENTAERYTHRITYL DISTEARATE-POLYACRYLATE-13-BRASSICA CAMPESTRIS (RAPESEED) STEROLS-CHLORPHENESIN-PIROCTONE OLAMINE-POLYISOBUTENE-SODIUM DEXTRAN SULFATE-O-CYMEN-5-OL-TOCOPHERYL ACETATE-XANTHAN GUM-CITRIC ACID-RASPBERRY SEED OIL/PALM OIL AMINOPROPANEDIOL ESTERS-POLYSORBATE 20-SORBITAN ISOSTEARATE-ASIATICOSIDE-PHYTOSPHINGOSINE-AMINO-GLYCEROL BORAGO OFFICINALIS FATTY AMIDE.

2.9. Statistics

2.9.1. *In Vitro* Studies

Data are expressed as means ± S.D. of 2 different experiments realized in duplicate (n = 2) and in triplicates (n = 3). The statistical significances were assessed by Student t-tests (*p < 0.05; **p < 0.01; ***p < 0.001).

2.9.2. *In Vivo* Studies

Data are expressed as means of the scores determined for each subject. The statistical significances were assessed by Paired Wilcoxon tests (as indicated).

3. Results and Discussion

As shown in **Figure 1**, in the selected experimental conditions, borage seed oil aminopropanediol amides at 0.005% (v/v) were able to significantly increase the cutaneous cell production of the pro-resolving mediators maresin 7 (R) MaR1 and lipoxins LxA4 and LxB4. We can then reasonably conclude that our BSOAA contain significant amounts of precursors of these mediators. Additionally, we can also logically expect in these conditions, that our BSOAA could afford for efficient anti-inflammatory effects. In order to test this hypothesis, we induced an inflammation in our co-culture model by the addition of phorbol myristate acetate (PMA) and the calcium ionophore A23187, and we evaluate the effect of our BSOAA on pro-inflammatory cytokines and PGE2 productions.

As shown in **Figure 2**, borage seed oil aminopropanediol amides at 0.005% (v/v) were able to significantly counteract the effect of PMA/A23187 in the cutaneous cells co-cultures. The production of the following pro-inflammatory cytokines was significantly reduced: IL-1β, 102.5% this (p < 0.05); IL-6, −109.5% (p < 0.001); IL-8, −90.3% (p < 0.001). PGE2 production, which is induced during inflammatory process, was also inhibited by BSOAA: −110.9% (p < 0.001). These results are in line with the work of Miller *et al.* showing that polyunsaturated fatty acids induce epidermal generation of local putative anti-inflammatory metabolites [9]. These results so clearly demonstrate the very potent anti-inflammatory effect of our borage seed oil aminopropanediol amides, which can be merely explained by the ability of BSOAA to induce pro-resolving lipid mediators like

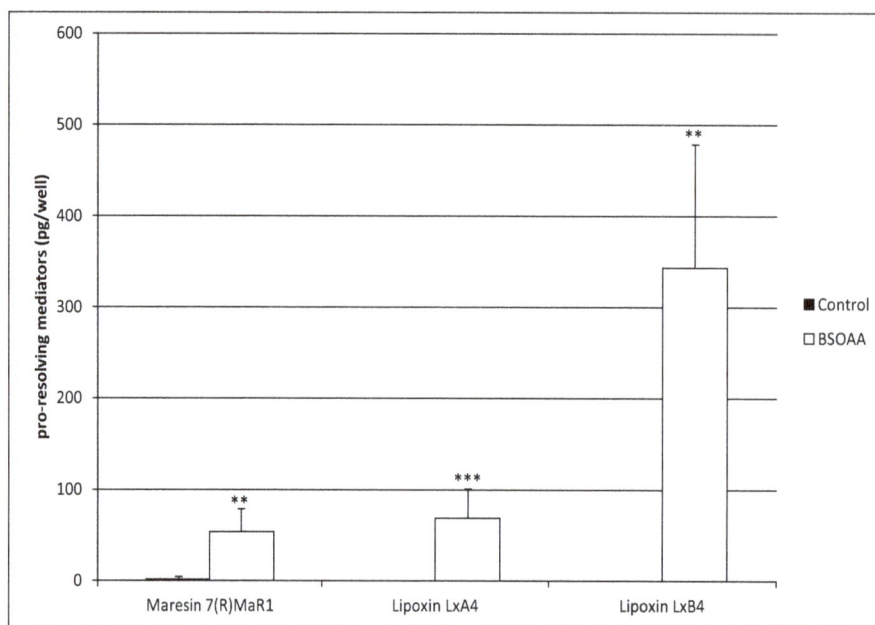

Figure 1. Effect of borage seed oil aminopropanediol amides at 0.005% (v/v) on the cutaneous cell production of resolvin RvD2, maresin 7(R) MaR1 and lipoxins LxA4 and LxB4. **Significantly different from the "control" (p < 0.01, Student t-test); ***Significantly different from the "control" (p < 0.001, Student t-test); n = 5, from 2 different experiments; NB: histogram for the "control" condition are not visible for the lipoxins measurements because the mean value is equal to 0.

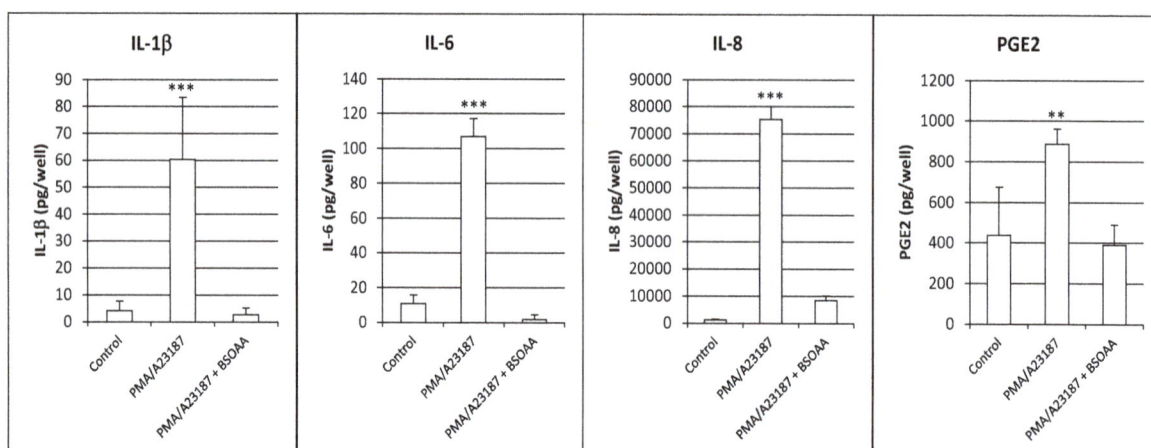

Figure 2. Effect of borage seed oil aminopropanediol amides at 0.005% (v/v) on the cutaneous cell production of IL-1b, IL-6, IL-8 and PGE2. **Significantly different from the "control" (p < 0.01, Student t-test). ***Significantly different from the "control" (p < 0.001, Student t-test). n = 5, from 2 different experiments.

lipoxins and maresin.

Psoriasis and atopic dermatitis are pathologies notably characterized by high skin levels of pro-inflammatory cytokines such as IL-1 and IL-8. Numerous therapeutic approaches so consider the targeting of the cytokine network as a promising therapeutic approach (for a review, see [24]).

Regarding the *in vitro* efficacy of our borage seed oil aminopropanediol amides, *i.e.* their ability to significantly reduce skin cells pro-inflammatory cytokines production, we were prompted in the second part of this work, to deepen our knowledge of our biotechnologically made product by evaluating its effect through *in vivo* study involving 36 subjects suffering from psoriasis and atopic dermatitis.

As shown in **Figure 3**, topical application of a formulation containing 1% of our borage seed oil aminopropanediol amides was able to significantly improve the xerosis of all the subjects' skins (suffering from psoriasis or atopic dermatitis): -67% ($p < 0.01$; visual scoring by dermatologists). As shown in **Figure 4**, the SRRC score of all the volunteers was also significantly improved: -69% ($p < 0.01$). In addition, the auto-evaluation of the product efficacy by the volunteers showed that sensations of itching, tightness and discomfort were also significantly reduced: -60% ($p < 0.01$), -68% ($p < 0.01$) and -74% ($p < 0.01$), respectively (**Figure 5**).

When we consider separately volunteers suffering from psoriasis or from atopic dermatitis, we can note (**Figure 6** and **Figure 7**) that the formulation containing the borage seed oil aminopropanediol amides significantly improve the severity of both psoriasis (PGA scale) and atopic dermatitis (SCORAD index): -13% ($p < 0.01$) and -65% ($p < 0.01$), respectively.

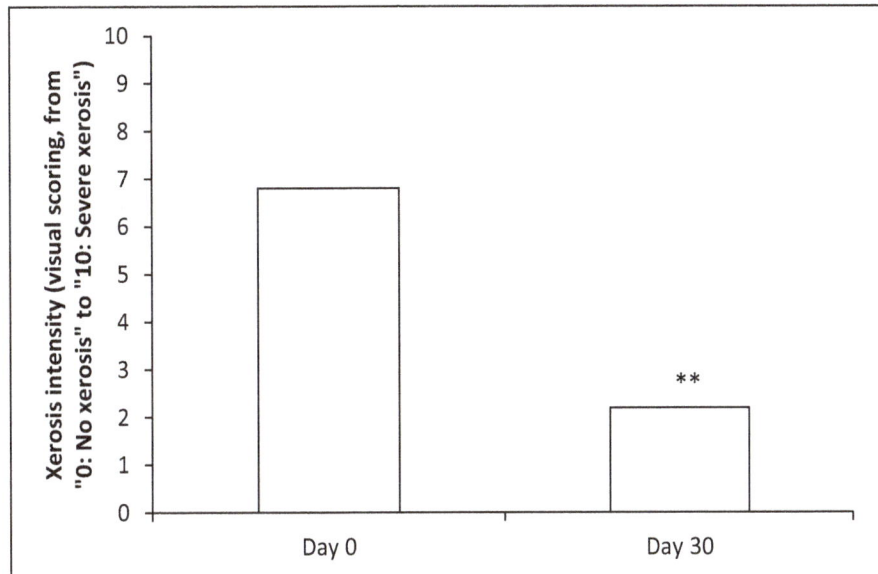

Figure 3. Effect of a formulation containing borage seed oil aminopropanediol amides on skin xerosis. **Significantly different from the "Day 0" ($p < 0.01$, paired Wilcoxon test). n = 36 subjects.

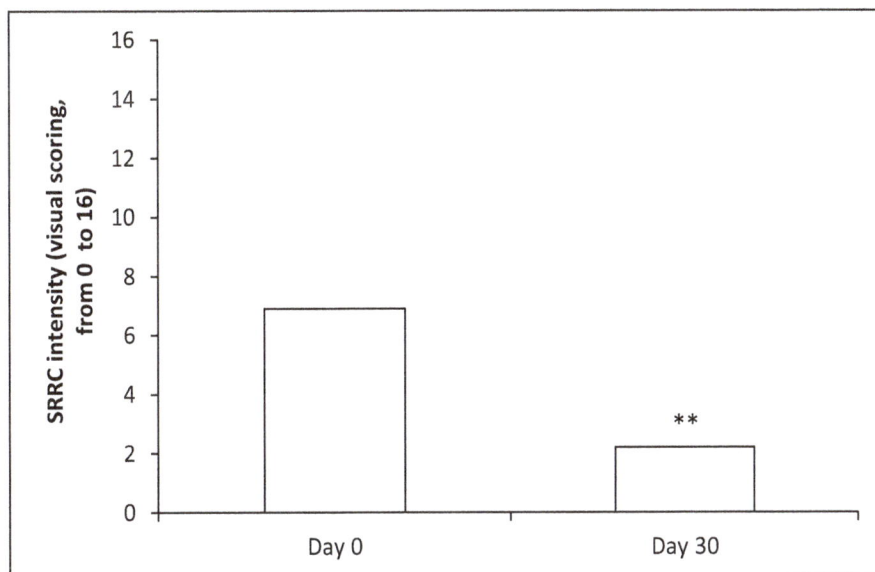

Figure 4. SRRC score after 30 days of use of a formulation containing borage seed oil aminopropanediol amides. **Significantly different from the "Day 0" ($p < 0.01$, paired Wilcoxon test). n = 36 subjects.

At last, as shown in the **Figure 8**, quality of life of the volunteers was significantly improved: the Infant's dermatitis Quality of Life Index (IDQOL) and the Dermatology Life Quality Index (DLQI) were reduced by 65 (p < 0.01) and 75% (p < 0.01), respectively.

All the results obtained in this *in vivo* study are in line with the works of numerous authors showing that targeting the cytokine network could consist in a very helpful therapeutic approach for the treatment of inflammatory diseases in human skin (for a review, see [24] and [25]).

Our *in vitro* and *in vivo* studies also permit us to demonstrate that pro-resolving lipid mediators, or active compounds able to increase their production in skin, could offer pertinent and efficient tools to improve the skin and the life quality of patients suffering from psoriasis or atopic dermatitis notably.

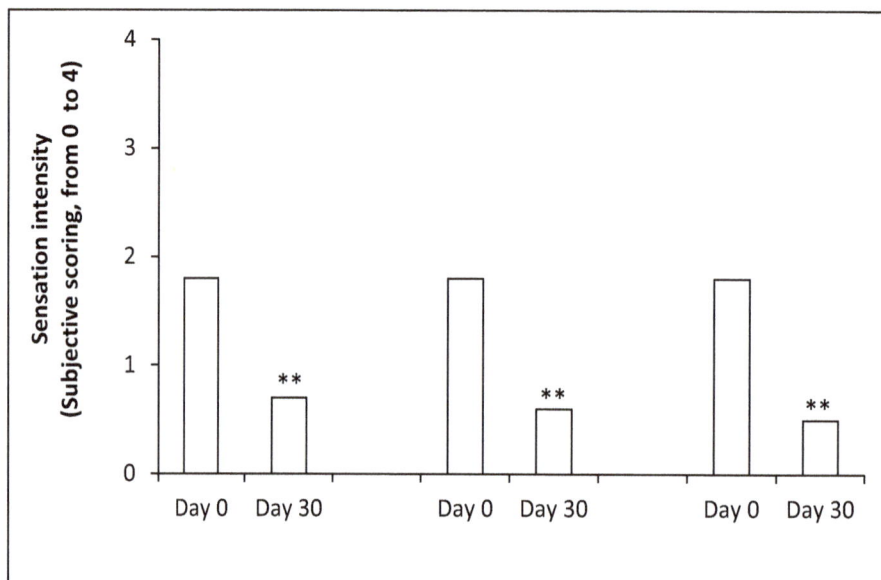

Figure 5. Sensations of tightness, itching and discomfort after 30 days of use of a formulation containing borage seed oil aminopropanediol amides-Auto-evaluation by the volunteers. **Significantly different from the "Day 0" (p < 0.01, paired Wilcoxon test). n = 36 subjects.

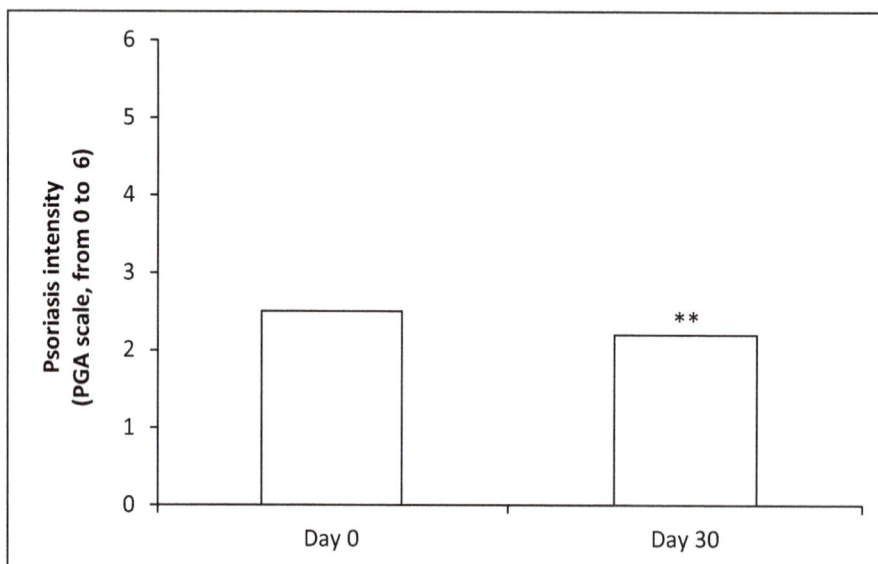

Figure 6. Effect of a formulation containing borage seed oil aminopropanediol amides on psoriasis severity. **Significantly different from the "Day 0" (p < 0.01, paired Wilcoxon test). n = 18 subjects.

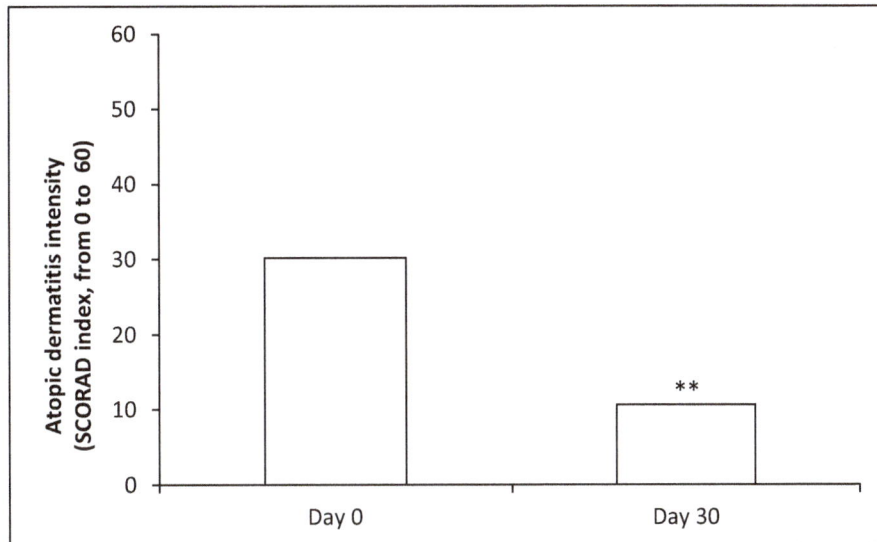

Figure 7. Effect of a formulation containing borage seed oil aminopropanediol amides on atopic dermatitis severity. **Significantly different from the "Day 0" ($p < 0.01$, paired Wilcoxon test) n = 18 subjects.

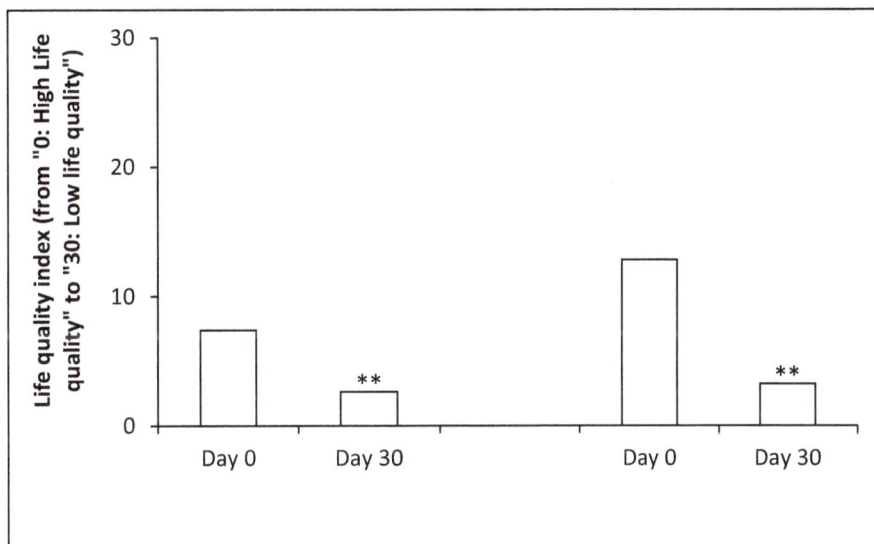

Figure 8. Effect of a formulation containing borage seed oil aminopropanediol amideson the Infant's dermatitis Quality of Life Index (IDQOL) and the Dermatology Life Quality Index (DLQI). **Significantly different from the "Day 0" ($p < 0.01$, paired Wilcoxon test) n = 36 subjects.

4. Conclusion

At last, we show that biotechnologies can be very useful for the generation and/or the amelioration of new therapeutics in human.

References

[1] Serhan, C.N. (2014) Pro-Resolving Lipid Mediators Are Leads for Resolution Physiology. *Nature*, **510**, 92-101. http://dx.doi.org/10.1038/nature13479

[2] Masoodi, M., Kuda, O., Rossmeisl, M., Flachs, P. and Kopecky, J. (2015) Lipid Signaling in Adipose Tissue: Connecting Inflammation & Metabolism. *Biochimica et Biophysica Acta*, **1851**, 503-518.

http://dx.doi.org/10.1016/j.bbalip.2014.09.023

[3]   Ono, E., Dutile, S., Kazani, S., Wechsler, M.E., Yang, J., Hammock, B.D., Douda, D.N., Tabet, Y., Khaddaj-Mallat, R., Sirois, M., Sirois, C., Rizcallah, E., Rousseau, E., Martin, R., Sutherland, E.R., Castro, M., Jarjour, N.N., Israel, E. and Levy, B.D. (2014) Lipoxin Generation Is Related to Soluble Epoxide Hydrolase Activity in Severe Asthma. *American Journal of Respiratory and Critical Care Medicine*, **190**, 886-897. http://dx.doi.org/10.1164/rccm.201403-0544OC

[4]   Giudetti, A.M. and Cagnazzo, R. (2012) Beneficial Effects of n-3 PUFA on Chronic Airway Inflammatory Diseases. *Prostaglandins Other Lipid Mediators*, **99**, 57-67. http://dx.doi.org/10.1016/j.prostaglandins.2012.09.006

[5]   Hsiao, H.M., Sapinoro, R.E., Thatcher, T.H., Croasdell, A., Levy, E.P., Fulton, R.A., Olsen, K.C., Pollock, S.J., Serhan, C.N., Phipps, R.P. and Sime, P.J. (2013) A Novel Anti-Inflammatory and Pro-Resolving Role for Resolvin D1 in Acute Cigarette Smoke-Induced Lung Inflammation. *PLoS ONE*, **8**, e58258. http://dx.doi.org/10.1371/journal.pone.0058258

[6]   Uddin, M. and Levy, B.D. (2011) Resolvins: Natural Agonists for Resolution of Pulmonary Inflammation. *Progress in Lipid Research*, **50**, 75-88. http://dx.doi.org/10.1016/j.plipres.2010.09.002

[7]   Kennedy, A., Fearon, U., Veale, D.J. and Godson, C. (2011) Macrophages in Synovial Inflammation. *Frontiers in Immunology*, **2**, 52. http://dx.doi.org/10.3389/fimmu.2011.00052

[8]   Janakiram, N.B. and Rao, C.V. (2009) Role of Lipoxins and Resolvins as Anti-Inflammatory and Proresolving Mediators in Colon Cancer. *Current Molecular Medicine*, **9**, 565-571. http://dx.doi.org/10.2174/156652409788488748

[9]   Saevik, B.K., Bergvall, K., Holm, B.R., Saijonmaa-Koulumies, L.E., Hedhammar, A., Larsen, S. and Kristensen, F. (2004) A Randomized, Controlled Study to Evaluate the Steroid Sparing Effect of Essential Fatty Acid Supplementation in the Treatment of Canine Atopic Dermatitis. *Veterinary Dermatology*, **15**, 137-145. http://dx.doi.org/10.1111/j.1365-3164.2004.00378.x

[10] Bahmer, F.A. and Schäfer, J. (1992) Treatment of Atopic Dermatitis with Borage Seed Oil (Glandol)—A Time Series Analytic Study. *Kinderärztliche Praxis*, **60**, 199-202.

[11] Lopes, C., Silva, D., Delgado, L., Correia, O. and Moreira, A. (2013) Functional Textiles for Atopic Dermatitis: A Systematic Review and Meta-Analysis. *Pediatric Allergy and Immunology*, **24**, 603-613. http://dx.doi.org/10.1111/pai.12111

[12] Kanehara, S., Ohtani, T., Uede, K. and Furukawa, F. (2007) Undershirts Coated with Borage Oil Alleviate the Symptoms of Atopic Dermatitis in Children. *European Journal of Dermatology*, **17**, 448-449.

[13] Foster, R.H., Hardy, G. and Alany, R.G. (2009) Borage Oil in the Treatment of Atopic Dermatitis. *Nutrition*, **26**, 708-718. http://dx.doi.org/10.1016/j.nut.2009.10.014

[14] Bamford, J.T., Ray, S., Musekiwa, A., van Gool, C., Humphreys, R. and Ernst, E. (2013) Oral Evening Primrose Oil and Borage Oil for Eczema. *Cochrane Database of Systematic Reviews*, **4**, Article ID: CD004416. http://dx.doi.org/10.1002/14651858.cd004416.pub2

[15] Bath-Hextall, F.J., Jenkinson, C., Humphreys, R. and Williams, H.C. (2012) Dietary Supplements for Established Atopic Eczema. *Cochrane Database of Systematic Reviews*, **2**, Article ID: CD005205. http://dx.doi.org/10.1002/14651858.cd005205.pub3

[16] Rahman, M., Beg, S., Ahmad, M.Z., Kazmi, I., Ahmed, A., Rahman, Z., Ahmad, F.J. and Akhter, S. (2013) Omega-3 Fatty Acids as Pharmacotherapeutics in Psoriasis: Current Status and Scope of Nanomedicine in Its Effective Delivery. *Current Drug Targets*, **14**, 708-722. http://dx.doi.org/10.2174/1389450111314060011

[17] Brosche, T. and Platt, D. (2000) Effect of Borage Oil Consumption on Fatty Acid Metabolism, Transepidermal Water Loss and Skin Parameters in Elderly People. *Archives of Gerontology and Geriatrics*, **30**, 139-150. http://dx.doi.org/10.1016/S0167-4943(00)00046-7

[18] Zhang, M.J. and Spite, M. (2012) Resolvins: Anti-Inflammatory and Proresolving Mediators Derived from Omega-3 Polyunsaturated Fatty Acids. *Annual Review of Nutrition*, **32**, 203-227. http://dx.doi.org/10.1146/annurev-nutr-071811-150726

[19] Langley, R.G. and Ellis, C.N. (2004) Evaluating Psoriasis with Psoriasis Area and Severity Index, Psoriasis Global Assessment, and Lattice System Physician's Global Assessment. *Journal of the American Academy of Dermatology*, **51**, 563-569. http://dx.doi.org/10.1016/j.jaad.2004.04.012

[20] Stalder, J.F. and Taïeb, A. (1993) Severity Scoring of Atopic Dermatitis: The SCORAD Index. Consensus Report of the European Task Force on Atopic Dermatitis. *Dermatology*, **186**, 23-31. http://dx.doi.org/10.1159/000247298

[21] Serup, J. (1995) EEMCO Guidance for Assessment of Dry Skin (Xerosis) and Ichthyosis. *Skin Research and Technology*, **1**, 109-114. http://dx.doi.org/10.1111/j.1600-0846.1995.tb00029.x

[22] Lewis-Jones, M.S., Finlay, A.Y. and Dykes, P.J. (2001) The Infants' Dermatitis Quality of Life Index. *British Journal of Dermatology*, **144**, 104-110.

[23] Finlay, A.Y. and Khan, G.K. (1994) Dermatology Life Quality Index (DLQI)—A Simple Practical Measure for Routine Clinical Use. *Clinical and Experimental Dermatology*, **19**, 210-216. http://dx.doi.org/10.1111/j.1365-2230.1994.tb01167.x

[24] Numerof, R.P. and Asadullah, K. (2006) Cytokine and Anti-Cytokine Therapies for Psoriasis and Atopic Dermatitis. *BioDrugs*, **20**, 93-103. http://dx.doi.org/10.2165/00063030-200620020-00004

[25] Wittmann, M., McGonagle, D. and Werfel, T. (2014) Cytokines as Therapeutic Targets in Skin Inflammation. *Cytokine Growth Factor Reviews*, **25**, 443-451. http://dx.doi.org/10.1016/j.cytogfr.2014.07.008

8

Effects of Makeup Application on Diverting the Gaze of Others from Areas of Inflammatory Lesions in Patients with Acne Vulgaris

Yumi Murakami-Yoneda[1], Mieko Hata[2], Yoshie Shirahige[1], Kozo Nakai[1], Yasuo Kubota[1*]

[1]Department of Dermatology, Faculty of Medicine, Kagawa University, Kagawa, Japan
[2]Department of Dermatology, Nippon Medical School, Tokyo, Japan
Email: [*]kubotay@med.kagawa-u.ac.jp

Abstract

Skin manifestations can be major sources of stress for patients with skin diseases; hence, the effective use of makeup and cosmetic products for these patients has been established. The objective of this study was to determine if makeup can divert observers' gaze from areas of inflammatory acne lesions. Both base and point makeup were applied to two Japanese female patients with mild to moderate acne vulgaris to hide skin manifestations, as well as to accentuate the eyes and lips. Photographs of their faces were shown, at various stages of makeup application, to 22 observers (11 men and 11 women). The effects of makeup application, and other eye-diverting strategies (e.g., clothing, accessories, and hairstyle), used to draw observers' gaze away from acne lesions, were evaluated by analyzing observers' eye movements. As base makeup application proceeded, time to first fixation, total fixation duration, and fixation count changed. Compared to "no makeup", the time to first fixation, total fixation duration, and fixation count also decreased significantly after point makeup application. The additional eye-diverting strategies used also had significant gaze-diverting effects. Therefore, makeup can be useful for patients with acne to divert others' gaze from lesions. Therefore, it should be actively integrated into acne management.

Keywords

Acne Vulgaris, Eye Tracking, Base Makeup, Point Makeup, Gaze Diversion

---

[*]Corresponding author.

1. Introduction

In dermatological therapy, cosmetic makeup is considered to exacerbate skin problems on the face. Therefore, patients are generally advised not to use it. However, patients with skin diseases and lesions that are difficult to treat or are incurable, such as vitiligo and scars, can achieve improved quality of life (QOL) when instructed to apply makeup to make skin manifestations less noticeable. The usefulness and safety of makeup and cosmetic products for patients with some skin diseases have been reported [1] [2]. For example, patients with atopic dermatitis and acne vulgaris, who apply makeup under the instruction of dermatologists, report improved QOL [3]-[5]. For patients with skin diseases, the skin manifestations themselves and other people looking at them can be major sources of psychological stress, negatively affecting patient QOL. Moreover, for adult women, the dermatologist-directed prohibition of makeup, which is a part of their personal daily grooming routine, can also become another source of stress.

Makeup can be broadly classified as base makeup and point makeup. Base makeup application can hide skin manifestations, while using point makeup, to accentuate the eyes and lips, can divert the gaze of other people from skin lesions and the affected areas. Thus, patients who are aware of this potential benefit of makeup can improve their QOL [5]. Although previous studies have verified the positive effects of makeup application on the QOL of patients with skin diseases, whether makeup can divert the gaze of other people from skin lesions has not been examined in detail.

Eye-tracking systems have recently enabled the recording and analysis of eye gaze movements and are already being applied in consumer psychology and public marketing research [6] [7]. Eye-tracking systems have also been used to evaluate skin features, such as pigmented lesions and acne vulgaris [8] [9].

Therefore, the present study investigated the ability of makeup application and other diversion strategies, such as hairstyle, to divert the gaze of others from areas affected by skin diseases.

2. Methods

2.1. Patients and Photography

Makeup was applied to a 25-year-old Japanese woman with moderate acne (woman A) and a 23-year-old Japanese woman with mild acne (woman B) in May 2012. Acne severity was determined on the basis of the Japanese Dermatological Association's criteria for acne severity [10]. The women were photographed at different stages of base and point makeup application. They were also photographed wearing different clothes, accessories, or a different hairstyle, or with all of these elements combined. For photography, the women were positioned away from windows to avoid exposure to direct natural light; indoor lighting, from below and above, was used so their faces were unshaded when photographed. They sat facing forward and looked directly into the camera (Canon Inc., Tokyo, Japan) viewfinder to adjust the observer's line of sight. Afterward, Casmatch® (Medical Bear Co., Ltd., Gunma, Japan) in Adobe Photoshop® (Adobe Systems Incorporated, San Jose, CA, USA) was used to edit image color for uniformity of tone and to ensure equal sizing. Written informed consent was obtained from both women, after receiving oral and written explanations of the study. The study was approved by the ethics committee.

2.2. Base and Point Makeup

All makeup products were made by Tokiwa Pharmaceutical Co., Ltd. (Tokyo, Japan). The base makeup consisted of a base control color that corrects for redness and skin rash (NOV® base control color, natural yellow), a concealer that covers areas of particularly strong redness (NOV concealer), and a powder foundation (NOV powdery foundation UV) used to prepare the texture of the skin. Successive images were taken at each stage (A-1 to A-4, respectively). The point makeup consisted of an eyebrow pencil (NOV eyebrow), an eye color product (NOV eye color), and a lipstick (NOV lipstick).

2.3. Observation Subjects

The observation study was performed in July 2012. There were a total of 22 observers (11 men and 11 women). The intent of the evaluation was not explained to the observers. The observers were instructed to look at the images of the women as if they were meeting them for the first time.

2.4. Gaze Movement Measurement

Points of gaze fixation were detected by using an eye tracker attached to an LCD (Tobii T120; Tobii Technology AB, Danderyd, Sweden) in order to measure the movements of the observers' eyes while they evaluated the women's faces. During the measurements, a blue cloth covered the left and right sides of the display so that only the women's face was in the field of view. The display was placed 600 mm in front of the observers' eyes. The images were displayed for 8 s each, at 2s-intervals. Four images were examined per session.

A region of interest analysis was performed. Briefly, several parts of the image of the women's faces were sectionalized, and the area with the most acne (*i.e.*, the right cheek) was established for the analysis. Tobii Studio analysis software (Tobii Technology AB) was used for the analysis. To verify gaze movements away from areas of acne eruption, the right cheek, which had no moles or other marks, was defined as the acne area. In this eye tracker system, green circles on the photographs of the women's faces indicate an observer looked at the area, while red circles indicate observers gazed at the area with greater attention. These "green" and "red" areas were defined as a "visit" and a "fixation", respectively. An image of the heat map is shown in **Figure 1**.

The following markers were analyzed: a) the number of observers who fixed their gaze on the acne area; b) the time to first fixation (*i.e.*, the time elapsed before the observer fixed their gaze on the acne area for the first time); c) total fixation duration (*i.e.*, the total amount of time the observer's gaze remained fixed on the acne area); and d) fixation count (*i.e.*, the number of times the observer fixed their gaze on the acne area).

2.5. Statistical Analysis

Data were analyzed using the Wilcoxon signed-rank test. The Steel-Dwass test was used for multiple comparisons. The level of significance was set at $P < 0.05$.

3. Result

3.1. Effects of Base Makeup Application (Figure 2, Table 1)

- *Number of observers*

As the base makeup process proceeded from A-1 to A-4, the number of observers who fixed their gaze at the acne-affected area decreased slightly: 22, 20, 18, and 19 observers fixated their gaze on the acne-affected area in A-1 through A-4, respectively.

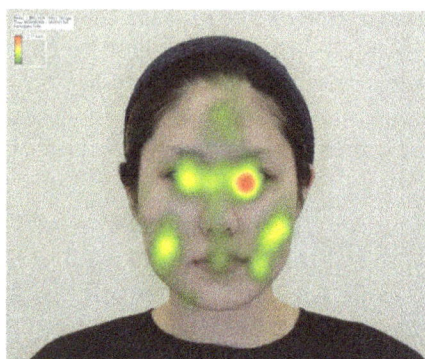

Indicating the concentration of the gaze.

green—yellow—red

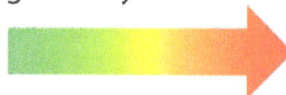

Figure 1. Heat map image.

- **Time to first fixation**

Greater time to first fixation indicates the observers' gaze was fixated less on the acne-affected area on the right cheek. The times to first fixation from A-1 to A-4 tended to increase, but the differences were not significant ($P > 0.05$).

- **Total fixation duration**

Shorter total fixation duration indicates less time was spent with the gaze fixed at the inflammatory acne eruptions. The total fixation from A-1 to A-4 tended to decrease. The total fixation duration in A-4 was significantly shorter than that in A-1 (no makeup) ($P = 0.045$).

- **Fixation count**

A lower fixation count indicates the observers' gaze was fixed at the acne-affected area on the right cheek fewer times. The fixation count tended to decrease from A-1 to A-4, but the differences were not significant ($P > 0.05$).

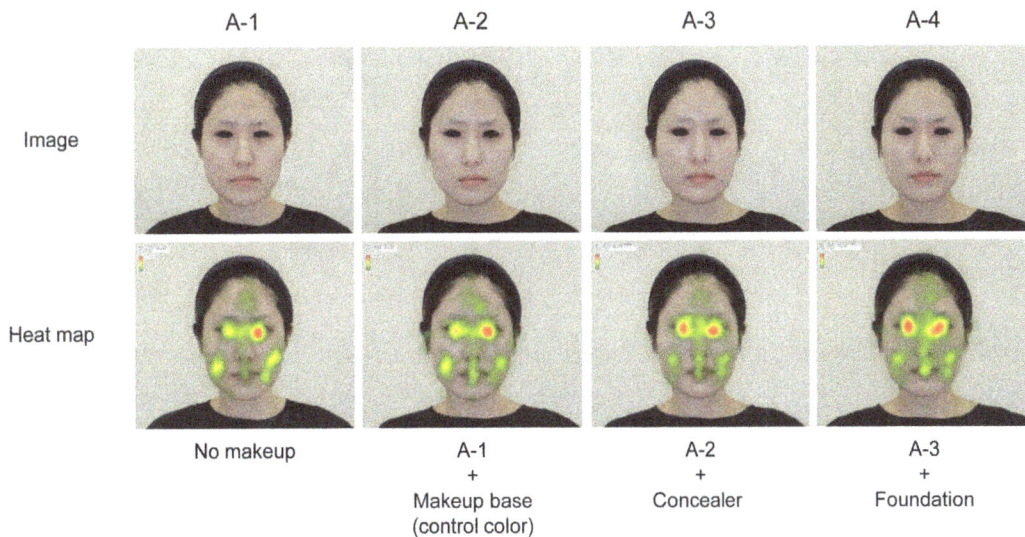

Figure 2. Base makeup images.

Table 1. Effects of base makeup.

		Fixation number (n)	Time to first fixation (s)		Total fixation duration (s)		Fixation count (n)	
			Mean	SE	Mean	SE	Mean	SE
A-1	No makeup	22/22	2.26	0.22	0.74	0.09	2.59	0.29
A-2	A-1 + makeup base (control color)	20/22	2.96	0.36	0.69	0.13	2.18	0.31
A-3	A-2 + concealer	18/22	2.74	0.35	0.47	0.13	1.68	0.35
A-4	A-3 + foundation	19/22	3.40	0.41	0.46	0.11	1.59	0.28
P value	A-1 vs. A-2		0.627	N.S.	0.839	N.S.	0.775	N.S.
	A-1 vs. A-3		0.571	N.S.	0.057	N.S.	0.125	N.S.
	A-1 vs. A-4		0.087	N.S.	0.045	*	0.053	N.S.
	A-2 vs. A-3		0.998	N.S.	0.351	N.S.	0.573	N.S.
	A-2 vs. A-4		0.691	N.S.	0.353	N.S.	0.457	N.S.
	A-3 vs. A-4		0.745	N.S.	0.997	N.S.	1.000	N.S.

**$P < 0.01$, *$P < 0.05$.

3.2. Effects of Point Makeup Application (Figure 3, Table 2)

- *Number of observers*

There were 22, 19, 9, and 15 observers who fixated on the acne-affected area in A-1, A-4, A-5, and A-6, respectively; 15 and 8 observers fixated on the acne-affected area in B-1 and B-2, respectively. Thus, the application of point makeup resulted in fewer observers fixing their gaze on the acne-affected area in both woman A and B.

- *Time to first fixation*

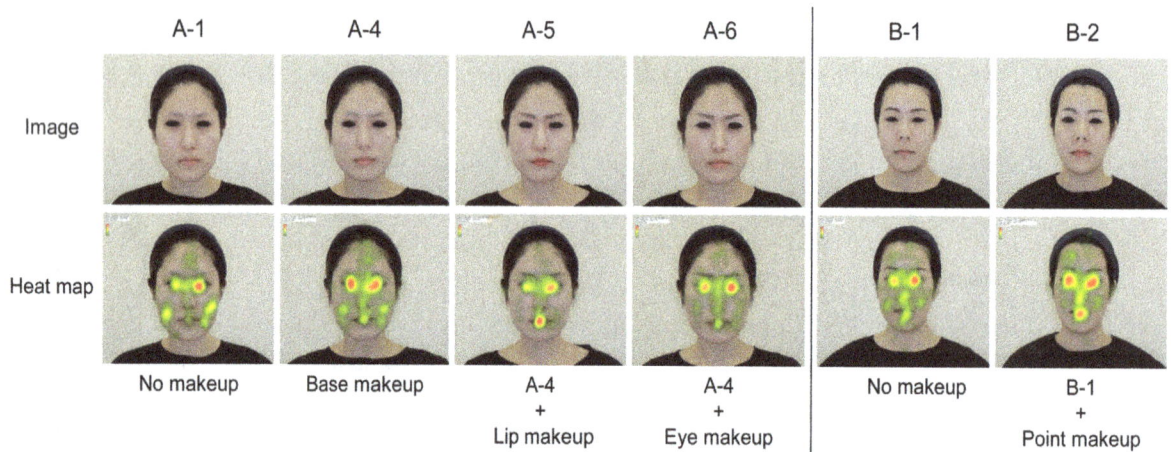

Figure 3. Point makeup images.

Table 2. Effects of point makeup.

		Fixation number (n)	Time to first fixation (s)		Total fixation duration (s)		Fixation count (n)	
			Mean	SE	Mean	SE	Mean	SE
A-1	No makeup	22/22	2.26	0.22	0.74	0.09	2.59	0.29
A-4	Base makeup	19/22	3.40	0.41	0.46	0.11	1.59	0.28
A-5	A-4 + lip makeup	9/22	3.73	0.74	0.17	0.06	0.73	0.22
A-6	A-4 + eye makeup	15/22	3.61	0.44	0.34	0.07	1.19	0.25
P value	A-1 vs. A-4		0.079	N.S.	0.045	*	0.053	N.S.
	A-1 vs. A-5		0.106	N.S.	<0.001	**	<0.001	**
	A-1 vs. A-6		0.035	*	0.012	*	0.008	**
	A-4 vs. A-5		0.961	N.S.	0.045	*	0.053	N.S.
	A-4 vs. A-6		0.900	N.S.	0.983	N.S.	0.756	N.S.
	A-5 vs. A-6		1.000	N.S.	0.218	N.S.	0.379	N.S.
		Fixation number (n)	Time to first fixation (s)		Total fixation duration (s)		Fixation count (n)	
			Mean	SE	Mean	SE	Mean	SE
B-1	No makeup	15/22	4.03	0.50	0.31	0.07	1.41	0.32
B-2	B-1 + point makeup	8/22	4.84	0.49	0.16	0.06	0.45	0.14
P value	B-1 vs. B-2		0.173	N.S.	0.084	N.S.	0.006	**

**$P < 0.01$, *$P < 0.05$.

Compared with the time to first gaze fixation for A-1, that for A-6 was significantly longer ($P = 0.035$). For woman B, the application of point makeup (B-2) tended to extend the time until the first gaze fixation compared to that without makeup (B-1), although the difference was not significant.

- **Total fixation duration**

The total fixation duration at the acne-affected area was significantly shorter in A-4, A-5, and A-6 than in A-1 ($P = 0.045$, < 0.001, and 0.012, respectively). Fixation duration was also significantly shorter in A-5 than A-4 ($P = 0.045$). Similarly, for woman B, the total fixation time was shorter in B-2 than B-1, but the difference was not significant.

- **Fixation count**

The observers looked at the acne-affected cheek significantly fewer times in A-5 and A-6 than A-1 ($P = <$ 0.001, and 0.008, respectively). The fixation count was also lower in A-5 and A-6 than A-4. Similarly, the fixation count was significantly lower in B-2 than B-1 ($P = 0.006$).

3.3. Effects of Point Makeup Application and Other Strategies (Figure 4, Table 3)

- **Number of observers**

Out of 22 observers, 15 and 8 fixated on the acne-affected area in the images without makeup (B-1) and with point makeup, different clothing and hairstyle, and accessories (B-3), respectively.

- **Time to first fixation**

The time to first fixation was shorter in B-3 than B-1, but the difference was not significant. There was no significant difference between B-2 and B-3.

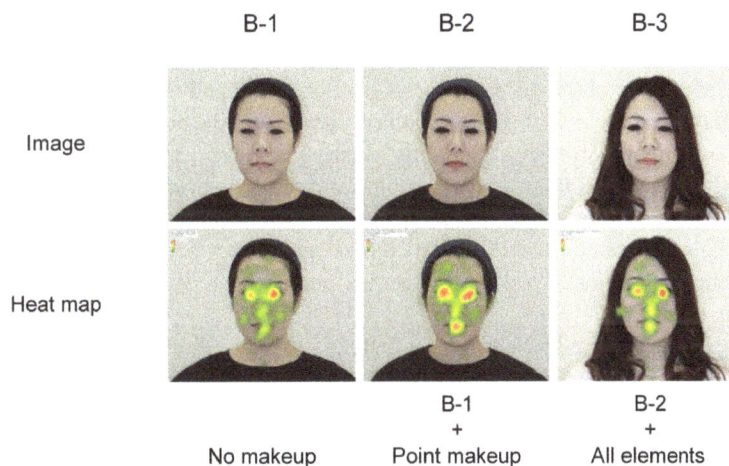

Figure 4. Combinations of makeup and non-makeup elements.

Table 3. Effects of makeup and non-makeup elements.

		Fixation number (n)	Time to first fixation (s)		Total fixation duration (s)		Fixation count (n)	
			Mean	SE	Mean	SE	Mean	SE
B-1	No makeup	15/22	4.03	0.48	0.31	0.07	1.41	0.32
B-2	B-1 + point makeup	8/22	4.84	0.49	0.16	0.06	0.45	0.14
B-3	B-2 + all elements	8/22	3.41	0.47	0.12	0.07	0.64	0.28
	B-1 vs. B-2		0.453	N.S.	0.157	N.S.	0.033	*
P value	B-1 vs. B-3		0.920	N.S.	0.018	*	0.049	*
	B-2 vs. B-3		0.172	N.S.	0.800	N.S.	0.999	N.S.

**$P < 0.01$, *$P < 0.05$.

- *Total fixation duration*

The total fixation duration at the acne-affected area was significantly shorter in B-3 than B-1 ($P = 0.018$), but there was no significant difference between B-2 and B-3.

- *Fixation count*

The fixation count was significantly lower in B-3 than B-1 ($P = 0.049$). There was also no significant difference between B-2 and B-3.

4. Discussion

Although patients with facial dermatologic diseases are generally advised not to use cosmetics in order to avoid exacerbating their skin problems, applying makeup to cover skin manifestations improves their QOL. Hence, the usefulness of makeup is being reevaluated. However, how other people observe patients' skin manifestations and whether makeup, and other strategies, can divert others' gaze from skin lesions have not been verified.

Woman A had moderate acne and noticeable inflammatory acne lesions. Hence, the gradual application of color-correcting base makeup, particularly the concealer, which covered up noticeable acne, and the skin foundation, which adjusted the skin texture, reduced the number of observers who fixed their gaze on the acne-affected area on the right cheek, as well as extended the amount of time until the first fixation. Base makeup also tended to reduce the length of time the observers gazed at the acne-affected area. After completing the steps of successive base makeup application, nearly all variables were equivalent between woman A and woman B, who had mild acne, without makeup.

For point makeup, either eye or lip makeup was applied in addition to the base makeup for woman A. Compared with no makeup, the time until the first gaze fixation was significantly extended, and both the number and duration of gazes were significantly reduced. When lip makeup was applied in addition to base makeup, the duration of gazes as well as the number and duration of fixation were significantly reduced. Because a significant gaze-diverting effect was observed with the application of lip and eye makeup, the choice of lipstick color and degree of eye makeup might also help divert others' gaze from the acne-affected area.

Moreover, non-makeup strategies including wearing different clothing, accessories, and having a different hairstyle tended to divert the gaze of other people from the acne-affected area. These non-makeup strategies significantly reduced the number of gazes, indicating that even when makeup cannot be fully applied, clothing, accessories, and hairstyle can be used to divert others' gaze from acne-affected areas. Accordingly, in women's daily life, makeup application, clothing, accessories, and hairstyle are generally used in combination, resulting in a gaze-diverting effect.

While other people may be less aware of a patient's skin eruptions than the patient believes them to be, acne patients who worry about their skin eruptions may try to hide these areas with their hair, by facing downward, or even by withdrawing and avoiding social encounters. As in other countries, acne is a common problem in Japan that causes personal and social difficulties, as well as reduced QOL. Eruptions on the face can hinder the social lives of young people [9] [11]. Acne eruptions can be a potential barrier in social relationships, particularly for young people [12] [13].

Designated therapeutic guidelines for treating acne have been established in Japan. The combined use of cosmetic moisturizer is reported to increase treatment adherence [14], and various other therapeutic modifications have been tried. Accordingly, the use of makeup does not appear to hinder acne treatments but actually improves patients' QOL [4]. However, applying makeup to cover skin diseases requires skills that can be taught by dermatologists and professional makeup artists [15] [16]; therefore, clinicians need to arrange proper circumstances in which guidance on makeup can be given to acne patients.

5. Conclusion

In conclusion, makeup can be useful for acne patients by diverting others' gaze from lesions. Considering this behavioral change in observers and the resultant psychological effect on the person, makeup may be useful for acne patients. Therefore, it should be actively integrated into acne management.

References

[1]   Tanioka, M. and Miyachi, Y. (2008) Waterproof Camouflage Age for Vitiligo of the Face using Cavilon 3M as a Spray.

European Journal of Dermatology, **18**, 93-94.

[2]   Tanioka, M., Yamamoto, Y., Kato, M. and Miyachi, Y. (2010) Camouflage for Patients with Vitiligo Vulgaris Improved their Quality of Life. *Journal of Cosmetic Dermatology*, **9**, 72-75. http://dx.doi.org/10.1111/j.1473-2165.2010.00479.x

[3]   Hayashi, N., Imori, M., Yanagisawa, M., Seto, Y., Nagata, O. and Kawashima, M. (2005) Make-Up Improves the Quality of Life of Acne Patients without Aggravating Acne Eruptions during Treatments. *European Journal of Dermatology*, **15**, 284-287.

[4]   Matsuoka, Y., Yoneda, K., Sadahira, C., Katsuura, J., Moriue, T. and Kubota, Y. (2006) Effects of Skin Care and Makeup under Instructions from Dermatologists on the Quality of Life of Female Patients with Acne Vulgaris. *The Journal of Dermatology*, **33**, 745-752. http://dx.doi.org/10.1111/j.1346-8138.2006.00174.x

[5]   Levy, L.L. and Emer, J. (2012) Emotional Benefit of Cosmetic Camouflage in the Treatment of Facial Skin Conditions: Personal Experience and Review. *Clinical, Cosmetic and Investigational Dermatology*, **5**, 173-182.

[6]   Maner, J.K., Kenrick, D.T., Becker, D.V., Delton, A.W., Hofer, B., Wilbur, C.J., *et al.* (2003) Sexually Selective Cognition: Beauty Captures the Mind of the Beholder. *Journal of Personality and Social Psychology*, **85**, 1107-1120. http://dx.doi.org/10.1037/0022-3514.85.6.1107

[7]   Kang, O.S., Chang, D.S., Jahng, G.H., Kim, S.Y., Kim, H., Kim, J.W., *et al.* (2012) Individual Differences in Smoking-Related Cue Reactivity in Smokers: An Eye-Tracking and fMRI Study. *Progress in Neuro-Psychopharmacology and Biological Psychiatry*, **38**, 285-293. http://dx.doi.org/10.1016/j.pnpbp.2012.04.013

[8]   Dreiseitl, S., Pivec, M. and Binder, M. (2012) Differences in Examination Characteristics of Pigmented Skin Lesions: Results of an Eye Tracking Study. *Artificial Intelligence in Medicine*, **54**, 201-205. http://dx.doi.org/10.1016/j.artmed.2011.11.004

[9]   Lee, I.S., Lee, A. R., Lee, H., Park, H. J., Chung, S. Y., Wallraven, C., *et al.* (2013) Psychological Distress and Attentional Bias toward Acne Lesions in Patients with Acne. *Psychology, Health & Medicine*, **19**, 680-686. http://dx.doi.org/10.1080/13548506.2014.880493

[10] Hayashi, N., Akamatsu, H. and Kawashima, M. (2008) Establishment of Grading Criteria for Acne Severity. *The Journal of Dermatology*, **35**, 255-260. http://dx.doi.org/10.1111/j.1346-8138.2007.00403.x-i1

[11] Timms, R.M. (2013) Moderate Acne as a Potential Barrier to Social Relationships: Myth or Reality? *Psychology, Health & Medicine*, **18**, 310-320. http://dx.doi.org/10.1080/13548506.2012.726363

[12] Hayashi, N., Higaki, Y., Kawamoto, K., Kamo, T., Shimizu, S. and Kawashima, M. (2004) A Cross-Sectional Analysis of Quality of Life in Japanese Acne Patients Using the Japanese Version of Skindex-16. *The Journal of Dermatology*, **31**, 971-976. http://dx.doi.org/10.1111/j.1346-8138.2004.tb00639.x

[13] Kubota, Y., Shirahige, Y., Nakai, K., Katsuura, J., Moriue, T. and Yoneda, K. (2010) Community-based Epidemiological Study of Psychosocial Effects of Acne in Japanese Adolescents. *The Journal of Dermatology*, **37**, 617-622. http://dx.doi.org/10.1111/j.1346-8138.2010.00855.x

[14] Munehiro, A., Murakami, Y., Shirahige, Y., Nakai, K., Moriue, T., Matsunaka, H., *et al.* (2012) Combination Effects of Cosmetic Moisturisers in the Topical Treatment of Acne Vulgaris. *Journal of Dermatological Treatment*, **23**, 172-176. http://dx.doi.org/10.3109/09546634.2010.551109

[15] Seite, S., Deshayes, F., Dréno, B., Misery, L., Reygagne, F., Saiag, F., *et al.* (2012) Interest of Corrective Makeup in the Management of Patients in Dermatology. *Clinical, Cosmetic and Investigational Dermatology*, **5**, 123-128.

[16] Peuvrel, L., Quéreux, G., Brocard, A., Saint-Jean, M., Vallet, C., Mère, A., *et al.* (2012) Evaluation of Quality of Life after a Medical Corrective Make-Up Lesson in Patients with Various Dermatoses. *Dermatology*, **224**, 374-380. http://dx.doi.org/10.1159/000339478

9

A Comparative Study of Topical Azailic Acid Cream 20% and Active Lotion Containing Triethyl Citrate and Ethyl Linoleate in the Treatment of Mild to Moderate Acne Vulgaris

Hayder R. Al-Hamamy[1*], Adil A. Noaimi[2,3], Ihsan A. Al-Turfy[2], Adil Ibrahim Rajab[4]

[1]Scientific Council of Dermatology and Venereology-Iraqi Board for Medical Specializations, Baghdad, Iraq
[2]Department of Dermatology, College of Medicine, University of Baghdad, Baghdad, Iraq
[3]Arab Board for Dermatology and Venereology, Baghdad Teaching Hospital, Medical City, Baghdad, Iraq
[4]Department of Dermatology, Baghdad Teaching Hospital, Baghdad, Iraq
Email: [*]hayder317@gmail.com, adilnoaimi@yahoo.com, dr_ihssanalturfi@yahoo.com, rajabadil729@yahoo.com

Abstract

Background: Acne vulgaris is a common disorder affecting 79% - 95% of the adolescent population. The choice of treatment depends on the severity, patients with mild to moderate acne should receive topical therapy such as azelaic acid. Rising antibiotic drug resistance consequent to the widespread use of topical antibiotics is causing concern and effective non-antibiotic treatments are needed. Objective: To compare the efficacy and side effects of topical azelaic acid cream 20% versus active lotion containing triethyl citrate and ethyl linoleate (TCEL) in treatment of mild to moderate acne vulgaris. Patients and Methods: This single, blinded, comparative, therapeutic study was done in the Department of Dermatology-Baghdad Teaching Hospital, Baghdad, Iraq; from May 2013-July 2014. Scoring of acne was carried out and the patients were examined every 2 weeks for 10 weeks of treatment. One month after stopping drugs, patients were evaluated for drug complications and disease recurrence. Sixty patients fulfilling enrollment criteria were included in this study. Patients were divided into 2 groups: *Group A* (30 patients) treated twice daily with TCEL lotion and *Group B* (30 patients) treated twice daily with topical azelaic acid cream 20%. Results: Both topical TCEL lotion and azelaic acid cream were statistically an effective therapy for treatment of mild to moderate acne vulgaris. TCEL lotion was more effective and act earlier than

---

[*]Corresponding author.

azelaic acid cream starting from 4 weeks of therapy till the end of treatment (after 10 weeks) and even after 4 weeks after stopping the treatment (P-value < 0.04). No systemic side effect for both groups was noted while the following side effects were reported; burning, pruritus and erythema, all these side effects disappeared after 8 weeks from starting treatment. After one month of follow up there was no significant relapse in both groups. Conclusion: The TCEL is non-antibiotic based, it had quicker onset of action and observable improvement of both inflammatory and non-inflammatory acne lesions. Its use would reduce the risk of antibiotic resistance developing within the skin flora.

Keywords

Acne Vulgaris, Inflammatory, Aknicare, Azelaic Acid

---

1. Introduction

Acne vulgaris is the most common chronic inflammatory skin disease. It affects mainly young people at the sensitive period of puberty and can have an adverse effect on their psychological development, which may lead to social phobias, withdrawal from society and clinical depression [1]-[3].

Current treatments for acne include topical and oral antibiotics, topical antimicrobials and topical and oral retinoids. All acne treatments have potential side-effects, some of which may be severe. Topical and oral antibiotics generally need to be used for several months to achieve a response, which leads to major problems with patient compliance. In addition to possible side-effects, long-term exposure to antibiotics has exerted enormous selective pressure on the bacterial skin flora of patients with acne, with the emergence of antibiotic-resistant *propioni bacteria* [4]-[6].

This has emphasized the need to develop new therapeutic options for the treatment of acne which are preferably non-antibiotic. Therefore, this study was arranged to investigate the efficacy and tolerability of a topical lotion composed of triethyl citrate and ethyl linoleate (TCEL lotion) as the active agents in the treatment of mild to moderate acne vulgaris.

2. Patients and Methods

This single, blinded, comparative, therapeutic study was carried out at the Department of Dermatology and Venereology-Baghdad Teaching Hospital, Baghdad, Iraq from May 2013-July 2014. Sixty patients were included in this study.

Full history was taken from each patient including: age, gender, duration of disease and previous treatment. Physical examination was done to evaluate the severity of acne.

Inclusion criteria were mild to moderate acne vulgaris. Exclusion criteria were severe and nodulocystic acne, coexistence of any other dermatoses involving the face and allergy to medications, plus patients who had used any topical and systemic treatments in the previous 2 months, pregnant and lactating women.

Acne was scored according to Global Acne Grading System (GAGS) [7].

Formal consent was taken from each patient before starting the trial of treatment, after full explanation for the nature of the disease, course of treatment, prognosis and complications, the target of the present work regarding the drug, its efficacy, side effects, the method and duration of treatment and follow up. Ethical approval was confirmed from Scientific Council of Dermatology and Venereology Iraqi Board for Medical Specializations.

Patients with mild to moderate acne vulgaris were divided into two groups (**Figure 1, Figure 2**):

Group A: Patients were treated with TCEL (Aknicare) lotion® (Active lotion containing triethyl citrate and ethyl linoleate) Produced by: General Topics s.r.l, Salo' Italy. In this group 30 patients were instructed to apply Aknicare lotion twice daily for 10 weeks. Clinical evaluation was done every 2 weeks till the end of the 10th week. Then patients were asked to stop the use of medication to be re-evaluated again after one month without any treatment to show any relapse. The assessment was carried out by (GAGS).

Group B: Patients treated with 20% Azelaic acid cream [(AZELEC)R Produced by: Domina Pharmaceuticals Company, Damascus, Syria, 20% cream]. In this group 30 patients were treated in the same manner as in *Group*

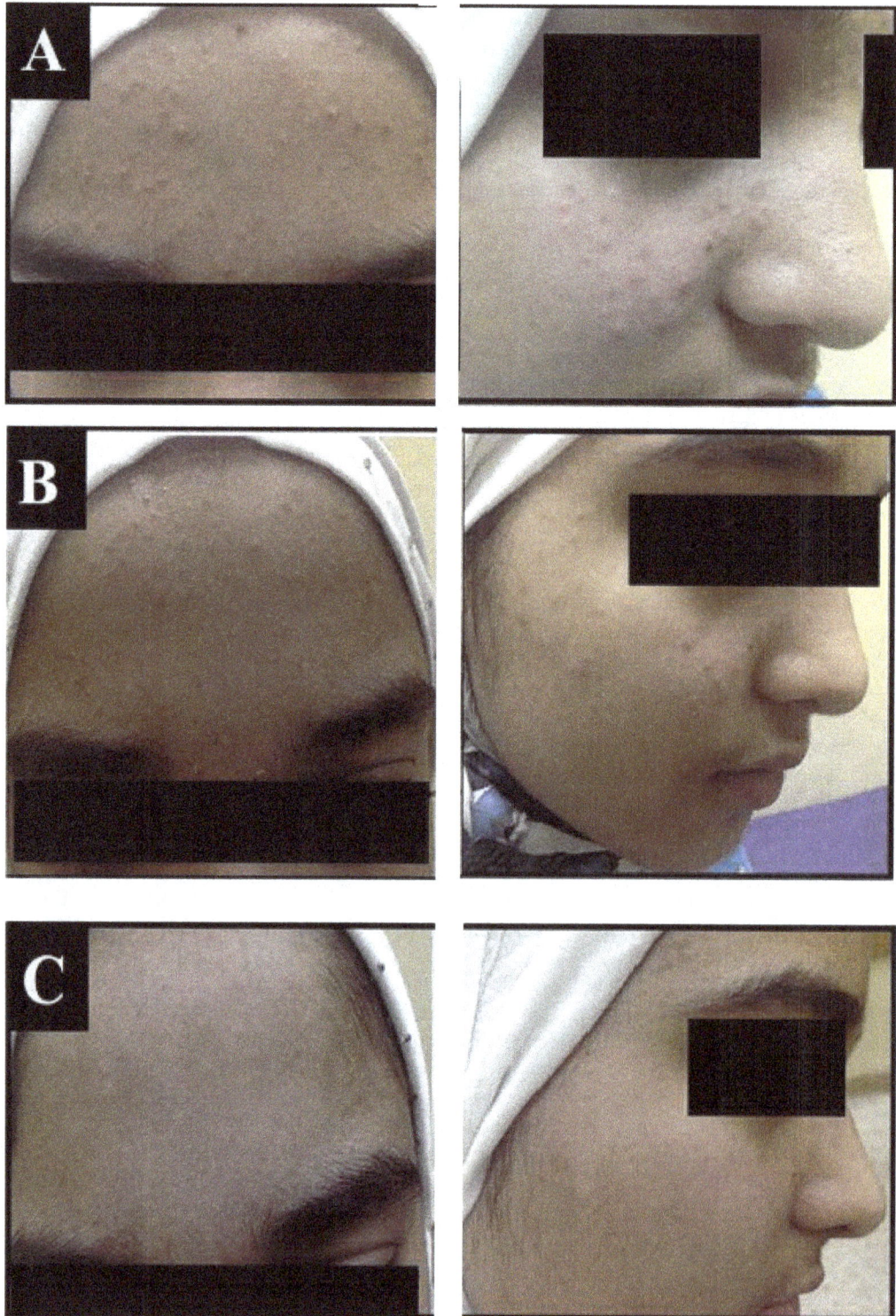

Figure 1. Seventeen years old female with moderate acne vulgaris (A) Before treatment; (B) after 4 weeks and (C) 10 weeks after treatment with topical TCEL lotion.

A patients. Any local or systemic side effects were recorded at each visit for both groups.

Quality of life before and at the end of therapy was measured using the Cardiff Acne Disability Index (CADI) [4].

Color photographs for each patient were obtained by using Sony-digital, high sensitivity, 16.1 megapixel

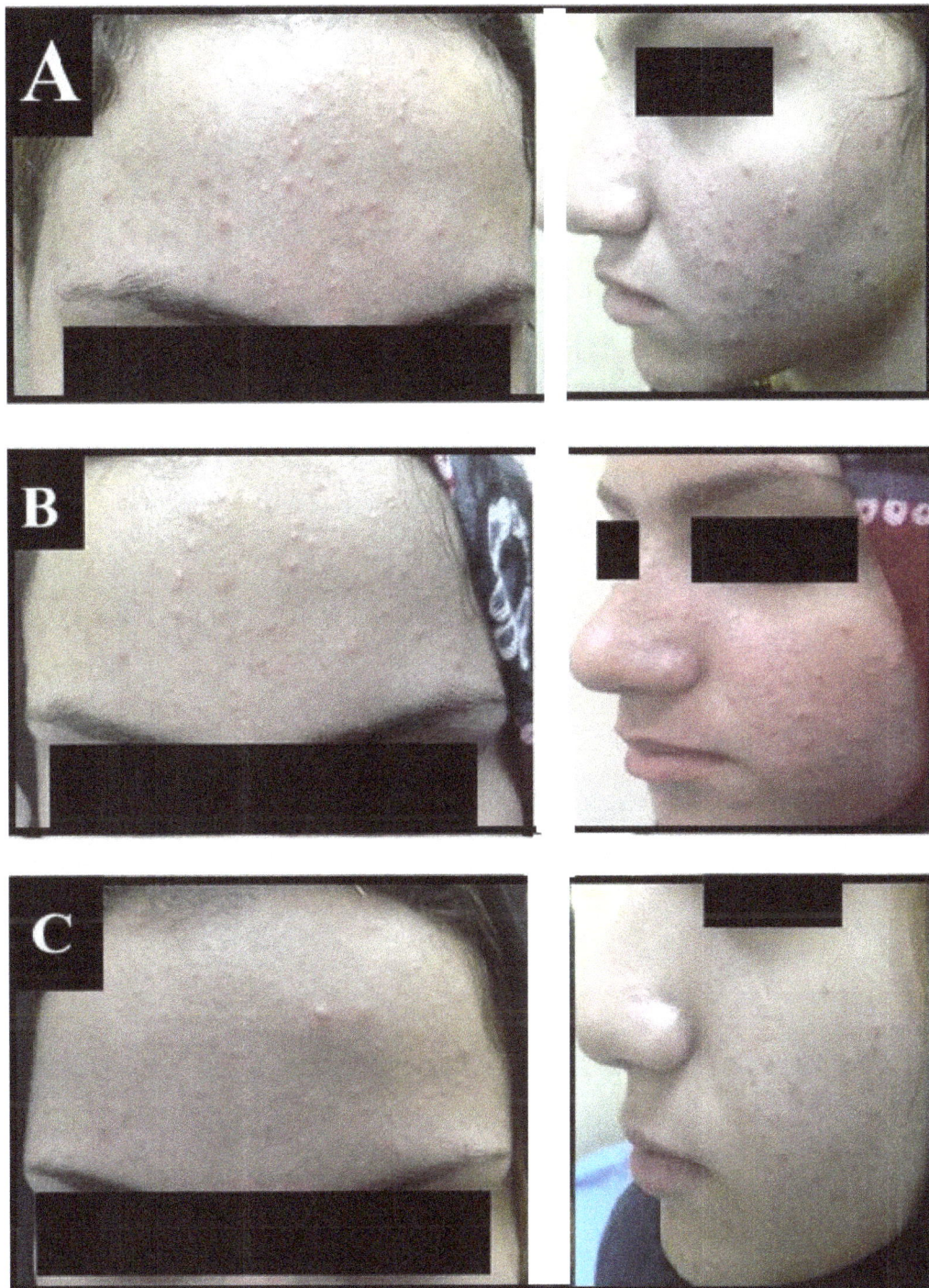

Figure 2. Twenty one years old female with moderate acne (A) Before treatment; (B) after 4 weeks and (C) 10 weeks after treatment with topical Azeliac acid cream 20%.

camera with fixed illumination and distance and the same place.

Statistical analysis of data was carried out using the statistical package of SPSS-20 (Statistical Packages for Social Sciences-version 20). Data were presented in simple measures of frequency, percentage, mean and standard deviation. Comparison between groups was done by using independent sample t-test. Comparison before and after treatment in each group was done by using paired t-test, comparison of reduction rate of the lesions in both groups was done by using chi-square, and P-value < 0.05 was considered as the level of significance.

3. Results

- **Demographic data:**

Patients in *Group A*, their mean age ± SD was 20.33 ± 3.85 years, 21 were females and 9 were males with female to male ratio 2.3:1; *Group B*, their mean age ± SD was 21.53 ± 3.72 years, 19 were females and 11 were female to male ratio 1.7:1.

The mean ± SD of duration of acne in patients within *Group A* was 11.1 ± 5.58 months, and the mean ± SD for those in *Group B* was 11.50 ± 5.24 months. Both groups were statistically matched regarding age, gender and duration of the disease.

- **GAG Score**

In *Group A* (TCEL lotion), the GAG score diminished after 2 weeks of treatment from 24.03 ± 5.07 to 22.10 ± 5.28 but this reduction was not statistically significant (P-value 0.15). At the 4th week the GAG score was 19.53 ± 5.35 which was statistically significant when compared to baseline (P-value 0.04). The GAG score continued to decrease till it became 18.23 ± 6.03 at 6th week, 17.47 ± 6.73 at 8th week and 16.00 ± 6.13 at 10th week (P-value 0.016, 0.001, 0.0001 respectively).

In *Group B* (Azelaic acid cream), the GAG score diminished after 2 weeks of treatment from 24.60 ± 5.16 to 23.33 ± 5.08 but this reduction was not statistically significant (P-value 0.36). At the 4th week the GAG score was 20.47 ± 5.32 which was statistically not significant when compared to baseline (P-value 0.056). The GAG score continued to decrease till it became 18.90 ± 5.55 at 6th week, 17.83 ± 6.35 at 8th week and 15.37 ± 6.16 at 10th week and in all these 3 visits were statistically significant when compared to baseline (P-value 0.032, 0.001, 0.0001 respectively) (**Table 1**).

- **Percent reduction:**

The percent reduction rate of GAG score from baseline visit up to 10 weeks of treatment for *Group A* were 33.4%, *Group B* were 27.5% (**Table 2**).

- **Patient satisfaction:**

Subjective improvement of acne was measured by using Cardiff Acne Disability Index (CADI); quality of life of patients in all groups showed less impairment at end of treatment in comparison with that at the beginning of therapy (P-value < 0.014 for *Group A*, 0.023 for *Group B*. When comparing both groups, patients treated with TCEL lotion had lower CADI than azelaic acid cream but both were statistically significant (**Table 3**).

Table 1. Global Acne Grading system for patients in *Group A* (TCEL lotion) and *Group B* (Azelaic acid) at each visit (2 weeks interval).

Visits	GAG Score (Mean ± SD)	
	Group A	**Group B**
Baseline	24.03 ± 5.07	24.60 ± 5.16
After 2 weeks	22.10 ± 5.28	23.33 ± 5.08
	*P = 0.15	*P = 0.36
After 4 weeks	19.53 ± 5.35	20.47 ± 5.32
	*P = 0.04	*P = 0.056
After 6 weeks	18.23 ± 6.03	18.90 ± 5.55
	*P = 0.016	*P = 0.032
After 8 weeks	17.47 ± 6.73	17.83 ± 6.35
	*P = 0.001	*P = 0.001
After 10 weeks	16.00 ± 6.13	15.37 ± 6.16
	*P = 0.0001	*P = 0.0001

*Statistically different from the 1st visit within the same group (paired t test).

Table 2. Showing percent reduction rate for *Group A* (TCEL lotion) and *Group B* (Azelaic acid cream) at each visit (2 weeks interval).

Visits	Group A	Group B
Baseline	0	0
After 2 weeks	8%	5.2%
After 4 weeks	18.7%	16.8%
After 6 weeks	24.1%	23.8%
After 8 weeks	27.3%	27.5%
After 10 weeks	33.4%	27.5%

*Percent Reduction = (X-Y)/X*100, X is an initial value, Y is a final value.

Table 3. The Cardiff Acne Disability Index for *Group A* (TCEL lotion) and *Group B* (Azelaic acid cream) before and at the end of treatment.

Cardiff Acne Disability Index		CADI Pre-treatment		CADI Post-treatment		*P value
		N	%	N	%	
Aknicare (TCEL lotion)	Mild impairment	0	0.0%	12	40.0%	
	Moderate impairment	15	50.0%	18	60.0%	0.014
	Severe impairment	15	50.0%	0	0.0%	
Azelaic acid cream	Mild impairment	0	0.0%	12	40.0%	
	Moderate impairment	14	46.7%	15	50.0%	0.023
	Severe impairment	16	53.3%	3	10.0%	

*Using Mann-Whitney Test for ordinal data.

- **Relapse rate:**

After one month of follow up, there was no significant relapse in *Group A* the CADI score was 16.00 ± 6.13 at the end of the 10 weeks of treatment and became 16.27 ± 5.84 four weeks following stopping treatment. In *Group B* the CADI score was 15.37 ± 6.16 and became 15.47 ± 6.03. In both groups they did not increased significantly (P-value= 0.43 in *Group A*, and 0.91 in *Group B*).

- **Side effects:**

The assessment of local side effects for *Group A* showed burning in 10 (33.3%) patients, flare-up in 2 (6%), dry skin in 9 (30%), pruritus in 12 (40%) and erythema in 6 (20%) patient. All these symptoms disappeared after 8 weeks from starting treatment. The assessment of local side effects for *Group B* showed burning in 21 (70%) of patients, erythema 18 (60%), scaling 13 (43.3%), flare-up in 2 (6%), dry skin 20 (66.7%) and pruritus 8 (26.7%). All these symptoms disappeared after 8 weeks from starting treatment.

4. Discussion

Acne vulgaris is a common skin disease, affecting about 70% - 80% of adolescents and young adults. It is a multifactorial disease of the pilosebaceous unit. The influence of androgens at the onset of adolescence leads to an enlargement of the sebaceous gland and a rise in sebum production. Additional increased proliferation and altered differentiation of the follicular epithelium eventually blocks the pilosebaceous duct, leading to development of the micro-comedones as the primary acne lesion. Concomitantly and subsequently, colonization with *Propioni bacterium* acnes increases, followed by induction of inflammatory reactions from bacteria, ductal corneocytes, and sebaceous pro-inflammatory agents [1]-[3]. Topical antibiotics are the main stay for mild to moderate inflammatory acne vulgaris [6].

This study demonstrates that this new lotion containing triethyl citrate and ethyl linoleate (TCEL lotion) (Aknicare) is an effective and well-tolerated topical agent in the treatment of mild to moderate acne vulgaris. The use of lotion twice daily for 10 weeks was associated with significant improvement in acne severity.

In the present study, both TCEL lotion cream and azelaic acid cream were shown to be effective in the treatment of mild to moderate acne vulgaris with significant improvement in GAG score after 6 weeks of treatment, while Aknicare acts quicker and was more effective in reduction of GAG score after 4 weeks of therapy.

No relapse was recorded in patients treated with TCEL lotion, and azelaic acid cream one month after stopping the treatment.

These results are comparable to other studies. As Charakida A *et al.* showed that TCEL lotion had significant reduction of inflammatory acne lesions within 4 weeks of treatment [8]. Akamatsu H *et al.* also showed significant reduction in inflammatory lesion count within the same period [9].

Elewski *et al.* [10] and Nazzaro-Porro M *et al.* [11] found that azelaic acid 15% provided a significant reduction in the mean inflammatory lesion count. In the study of Thiboutot *et al.* [12], the mean reductions of inflammatory lesions in the azelaic acid 15% gel treated patients were 58% at the end of therapy, but the present study showed 36.4% decrement in GAG score and this difference may be due to different acne scoring in these studies.

The combination of ethyl linoleate and triethyl citrate can reduce the hyperkeratinization of the pilosebaceous duct, the bacterial colonization of the infundibulum by *Propioni bacterium* acnes and seborrhea, targeting the different steps in the pathogenesis of acne [13]-[15].

The exact mechanism of action in the treatment of acne is not yet known. The antimicrobial, anti-keratinization, and anti-inflammatory effects have been implicated. The antimicrobial action may be related to inhibition of microbial cellular protein synthesis. Azelaic acid is bactericidal against *Propioni bacterium acnes*, *Staphylococcus epidermidis* and possesses bacteriostatic properties against many other aerobic microorganisms [11] [12]. Effects of azelaic acid on neutrophils function have been studied by Akamatsu *et al.* [9] in 1991, and its ability to inhibit of the production of reactive oxygen species have been shown which may contribute the anti-inflammatory effects of azelaic acid. It has been reported that azelaic acid treatment achieved a reduction in the thickness of the stratum corneum, a reduction in the number and size of keratohyalin granules, and a reduction in the amount and distribution of filaggrin in epidermal layers [16].

Local side effects were more common in Azelaic acid. In spite of these side effects, both drugs were tolerable and no patient stopped treatment because of side effects.

The limitations of this study include small sample size and short duration of therapy.

5. Conclusion

In conclusion, the TCEL is non-antibiotic based; it had quicker onset of action and observable improvement of both inflammatory and non-inflammatory acne lesions. Its use would reduce the risk of antibiotic resistance developing within the skin flora.

Disclosure

This study is an independent study and not funded by any drug companies.

References

[1]   Simpson, N.B. and Cunliffe, W.J. (2004) Disorders of the Sebaceous Glands. In: Burns, T., Breathnach, S., Cox, N., Griffiths, C., Eds., *Rook's Text Book of Dermatology*, 7th Edition, Blackwell Science, **43**, 1-7. http://dx.doi.org/10.1002/9780470750520.ch43

[2]   Habif, T.P. (2010) Acne and Related Disorder. *Clinical Dermatology: A Color Guide to Diagnosis and Therapy*, 5th Edition, Edinburgh, **7**, 217-247.

[3]   Dreno, B. and Poli, F. (2003) Epidemiology of Acne. *Dermatology*, **206**, 7-10. http://dx.doi.org/10.1159/000067817

[4]   Sharquie, K.E., Gumar, A. and Al-Kodsi, Z. (1991) Acne Vulgaris Epidemiology and Grading. *Saudi Medical Journal*, **12**, 44-47.

[5]   Kurokawa, I., Danby, F.W., Ju, Q., Wang, X., Xiang, L.F., Xia, L., Chen, W., Nagy, I., Picardo, M., Suh, D.H., Ganceviciene, R., Schagen, S., Tsatsou, F. and Zouboulis, C.C. (2009) New Developments in Our Understanding of Acne Pathogenesis and Treatment. *Experimental Dermatology*, **18**, 821-832.

http://dx.doi.org/10.1111/j.1600-0625.2009.00890.x

[6] Katsamba, A. and Dessinioti, C. (2008) New and Emerging Treatments in Dermatology: Acne. *Dermatology and Therapy*, **21**, 86-95. http://dx.doi.org/10.1111/j.1529-8019.2008.00175.x

[7] Doshi, A., Zaheer, A. and Stiller, M.J. (1997) A Comparison of Current Acne Grading Systems and Proposal of a Novel System. *International Journal of Dermatology*, **36**, 416-418. http://dx.doi.org/10.1046/j.1365-4362.1997.00099.x

[8] Charakida, A., Charakida, M. and Chu, A.C. (2007) Double-Blind, Randomized, Placebo-Controlled Study of a Lotion Containing Triethyl Citrate and Ethyl Linoleate in the Treatment of Acne Vulgaris. *British Journal of Dermatology*, **157**, 569-574. http://dx.doi.org/10.1111/j.1365-2133.2007.08083.x

[9] Akamatsu, H., Komura, J., Miyachi, Y., *et al.* (1990) Suppressive Effects of Linoleic Acid on Neutrophil Oxygen Metabolism and Phagocytosis. *Journal of Investigative Dermatology*, **95**, 271-274. http://dx.doi.org/10.1111/1523-1747.ep12484890

[10] Elewski, B.E., Fleischer Jr., A.B. and Pariser, D.M. (2003) A Comparison of 15% Azelaic Acid Gel and 0.75% Metronidazole Gel in the Topical Treatment of Papulopustular Rosacea: Results of a Randomized Trial. *Archives of Dermatology*, **139**, 1444-1450. http://dx.doi.org/10.1001/archderm.139.11.1444

[11] Nazzaro-Porro, M., Passi, S., Picardo, M., Breathnach, A., Clayton, R. and Zina, G. (1983) Beneficial Effect of 15% Azelaic Acid Cream on Acne Vulgaris. *British Journal of Dermatology*, **109**, 45-48. http://dx.doi.org/10.1111/j.1365-2133.1983.tb03990.x

[12] Thiboutot, D., Thieroff-Ekerdt, R. and Graupe, K. (2003) Efficacy and Safety of Azelaic Acid (15%) Gel as a New Treatment for Papulopustular Rosacea: Results from Two Vehicle-Controlled, Randomized Phase III Studies. *Journal of the American Academy of Dermatology*, **48**, 836-845. http://dx.doi.org/10.1067/mjd.2003.308

[13] Namazi, M.R. (2004) Further Insight into the Patho-Mechanism of Acne by Considering the 5-Alpha-Reductase Inhibitory Effect of Linoleic Acid. *International Journal of Dermatology*, **43**, 701. http://dx.doi.org/10.1111/j.1365-4632.2004.02200.x

[14] Charakida, A., Charakida, M. and Chu, A.C. (2007) Double-Blind, Randomized, Placebo-Controlled Study of a Lotion Containing Triethyl Citrate and Ethyl Linoleate in the Treatment of Acne Vulgaris. *British Journal of Dermatology*, **157**, 569-574. http://dx.doi.org/10.1111/j.1365-2133.2007.08083.x

[15] Park, S.Y., Seetharaman, R., Ko, M.J., Kim do, Y., Kim, T.H., Yoon, M.K., Kwak, J.H., Lee, S.J., Bae, Y.S. and Choi, Y.W. (2014) Ethyl Linoleate from Garlic Attenuates Lipopolysaccharide-Induced Pro-Inflammatory Cytokine Production by Inducing Heme Oxygenase-1 in RAW264.7 Cells. *International Immunopharmacology*, **19**, 253-261. http://dx.doi.org/10.1016/j.intimp.2014.01.017

[16] Fitton, A. and Goa, K.L. (1991) Azelaic Acid: A Review of Its Pharmacological Properties and Therapeutic Efficacy in Acne and Hyperpigmentary Skin Disorders. *Drugs*, **41**, 780-798. http://dx.doi.org/10.2165/00003495-199141050-00007

10

Peri-Orbital Non-Invasive and Painless Skin Tightening-Safe and Highly Effective Use of Multisource Radio-Frequency Treatment Platform

Isabelle Rousseaux

Cabinet de Dermatologie Esthétique, Lille Côté Sud, Loos, France
Email: irousseaux@wanadoo.fr

Abstract

The periorbital area is the third highest-ranking area for cosmetic surgery. However, surgery in this area presents a number of difficulties and safety concerns. First generation Monopolar RF treatments in this area were usually associated with considerable pain and long downtime. In the present clinical study, we used the iFine handpiece of the EndyMed PRO, multi-source phase-controlled radiofrequency (RF) for Non-invasive, pain free, skin rejuvenation of the periorbital area. The study included eleven (11) subjects, treated for periorbital signs of aging (iFine handpiece, EndyMed PRO platform, EndyMed Medical, Caesarea, Israel). The degree of clinical improvement was assessed by the global aesthetic improvement scale (GAIS) and subjects satisfaction by post treatment questionnaires. 91% of patients showed good to excellent improvement as a result of the treatment. Subjects satisfaction showed that 55% of patients reported that they were very satisfied, 45% were satisfied while none were dissatisfied. There were no incidences of infections, scarring, hypopigmentation, or any other serious complications.

Keywords

Facial Tightening, Radiofrequency, EndyMed, 3DEEP®, Periorbital

1. Introduction

The periorbital area is the third highest-ranking area for cosmetic surgery [1]. Blepharoplasty, eyelid surgery, has traditionally been used at a relatively early stage due to the limitations of non-surgical alternatives. However, surgery in this area presents a number of difficulties and safety concerns. In the present clinical study, we used the iFine handpiece of the Endymed PRO, multi-source phase-controlled radiofrequency (RF) for Non-invasive skin tightening around the eyes.

The periorbital area is one of the first areas to show the signs of ageing, laxity, fine lines and wrinkles. Treatment options are limited, due to the delicate nature of the skin in this area and safety concerns related to proximity to the eyeball. Blepharoplasty, whilst still being the third most common cosmetic surgical procedure, is not an option for many patients due to cost, risks associated with the general anesthesia, risks of scarring, and the post-operative recovery period [1]. Non-surgical options such as Botulinum toxin and dermal fillers can be effective, in the right hands, but also have inherent risks [2] [3]. Dermal fillers can lead to infection at the injection site as well as nodule formation or a bluish discoloration beneath the skin (the Tyndall phenomenon) due to superficial injection technique [2]. Complications of injecting Botulinum toxin include dry eye syndrome, which if unidentified can lead to eyelid swelling, epiphora (excessive tear production) and scleral show [3].

RF has been found to be effective in the safe delivery of energy into the skin, independent of skin color [4]. Resistance encountered by the RF energy flow causes a build-up of heat, which induces an immediate contraction of the collagen (an "instant lift") and stimulates a natural wound-healing response, production of new skin cells and collagen [6]. When focused in the dermis and hypodermis, non-ablative RF treatment can lead to improvements in the skin structure and tightening of lax and sagging skin. In addition to providing skin tightening, RF can be implemented for skin resurfacing and micro-needle dermal remodeling.

Due to the high safety profile of the treatment, it is suitable for most patient groups and all skin types [6]. Multiple RF technologies and devices are available, with varying levels of efficacy and safety [7].

Most RF devices use monopolar or bipolar technologies. Monopolar RF uses one RF generator and one electrode to deliver the RF energy into the skin, often using a grounding pad. Bipolar RF also uses one RF generator and the energy flows between two electrodes. Results with these technologies can be variable, patients are often exposed to high levels of energy, causes epidermal heating and discomfort, thus cooling must be implemented, and there are possible side effects including burns, purpura and hyperpigmentation [9]. Monopolar RF transmits RF from one electrode of the skin to a second electrode under the back. The flow of energy in this case in uncontrolled and may raise concerns especially when treating periorbital areas.

Multi-source phase-controlled RF is a sophisticated FDA-cleared RF technology that uses six RF generators and six electrodes. Proprietary software controls how the energy flows between the electrodes, with multiple fields of energy interacting and forcing the energy deep into the skin without overheating its surface. The result is a deep, volumetric heating of the dermis and hypodermis, which delivers high level and predictable clinical results with excellent patient comfort and a high safety profile [5]-[8].

Multi-source RF can also be implemented for fractional skin resurfacing, providing an epidermal and dermal skin rejuvenation effect. The multi-source RF micro-ablates up to 10% of the treated area with simultaneous volumetric heating of the dermis, resulting in good and predictable clinical outcomes [10] [11]. The downtime is shorter than traditional laser resurfacing procedures and the risk of side effects is minimal [10]. In comparison to monopolar technology in which the energy from the skin electrode to the back plate uncontrolled through the body, in the Multisource technology the emitting and return electrodes are in the handpiece and all energy will be confined to the skin .

Amy Patdu reported on her experience using multi-source RF for eye rejuvenation in Asian skin [4] about 19 patients who had completed a course of six treatments with the 3DEEP® iFine; a specially designed handpiece for the periorbital area that delivers heat to a depth of 2.8 mm. During each treatment the skin temperature was raised to approximately 40°C and sustained for three minutes.

The technology allows pain-free, safe and effective treatment of the delicate and hard-to-reach skin immediately around the eyes and will reduce under eye bags, smooth and tighten the skin and lift the upper eyelid to reveal a more open eye. There is an immediate visible improvement, which disappears after one to two days but is an indication of the long-lasting result and is a great hook for first-time patients. More recently we have significantly enhanced our protocol and results for periorbital rejuvenation.

Inglefield [12] reported the combination of 2 different multisource RF treatments, combining a single treatment periorbital skin tightening and fractional skin resurfacing. The skin tightening treatment was carried out according to the standard protocol, then after application of a topical anesthetic the Fractional RF skin resurfacing (FSR) handpiece was used over the area. A course of four treatments spaced four weeks apart was performed. Inglefield found that the addition of the FSR, provided an additional tightening effect and epidermal ablation for a smoother, brighter result. Inglefield reported in his study overall patient satisfaction of 94% of patients very satisfied or extremely satisfied with the results they have achieved.

2. Patients and Methods

Eleven subjects (10 females, 1 male, ages of 61.1 ± 8.6 years) with periorbital signs of aging were enrolled in the study. All patients were Caucasians, Fitzpatrick's skin types 1 - 4. Inclusion criteria were visible signs of periorbital skin aging and more specifically visible peri-orbital wrinkles and or lax skin.

We excluded patients that have cardiac arrhythmia or pacemakers and patients that had undergone surgery or injection in treated area in the last 6 months.

Patients were photographed using standardized methods before each session. In each treatment session, each patient received a periorbital non-ablative skin tightening treatment. iFine handpiece of the EndyMed PRO treatment platform (Endymed Medical Ltd., Caesarea, Israel) was used (**Figure 1**). A total number of 6 sessions were performed for each patient. The treatment sessions were repeated every 2 weeks for the first four sessions, then once a month for the 2 last sessions.

Treated areas were visually assessed for skin responses, including edema, erythema, hypopigmentation, hyperpigmentation, and textural changes following the treatment. Global Aesthetic Improvement Scale (GAIS), validated by Day *et al.* [13], is a five grade scale where "5" is "very much improved" (75% - 100% improvement), "4" is "much improved" (50% - 75% improvement), "3" is "improved" (25% - 50% improvement) 2 is minimal-no change (0% - 25% improvement) and "1" is "worse". Patients' photographs were graded according to the Global Aesthetic Improvement Scale (GAIS) by a board certified dermatologist in addition to subjective satisfaction questionnaires filled by the patients.

Patients' photographs were graded according to the Global Aesthetic Improvement Scale (GAIS) by a board certified dermatologist in addition to subjective satisfaction of the patients.

3. Results

Six subjects had 6 treatment sessions, 1 had 8 sessions and 3 others had 10 sessions. Mild to moderate eryhema and mild edema were noted following the non-ablative Skin Tightening procedure. No unexpected adverse effects were detected or reported. There were no incidences of infections, scarring, hypopigmentation, or any other serious complications.

Physician Evaluation

All patients showed improvement. Excellent improvement (>76%) was noted in 2 patients, very good improvement (50% - 75%) in 4 patients, good (26% - 50%) in 4 patients and minimal to no change in one patient (**Figure 2**, **Figure 3**, **Table 1**).

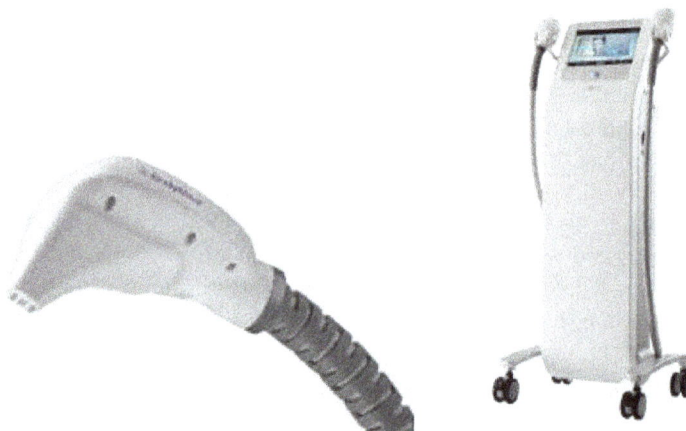

Figure 1. iFine Multisource RF for the periorbital and perioral areas. Rt. EndyMed Pro Multisource RF (3DEEP) treatment platform.

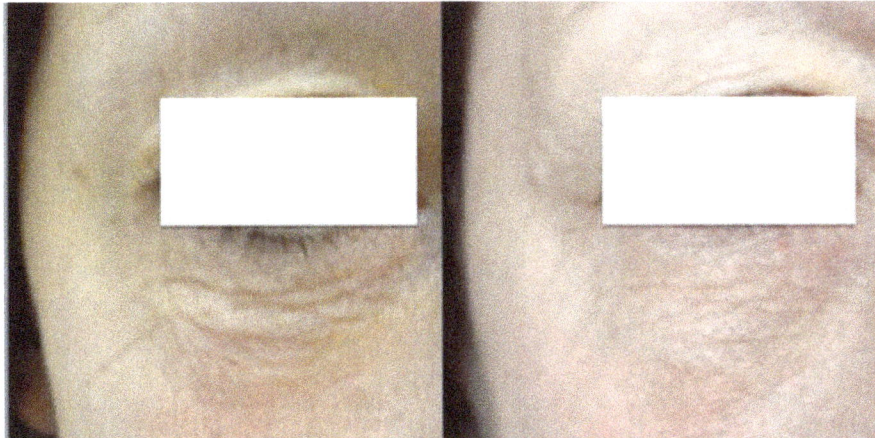

Figure 2. Before and after 6 sessions of EndyMed's iFine treatments. Significant improvement of texture, wrinkle reduction and tightening of the periorbital skin.

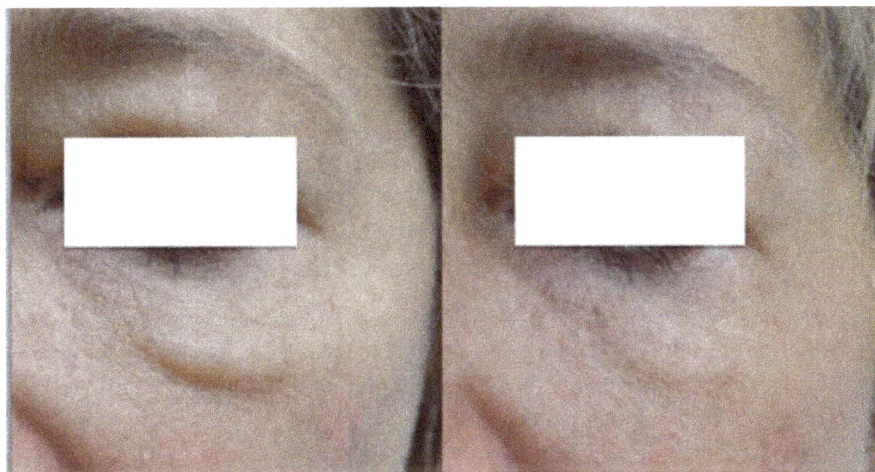

Figure 3. Before and after 4 sessions of EndyMed's iFine treatments. Significant improvement of texture, wrinkle reduction and tightening of the periorbital skin.

Table 1. Physician evaluation using the global aesthetic improvement scale (GAIS) showed improvement in 91% of patients.

Global aesthetic improvement scale (GAIS)	Improvement	Patients	Percent
Very much improved		2	18
Much improved	75% - 100%	4	37
Improved	50% - 75%	4	36
Minimal to no change	25% - 50%	1	9
Worse	0% - 25%	0	0

In addition to clinical evaluation of the results by the physician the patients were asked about their satisfaction with the treatment. The questionnaires suggested 5 grades of satisfaction. Very satisfied, satisfied, neutral, somewhat dissatisfied, and very dissatisfied. In our study, 55% of patients reported that they were very satisfied, 45% were satisfied while none were dissatisfied (**Figure 4**).

4. Discussion and Conclusions

Periorbital treatments were performed for the above study using multisource phase controlled system. iFine handpiece, used in this study, is specially designed to treat delicate areas such as periorbital and perioral.

Subjective Patient Satisfaction

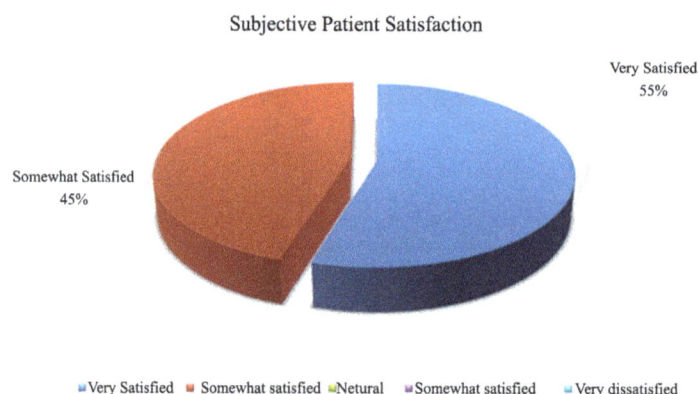

Very Satisfied
55%

Somewhat Satisfied
45%

Very Satisfied   ■ Somewhat satisfied ■Netural   ■Somewhat satisfied   ■ Very dissatisfied

Figure 4. Patient Satisfaction questionnaires. When asked about treatment satisfaction 55% of patients reported that they were very satisfied, 45% were satisfied while none were dissatisfied.

Body and face non-ablative skin tightening using multisource radiofrequency (EndyMed PRO) is one of the leading technologies for this purpose in France. In this present report, we describe for the first time in France a clinical study of periorbital area, showing significant improvement of skin texture, skin laxity and eye bags.

Blepharoplasty and other periorbital surgical procedures have increased in popularity over the past few decades, notably including new solutions in skin tightening and rejuvenation and the treatment of facial rhytides [12]. However, lots of patients prefer non-invasive treatments with no to minimal downtime.

In our current study, Dermatologist's evaluation using the global aesthetic improvement scale (GAIS) showed good to excellent improvement in 91% of the patients and mild improvement in additional 9%. Patients' subjective satisfaction was high.

The treatment was well accepted by the patients with minimal or no pain. There was no need for post therapy treatment and patients were able to return to work with makeup as soon as one hour after therapy.

Four to six weeks after treatment dermal changes were noted including significant improvement in skin texture, reduction of wrinkles and skin laxity.

Based on the above results, we believe the new EndyMed PRO iFine RF procedure provides an exciting new option for effective treatment of skin laxity around the eyes with minimal discomfort and downtime. To further explore this very promising technology there is a need for larger studies, with a larger range of skin types and longer follow up.

References

[1]   American Society of Plastic Surgeons (2013) Plastic Surgery Statistics Report.

[2]   Lafaille, P. and Benedetto, A. (2010) Fillers: Contraindications, Side Effects and Precautions. *Journal of Cutaneous and Aesthetic Surgery*, **3**, 16-19. http://dx.doi.org/10.4103/0974-2077.63222

[3]   Ozgur, O., Murariu, D., Parsa, A. and Parsa, F. (2012) Dry Eye Syndrome Due to Botulinum Toxin Type-A Injection: Guideline for Prevention. *Hawai'i Journal of Medicine & Public Health*, **7**, 120-123.

[4]   Patdu, A. (2014) Non-Invasive Eye Rejuvenation of Asian Skin Using a Novel Multi-Source Phase-Controlled Radiofrequency Device. *PRIME*, **2**, 19-27.

[5]   Elman, M. and Harth, Y. (2011) Novel Multi-Source Phase-Controlled Radiofrequency Technology for Nonablative and Micro-Ablative Treatment of Wrinkles, Lax Skin and Acne Scars. *Laser Therapy*, **20**, 139-144. http://dx.doi.org/10.5978/islsm.20.139

[6]   Harth, Y. (2015) Painless, Safe, and Efficacious Noninvasive Skin Tightening Body Contouring, and Cellulite Reduction Using Multisource 3DEEP Radiofrequency. *Journal of Cosmetic Dermatology*, **14**, 70-75. http://dx.doi.org/10.1111/jocd.12124

[7]   De la Torre, J.R., Moreno-Moraga, J., Muñoz, E. and Navarro, P.C. (2011) Multisource, Phase-Controlled Radiofrequency for Treatment of Skin Laxity. Correlation between Clinical and *In-Vivo* Confocal Microscopy Results and Real-Time Thermal Changes. *Journal of Clinical and Aesthetic Dermatology*, **4**, 28-35.

[8]   Harth, Y. and Lischinsky, D. (2011) A Novel Method for Real-Time Skin Impedance Measurement during Radiofre-

quency Skin Tightening Treatments. *Journal of Cosmetic Dermatology*, **10**, 24-29.
http://dx.doi.org/10.1111/j.1473-2165.2010.00535.x

[9]　Paasch, U., Bodendorf, M.O., Grunewald, S. and Simon, J.C. (2009) Skin Rejuvenation by Radiofrequency Therapy: Methods, Effects and Risks. *Journal der Deutschen Dermatologischen Gesellschaft*, **7**, 196-203.
http://dx.doi.org/10.1111/j.1610-0387.2008.06780.x

[10]　Dahan, S., Rousseaux, I. and Cartier, H. (2013) Multisource Radiofrequency for Fractional Skin Resurfacing-Significant Reduction of Wrinkles. *Journal of Cosmetic & Laser Therapy*, **15**, 91-97.
http://dx.doi.org/10.3109/14764172.2012.748205

[11]　Elman, M., Frank, I., Cohen-Froman, H. and Harth, Y. (2012) Effective Treatment of Atrophic and Icepick Acne Scars Using Deep Non-Ablative Radiofrequency and Multisource Fractional RF Skin Resurfacing. *Journal of Cosmetics, Dermatological Sciences and Applications*, **2**, 267-272. http://dx.doi.org/10.4236/jcdsa.2012.24051

[12]　Ingelfield, C. (2014) Radiofrequency Treatment for the Treatment of the Periorbital Region. *Aesthetic Journal*, **11**, 45-46.

[13]　Day, D.J., *et al.* (2004) The Wrinkle Severity Rating Scale: A Validation Study. *American Journal of Clinical Dermatology*, **5**, 49-52. http://dx.doi.org/10.2165/00128071-200405010-00007

Surgical Flap and Graft Reconstruction Workshop for Dermatology Residents[*]

Brandon Goodwin, Richard Wagner

Department of Dermatology, The University of Texas Medical Branch, Galveston, TX, USA
Email: bpgoodwi@utmb.edu

Abstract

Background: Traditional models for teaching surgical principles focus primarily on the apprenticeship theory; however there has been a trend in surgical education to certifying competency in a simulation environment prior to working with patients. Many surgical models emphasize learning the technical and manual dexterity skills necessary to be a surgeon, yet few focus on obtaining the theoretical and abstract skills needed for planning complex cutaneous surgical repairs with flaps and grafts. We developed and evaluated a novel surgical flaps and grafts workshop for residents through the Department of Dermatology. Methods: Participants received a 60 minute PowerPoint lecture focusing on the basic principles of cutaneous repair with flaps and grafts, with examples and explanation of each of the four main types of flaps and grafts. The participants then received nine photocopies of Mohs micrographic surgery defects with instructions to design three repairs, focusing on functional and aesthetic outcome. Hypothetical and actual repair designs were then discussed in an open forum format. Anonymous surveys administered to 11 dermatology residents assessed their knowledge level, confidence level, and likelihood of using flaps and grafts pre- and post-workshop using Likert scales. Overall experience was also assessed. A paired sample Wilcoxon Signed Rank Test was used for analysis, since the data was non-parametrically distributed. Results: There was a statistically significant increase in confidence performing flaps post workshop ($p = 0.0469$). There was also an increase in knowledge of flaps and grafts, confidence in planning flaps and grafts, and confidence in performing grafts post workshop, but these findings did not reach statistical significance. The workshop had no effect on expected future use of flaps and grafts. Conclusions: The surgical workshop is a novel simulation teaching tool for learning basic principles and design of flaps and grafts in cutaneous surgery.

Keywords

Surgical Skills Workshop, Flaps, Grafts, Dermatology, Resident Education

[*]Presented in part at the Dermatology Teachers Exchange Group, San Francisco, California, USA, March 23, 2015.

1. Introduction

Traditional teaching models in surgical training revolve around the apprenticeship theory, "see one, do one, teach one" [1]. Most residents still obtain cutaneous surgery skills by assisting attending surgeons during surgical procedures, not within formal training environments [2]. Concerns over the adequacy of traditional surgical training have stemmed from a climate of decreasing clinical exposure during residency secondary to work hour restrictions and patient safety concerns [3]. In a recent study by Lee and colleagues of US dermatology residency programs, third year dermatology residents assume the role of the primary surgeon during 49% of flap and graft reconstruction cases and during 18% of Mohs micrographic surgery cases [4]. As direct hands-on experience with flap and graft reconstruction of Mohs defects may be limited in some dermatology programs, exposure to learning through surgical apprenticeship is as well. Therefore it is imperative that new teaching models be developed to maximize learning these concepts.

The classic adult learner prefers learning activities that are experience oriented, self-directed, immediately applicable, internally motivated, and problem-centered [5]. A study assessing learning styles among US dermatology residents showed that active learning styles were significantly favored over passive teacher oriented learning styles overall and among male and female residents separately [5]. A surgical skills workshop incorporates many of the traditional active learning styles preferred by dermatology residents. Surgical skills workshops certify the competency of the learner in a stress free simulation environment thereby increasing confidence, knowledge and surgical ability prior to exposure to patients [6] [7]. While many surgical skills workshops have been developed to facilitate learning technical skills and manual dexterity essential in becoming a surgeon, few have been created to teach planning and design of complex repairs of surgical defects. We created a novel teaching tool for learning about and planning flap and graft reconstruction that is easy to use and assemble, inexpensive, incorporates a low-stress learning environment, and utilizes active learning.

2. Background

The Accreditation Council for Graduate Medical Education (ACGME) is the accrediting body for US post graduate medical training programs, including dermatology programs. According to the ACGME, a dermatology residency program must provide a clinical experience with significant exposure to Mohs micrographic surgery, and wound reconstruction, including flaps and grafts. Residents must be able to competently perform all surgical procedures considered essential for the area of practice including closures of surgical defects with attention to the patient outcome. Residents must also demonstrate knowledge of proper techniques for repairs of cutaneous surgical defects using flaps and grafts [8].

3. Materials and Methods

Eleven dermatology residents participated in the surgical flap and graft reconstruction workshop during the 2014-2015 academic year. The workshop started with an anonymous pre-workshop questionnaire (**Appendix 1**) followed by a 60-minute PowerPoint presentation that focused on the basic principles of flap and graft reconstruction with specific examples and explanations of the main types of flaps and grafts [9]. Identified learning objectives included: identify and know the four main types of flaps (advancement, rotation, transposition, and interpolation flaps); understand how each of the four main types of flaps move; understand how/when flaps may be used in dermatological surgery; identify and know the four main types of grafts (full thickness, split thickness, composite, and free cartilage grafts); and understand how/when grafts may be used in dermatological surgery. After the presentation, the participants were given nine photocopies of Mohs micrographic surgery defects (cheek, forehead, dorsal hand, nose {nasal sidewall-small/large, nasal tip}, upper cutaneous lip, ear {superior helix, lobule}) with instructions (**Appendix 2**) to design three repairs for each defect, focusing on functional and aesthetic outcome for the patient. Participants had one week to design their repairs. No repair was considered "off limits", but the participants were expected to be able to defend why one repair was chosen over another. On follow up, participants met in an open forum format to discuss both the hypothetical repairs (**Figure 1**) designed by residents and the actual repair performed following Mohs micrographic surgery. The attending Mohs surgeon was present to facilitate the dialogue and provide guidance and expertise when discussing repair options. The workshop concluded with an anonymous post-workshop questionnaire (**Appendix 3**). Internal departmental educational activities are not subject to Institutional Review Board review.

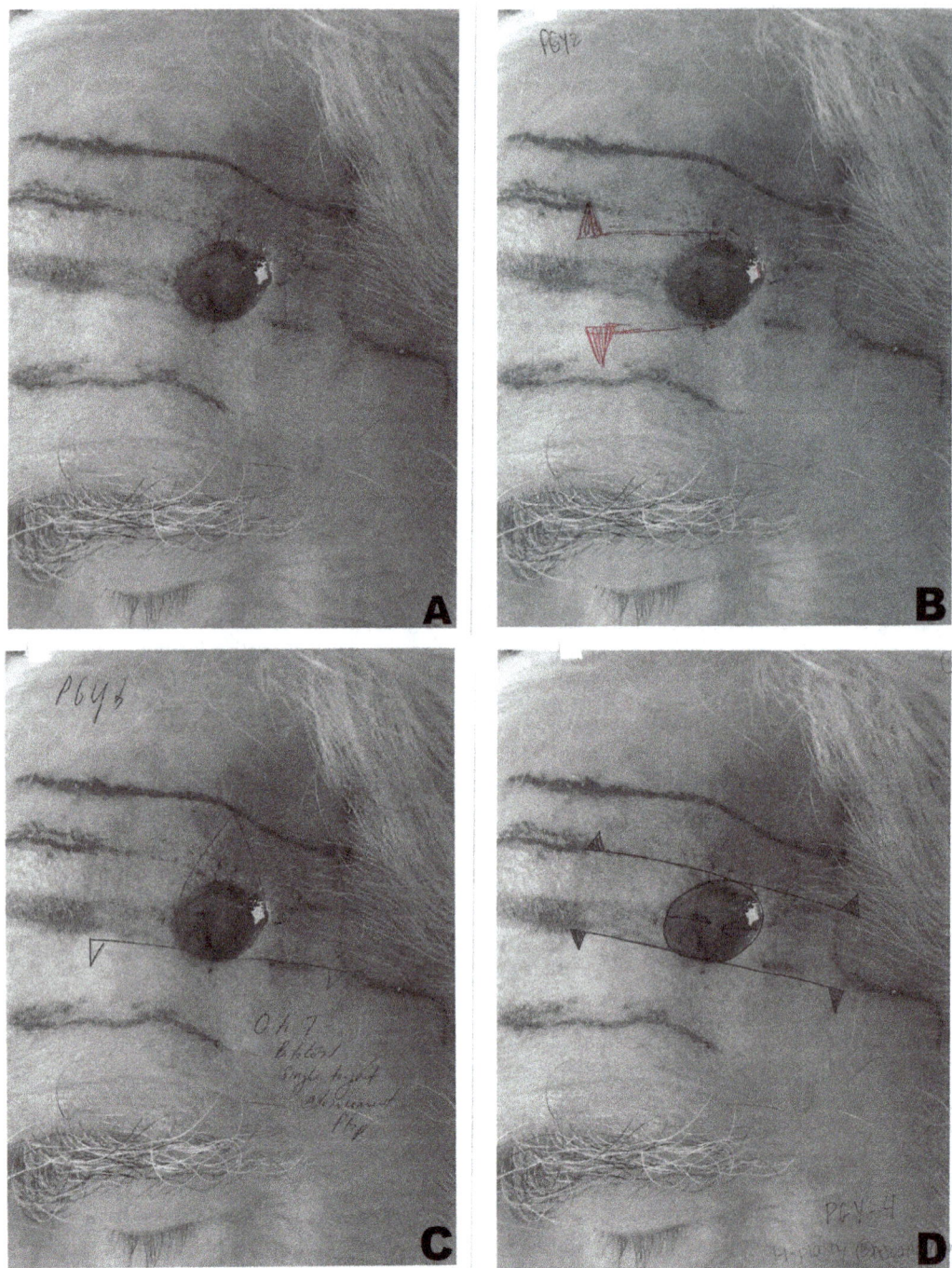

Figure 1. MMS forehead defect and repairs designed by different post graduate year (PGY) participants. (A) Mohs micrographic surgery forehead defect; (B) post graduate year 2 repair design; unilateral double tangent advancement flap; (C) post graduate year 3 repair design; O to T bilateral single tangent advancement flap; (D) post graduate year 4 repair design; H-plasty bilateral double tangent advancement flap.

In the anonymous surveys administered for the pre and post skills workshop, respondents were asked to assess their overall knowledge of flap and graft repairs, confidence level in both planning and performing flap and graft repairs, if the stated learning objectives were met during the workshop, if the workshop was a good educational experience and the likelihood of flap and graft use in future practice using Likert scales. Likert scale responses of four or higher (4 = somewhat agree, 5 = completely agree) were considered "positive", and a response of three or lower (3 = neutral, 2 = somewhat disagree, 1 = completely disagree) were considered "negative" in evaluating participant responses for assessment of the workshop obtaining its learning objectives and its overall educational experience. The participants were also asked to assess overall surgical experience with flaps and graft repair using yes/no response questions prior to the workshop. A paired sample Wilcoxon Signed Rank non-parametric test was used to compare the medians for pre- vs. post-workshop survey questions. This test was used to account for non-normal distribution of the data using SAS for window software, version 9.3.

4. Results

Ninety one percent (10/11) of respondents had witnessed a flap reconstruction and 73% (8/11) of respondents had performed a flap reconstruction prior to the surgical workshop. The percentage of flap repairs witnessed and performed increased with post graduate year of training. Of the 73% (8/11) of respondents who had performed a flap repair in the past, 50% (4/8) had performed less than five repairs and 50% (4/8) had performed greater than 10 repairs. The number of flap repairs increased with post graduate year training, with 100% (3/3) of PGY-4 residents performing greater than 10 flap repairs.

Ninety one percent (10/11) of respondents had witnessed a graft reconstruction and 55% (6/11) of respondents had performed a graft reconstruction prior to the surgical workshop. The percentage of graft repairs witnessed did not increase with post graduate year level, while the percent performed did increase with post graduate year of training. Of the 55% (6/11) of respondents who had performed a graft repair in the past, 50% (3/6) had performed less than five repairs and 50% (3/6) had performed greater than 10 repairs. The number of graft repairs increased with post graduate year training, with 100% (3/3) of PGY-4 residents performing greater than 10 graft repairs.

Results showed a statistically significant change in confidence with performing flap reconstruction (p = 0.0469) post workshop. There was an increase in knowledge of flaps and grafts, confidence in planning flaps and grafts, and confidence in performing grafts post workshop. The workshop had no effect on the likelihood of participant's future use of flap and graft reconstruction. However this data failed to reach statistical significance, most likely due to a small sample size (n = 11).

Positive response rates for each of the learning objectives are as follows: identify and know the 4 main types of flaps (100%, 11/11 positive); understand how each of the four main types of flaps move (73%, 8/11 positive); understand how/when flaps may be used in dermatological surgery (82%, 9/11 positive); identify and know the four main types of grafts (100%, 11/11 positive); and understand how/when grafts may be used in dermatological surgery (91%, 10/11 positive). Eighty two percent (9/11) of participants thought the flap and graft surgical workshop was a good educational experience.

5. Discussion

There was an increase in participant knowledge of flaps and grafts, confidence in planning flaps and grafts, and confidence in performing flaps and grafts post workshop, but only confidence in performance of flaps reached statistical significance. Research supports our above finding that surgical workshops increase participants' ability to perform procedural skills and their confidence [1] [2] [6]. Overall, the majority of participants found the workshop to be useful and a good educational experience for learning about flap and graft repairs.

Limitations of our study include a small number of participants (n = 11), focusing only on surgical theory while disregarding actual "hands-on" training for flap and graft reconstruction, and poor quality photocopies with lack of defect measurements, which may have influenced repair decisions. In the future, hands on training with surgical simulation models can be added to apply the concepts learned with the current flap and graft workshop.

6. Conclusion

Since dermatology residents must demonstrate knowledge of proper techniques for repairs of cutaneous surgical defects using flaps and grafts prior to graduation, an interactive surgical workshop focusing on the planning of defect repairs using flap and graft reconstruction may be a beneficial addition to a surgical curriculum [8]. As dermatology residents tend to prefer active teaching styles, implementing active teaching styles will often lead to a more enjoyable educational experience [5]. We present the surgical flap and graft reconstruction workshop as a novel teaching tool for learning flaps and grafts that is easy to use and assemble, inexpensive, incorporates a low stress learning environment, and utilizes active learning.

References

[1]   Banks, E., *et al.* (2006) A Surgical Skills Laboratory Improves Residents' Knowledge and Performance of Episiotomy Repair. *American Journal of Obstetrics and Gynecology*, **195**, 1463-1467. http://dx.doi.org/10.1016/j.ajog.2006.05.041

[2]   Altinyazar, H.C., Hosnuter, M., Unalacak, M., Koca, R. and Babuccu, O. (2003) A Training Model for Cutaneous Surgery. *Dermatological Surgery*, **29**, 1122-1124.

[3]   Nicholas, L., Toren, K., Bingham, J. and Marquart, J. (2013) Simulation in Dermatologic Surgery: A New Paradigm in Training. *Dermatological Surgery*, **39**, 76-81. http://dx.doi.org/10.1111/dsu.12032

[4]   Lee, E., Nehal, K., Dusza, S., Hale, E. and Levine, V. (2011) Procedural Dermatology Training during Dermatology Residency: A Survey of Third-Year Dermatology Residents. *Journal of the American Academy of Dermatology*, **64**, 475-483. http://dx.doi.org/10.1016/j.jaad.2010.05.044

[5]   Stratman, E., Vogel, C., Rick, S. and Mukesh, B. (2008) Analysis of Dermatology Resident Self-Reported Successful Learning Styles and Implications for Core Competency Curriculum Development. *Medical Teacher*, **30**, 420-425. http://dx.doi.org/10.1080/01421590801946988

[6]   Adams, C., Marquart, J., Nicholas, L., Sperling, L. and Meyerle, J. (2014) Survey of Medical Student Preference for Simulation Models for Basic Dermatologic Surgery Skills: Simulation Platforms in Medical Education. *Dermatological Surgery*, **40**, 427-435. http://dx.doi.org/10.1111/dsu.12445

[7]   Ghiabi, E. and Taylor, L. (2010) Teaching Methods and Surgical Training in North American Graduate Periodontics Programs: Exploring the Landscape. *Journal of Dental Education*, **74**, 618-627.

[8]   (2014) ACGME (Accreditation Council for Graduate Medical Education). http://www.acgme.org/acgmeweb/Portals/0/PFAssets/ProgramRequirements/080_dermatology_07012014_u06152014.pdf

[9]   Bolognia, J.L., Jorizzo, J.L. and Schaffer, J.V., Eds (2012) Bolognia Textbook of Dermatology. 3rd Edition, Mosby Elsevier Publishing, Spain, Chapters 147-148.

Appendix 1. Anonymous Pre Flap/Graft Surgical Workshop Survey

Year (PGY 2, PGY 3, PGY 4): _____
I have witnessed a surgical flap repair in the past
(1) Yes
(2) No
I have performed a surgical flap repair in the past
(1) Yes
(2) No
I have witnessed a surgical graft repair in the past
(3) Yes
(4) No
I have performed a surgical graft repair in the past
(1) Yes
(2) No
Regarding the number of surgical flap repair opportunities (performed and witnessed), I have participated in:
(1) < 5
(2) 5 - 10
(3) > 10
Regarding the number of surgical graft repair opportunities (performed and witnessed), I have participated in:
(1) < 5
(2) 5 - 10
(3) > 10

My surgical flap repair knowledge prior to participation in the flap/graft surgical workshop
1   2   3   4   5
(1 = no experience, 2 = below average, 3 = average, 4 = above average, 5 = excellent)

My surgical graft repair knowledge prior to participation in the flap/graft surgical workshop
1   2   3   4   5
(1 = no experience, 2 = below average, 3 = average, 4 = above average, 5 = excellent)

I feel confident planning surgical defect repairs with flap procedures
1   2   3   4   5
(1 = completely disagree, 2 = somewhat disagree, 3 = neutral, 4 = somewhat agree, 5 = completely agree)

I feel confident planning surgical defect repairs with graft procedures
1   2   3   4   5
(1 = completely disagree, 2 = somewhat disagree, 3 = neutral, 4 = somewhat agree, 5 = completely agree)

I feel confident performing surgical repairs with flap procedures
1   2   3   4   5
(1 = completely disagree, 2 = somewhat disagree, 3 = neutral, 4 = somewhat agree, 5 = completely agree)

I feel confident performing surgical repairs with graft procedures
1   2   3   4   5
(1 = completely disagree, 2 = somewhat disagree, 3 = neutral, 4 = somewhat agree, 5 = completely agree)

I am likely to use surgical flaps and graft repairs in the future
1   2   3   4   5
(1 = completely disagree, 2 = somewhat disagree, 3 = neutral, 4 = somewhat agree, 5 = completely agree)

Appendix 2. Anonymous Flap/Graft Surgical Workshop Instructions

• You are given nine Mohs micrographic surgery (MMS) defects with negative margins in need of repair.
   -Cheek, forehead, dorsal hand, nose (nasal sidewall-small/large, nasal tip), upper cutaneous lip, ear (supe-rior helix, lobule)

• Develop three different repair options for each MMS defect by drawing your planned repair on the handout.

• All methods for repair may be used (primary repair, split thickness skin graft, full thickness skin graft, ad-vancement flaps, rotational flaps, transposition flaps, interpolation flaps, etc...).

• All repairs must keep in mind both functional and aesthetic concerns for the patient (free margins, cosmetic subunits, relaxed skin tension lines, tissue laxity, surgical danger zones, etc...).

• After completing your three repairs for the MMS defect place your post graduate year level at the top of each handout. Avoid any other identifying factors.

• We will discuss repair options for each of the defects in one week with an open forum discussion.

• Remember, there is no one "right" way to repair a defect, but be prepared to discuss why one repair option was chosen over the other.

• At the end of the discussion, the anonymous MMS defect/repairs will be collected.

Appendix 3. Anonymous Post Flap/Graft Surgical Workshop Survey

Year (PGY 2, PGY 3, PGY 4): _____

My surgical flap repair knowledge after participation in the flap/graft surgical workshop
1   2   3   4   5
(1 = no experience, 2 = below average, 3 = average, 4 = above average, 5 = excellent)

My surgical graft repair knowledge after participation in the flap/graft surgical workshop
1   2   3   4   5
(1 = no experience, 2 = below average, 3 = average, 4 = above average, 5 = excellent)

I feel confident planning surgical defect repairs with flap procedures
1   2   3   4   5
(1 = completely disagree, 2 = somewhat disagree, 3 = neutral, 4 = somewhat agree, 5 = completely agree)

I feel confident planning surgical defect repairs with graft procedures
1   2   3   4   5
(1 = completely disagree, 2 = somewhat disagree, 3 = neutral, 4 = somewhat agree, 5 = completely agree)

I feel confident performing surgical repairs with flap procedures
1   2   3   4   5
(1 = completely disagree, 2 = somewhat disagree, 3 = neutral, 4 = somewhat agree, 5 = completely agree)

I feel confident performing surgical repairs with graft procedures
1   2   3   4   5
(1 = completely disagree, 2 = somewhat disagree, 3 = neutral, 4 = somewhat agree, 5 = completely agree)

I am likely to use surgical flaps and graft repairs in the future
1   2   3   4   5
(1 = completely disagree, 2 = somewhat disagree, 3 = neutral, 4 = somewhat agree, 5 = completely agree)

The surgical flap and grafts workshop was a good educational experience
1   2   3   4   5
(1 = completely disagree, 2 = somewhat disagree, 3 = neutral, 4 = somewhat agree, 5 = completely agree)

Were the following learning objectives met during the presentation and workshop?

1.   Identify and know the 4 main types of flaps   1   2   3   4   5
2.   Understand how each of the 4 main types of flaps move   1   2   3   4   5
3.   Understand how/when flaps may be used in dermatological surgery   1   2   3   4   5
4.   Identify and know the 4 main types of grafts   1   2   3   4   5
5.   Understand how/when grafts may be used in dermatological surgery   1   2   3   4   5
(1 = completely disagree, 2 = somewhat disagree, 3 = neutral, 4 = somewhat agree, 5 = completely agree)

Are there any changes you would recommend for future flap/graft workshops:
_____

Additional comments:
_____

12

Inter-Toe Cracks: A Cosmetic Response versus Excipient. Efficacy and Tolerance Evaluation

Adeline Jeudy[1,2,3], Thomas Lihoreau[1,2,3], Ferial Fanian[1,2,3], Rafat Messikh[1,2,3], Christine Lafforgue[1,2,3], Philippe Humbert[1,2,3]*

[1]Research and Studies Center on the Integument (CERT), Department of Dermatology, Besançon University Hospital, Besançon, France
[2]Clinical Investigation Center (CIC Inserm 1431), Besançon University Hospital, Besançon, France
[3]Inserm UMR1098, FED4234 IBCT, Besançon University Hospital, Besançon, France
Email: *philippe.humbert@univ-fcomte.fr

Abstract

A randomized, monocentric, double-blind, intra-individual excipient-controlled comparative study was performed to evaluate the efficacy and tolerance of an active peptide (laminin 5 fragment [LN-5]) formulated in cosmetic balm, versus excipient in inter-toe cracks. Two products were tested on 10 healthy volunteers. Each of them suffered from this particular superficial wound characterized by a peeling off a skin tab between at least two inter-toe spaces. The duration of this study belonged of 28 days with an intermediate visit to D14. Initial and outcome evaluation was performed using a 4-grade-scale depending on the severity of the inter-toe cracks. Tolerance and healing were assessed using macrophotographs. At D14 and D 28, the difference of cure between the 2 treatments was in favor of the peptide active product. The clinical score showed a best efficiency of the active compared with the excipient; indeed a significant difference between D28 and D0 was observed for the active ingredient. Active product repairs more quickly inter-toes cracks than the excipient and we noted the complete disappearance of the "severe" and "moderate" stages from the 14th day. This study showed clearly a fast (in 14 days) and beneficial effect of the application of LN-5 compared with the excipient, on the cutaneous repair of inter-toes cracks. Since LN-5 fragment is capable of producing immediate biological activity and reinforcing the dermal-epidermal junction, it can accelerate tissue repair.

Keywords

Formulation, Laminin 5, Inter-Toe Cracks, Healing Process, Double-Blind Clinical Study

---

*Corresponding author.

1. Introduction

The dermal-epidermal junction (DEJ) adheres to the epidermis thanks to the presence of anchoring fibres which allow it to withstand the various stresses [1] [2]. Among these, Laminin 5 (LN-5) is the skin's main and irreplaceable major adhesion protein [2]. LN-5 has a structural role and participates in maintaining skin cohesion. It also carries biological signals essential for keratinocyte adhesion [3].

In-vivo studies of skin healing showed increased expression of the various LN-5 chains by keratinocytes located in the colonization zone of the wound [3]. Laminin 5 is also affected by ageing as mature reconstructed skin produces only half as much laminin as young reconstructed skin [4].

Based on protocols [3], it has been shown that a peptide fragment of LN-5 causes cell adhesion and in a dose-dependent way. Experience shows that the cells are solidly anchored on this peptide, as they withstand repeated washing. This demonstrates that this major extract of LN-5 acts in a specific way on the DEJ.

The aim of the study was to evaluate the effect of a cosmetic product containing a fragment of laminin 5 (Genepep in Montpellier) on tissue repair. Thus, we assessed the effect of the product on the kinetics of healing of inter-toe cracks in a panel of ten volunteers, and to compare these results with those obtained using the product without the fragment of laminin 5 (excipient) on half-body (intra-individual comparison). The assessment was performed by clinical analysis of the status of the inter-toe cracks, as well as by macrophotographies.

2. Material and Methods

2.1. Study Design

This study was a randomized, monocentric, double-blind, excipient-controlled comparative study of 10 healthy volunteers with inter-toe cracks. The products (active and excipient) were applied to the crack of a foot, twice a day during 28 days. The study duration was 28 days with an intermediate visit to D14. The recruitment of 10 volunteers (healthy female or male volunteers) was conducted at the Department of Dermatology, University Hospital, Besançon, France (French Health Ministry authorization 09023 M and 09023 S for the conduct of clinical studies with drugs, medical devices, and cosmetic products). This investigation was approved by the internal ethics committee of Department of Dermatology, University Hospital, Besançon, France. All volunteers signed an informed consent after having carefully read the modalities and the aim of the study.

2.2. Subject Selection

The volunteers presented with one or more asymptomatic inter-toe cracks (not due to a dermatophytic infection) on every foot. The volunteers were 18 years old or older and considered as healthy after a medical exam.

Exclusion criteria concerned pregnant or breastfeeding women, patients presenting with acute or chronic illness and/or topical or systemic treatment (including cosmetic products), or any dermatitis that could influence the results of the study. Were also not included volunteers with "athlete's foot" (Interdigital intertrigo of the toes), volunteers having gone to the pool the week before the study, or volunteers who had a sunburn on the feet during the week before the beginning of the study.

2.3. Treatment Procedure

Application of the treatment (LCE Balm of CEBELIA or excipient) was randomized in split body (right or left foot). The INCI formula of product is: Aqua (water), Cyclopentasiloxane, Glycerin, Dipropylene Glycol, Nylon-12, Butylene Glycol, Cetyl PEG/PPG-10/1 Dimethicone, Dimethicone Crosspolymer, PEG/PPG-18/18 Dimethicone, Magnesium Sulfate, Tocopheryl Acetate, Salicylic Acid, Escin, Maltodextrin, Ribes Nigrum (Blackcurrant) Fruit Extract, Sodium Hydroxide, Sodium Carboxymethyl Betaglucan, Oligopeptide-69. The fragment is chemical and has been toxically tested: not irritant to skin (patch test), slightly irritant to eyes (HET CAM test), does not have any mutagenic activity (Ames test).

The products were applied twice daily, on a carefully dried foot skin, on the affected inter-toes spaces. A special care was brought to the massage, in order to allow good penetration of the creams (especially before putting on socks). No topical application of any other product onto the region of interest was permitted during the week before the beginning of the study. No treatment with corticosteroid, retinoïd, antimycotic agent (except for medical reasons) were permitted, as well as topical application of any cream, during the study.

Throughout the duration of the study, each volunteer was asked not to change their hygiene products, not to expose themselves to the sun or UV sessions, not to apply any other product (cream, exfoliation, self-tanner…) or drug onto their feet. Volunteers were asked to report to the investigator any new medication, or any product applied on the feet.

2.4. Treatment Evaluation

Evaluations were performed in a room with constant temperature (T°C) and hygrometry. The volunteers rested quietly for at least 15 minutes in stable environmental conditions prior any assessment. The skin was not subject to any strain or stress. All subjects were asked to wash their feet on the evening prior to the examination days (D0, D14, and D28) and to not apply anything on their feet (including water, soap, tested cream…) until the visit.

The primary outcome was the severity of the inter-toe crack based on 4 grades scale from 0 to 3, where 0 = absent, 1 = mild, 2 = moderate and 3 = severe.

Secondary criteria evaluated were illustrative macrophotographs and tolerance. Standardized photographs of each inter-toe crack were taken for each subject at each time of the study. Photographs were taken in normal light with Nikon D70 digital camera associated to an AF Micro-Nikkor 60 mm lens objective and two parallel NIKON Speedlight SB23 flashes. Intolerance and adverse events were recorded for the entire study duration.

2.5. Statistical Analysis

The analysis was performed on the intention-to-treat population. Descriptive statistics were reported for each parameter, *i.e.*, mean, standard deviation, minimum, maximum, and percentages. A Wilcoxon non-parametric test was performed to compare the active and excipient at D0. A Friedman non-parametric test was carried out to evaluate the evolution in time (D0, D14 and D28). The analysis was completed by a test for multiple comparisons (Dunn's test). A 2×2 table analysis was performed with a successful treatment considered as completed healing (Mc Nemar test). Statistical significance level was set at p-value ≤ 0.05.

3. Results

Ten healthy volunteers aged 34 - 59 years (mean 47 ± 7 years) were enrolled, including 9 women and 1 man, and tested on split-body (intra-individual comparison). No subject terminated the study prematurely. The compliance was reported to 5 missed applications on average, per volunteer (max = 10; min = 2).

3.1. Clinical Analysis

Descriptive data are presented in **Table 1** and **Figure 1**. Data are comparable on D0 ($p > 0.05$). The Friedman test showed a time effect for active ingredient and excipient ($p < 0.05$). Dunn's test showed a significant difference between D0 and D28 with active ingredient ($p < 0.05$). The percentage of volunteers improved at day 14 were 70% for active *versus* 40% for excipient and at D28, 80% for active versus 70% for excipient ($p > 0.05$).

The percentage of complete healing at day 14 were 40% for active *versus* 10% for excipient ($p > 0.05$) and at D28, 70% for active versus 20% for excipient ($p = 0.074$).

The clinical score showed a better efficiency of active compared with the excipient: A significant difference between D0 and D28 was only observed for the active ingredient and a percentage of complete healing in favor of active ingredient tends to be significant.

Figure 2 illustrates cracks evolution with active ingredient on one of the volunteers.

3.2. Safety Analysis

No adverse effect, intolerance or serious adverse events have been reported. Two mild adverse events were reported: headaches and urinary infection. These adverse events were minor, transient and resolved with medical treatment.

4. Discussion

Two products were blind tested, active cream being applied to the crack of a foot, the excipient on a crack of the other foot, twice a day during 28 days. Products allocation was randomized. The duration of this study was 28 days with an intermediate visit to day 14. The objectives were to assess the efficacy of active product on

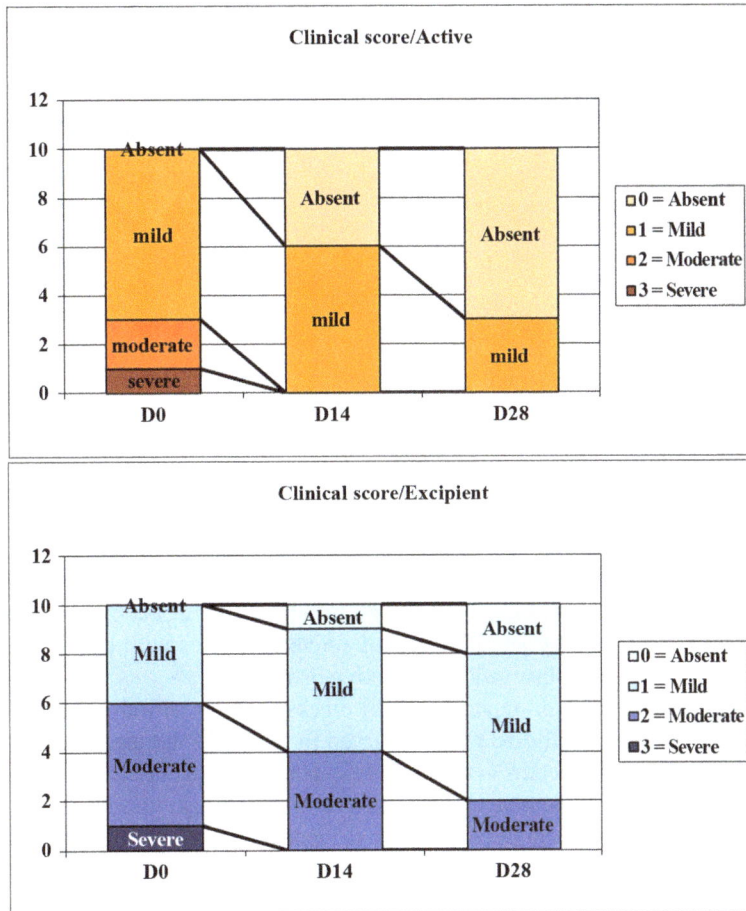

Figure 1. Evolution of clinical score for active and excipient with time.

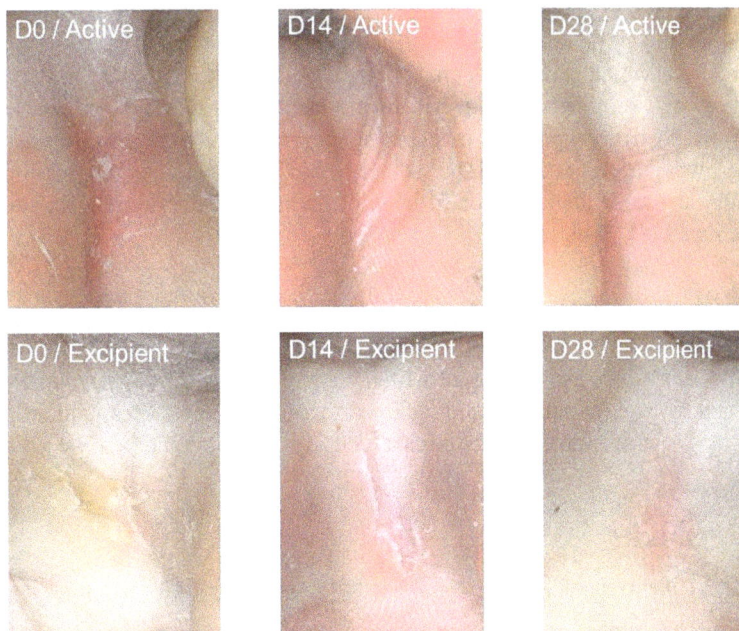

Figure 2. Cracks evolution with active product, compared with excipient in a volunteer.

Table 1. Clinical score: descriptive statistics.

		D0 Active	D0 Excipient	D14 Active	D14 Excipient	D28 Active	D28 Excipient
	N	10	10	10	10	10	10
	Min	1	1	0	0	0	0
	Mean	**1.4**	**1.7**	**0.6**	**1.3**	**0.3**	**1.0**
	Standard deviation	0.7	0.7	0.5	0.7	0.5	0.7
	Max	3	3	1	2	1	2
Prevalence in percentage (n)	0 = absent	0 (0)	0 (0)	40 (4)	10 (1)	70 (7)	20 (2)
	1 = mild	70 (7)	40 (4)	60 (6)	50 (5)	30 (3)	60 (6)
	2 = moderate	20 (2)	50 (5)	0 (0)	40 (4)	0 (0)	20 (2)
	3 = severe	10 (1)	10 (1)	0 (0)	0 (0)	0 (0)	0 (0)
	1 grade improvement			60 (6)	40 (4)	50 (5)	70 (7)
	2 grades improvement			10 (1)	0 (0)	30 (3)	0 (0)
	3 grades improvement			0 (0)	0 (0)	0 (0)	0 (0)

inter-toe cracks, based on severity clinical score and to illustrate its effect by macrophotographies.

The clinical score showed a better efficiency of active compared with the excipient: a significant difference between D0 and D28 was only observed for the active ingredient.

70% of volunteers presented an improvement of cracks severity with the active product versus 40% with excipient at day 14. This beneficial effect was observed in 80% of volunteers with active compared to 70% with excipient at day 28. The active seems to repair more quickly inter-toe cracks compared to excipient.

We noted the complete disappearance of the "severe" and "average" stages from the 14th day on active treated area, while with excipient only the "severe" stage disappears, and the "moderate" stage is still observed at 28th day. Complete cracks' healing was observed in 70% of volunteers with active product and 20% with excipient at day 28.

Only 3 volunteers did not heal within 28 days with the active product (versus 8 with excipient): 2 did not improve and there was an improvement from a "severe" stage (day 0) to a "mild" stage (day 28) for the 3rd one.

A good tolerance was observed. Two non-serious adverse events have been identified: one subject reported headaches and one subject reported urinary infection. These events were resolved with a medical treatment.

An LN-5 fragment, which is a peptide that is formulated in active product, is capable of producing immediate biological activity and reinforcing the Dermal-Epidermal Junction, and can accelerate tissue repair. This improvement may result from deposition of laminin 5 (extract of LN-5) into the basal membrane, leading to the epidermal outgrowth that migrates into the wound bed [5]. The activated expression of laminin 5 occurs within hours after injury and prior to expression of laminin 10/11 or type VII collagen, attesting to the import of laminin 5 for tissue repair [6].

5. Conclusion

This study, although on a small number of subjects, showed clearly a fast (14 days) and beneficial effect with the application of active product compared with the excipient, on the tissular repair of inter-toes cracks. An extract of LN-5 can replace its native homologous absent or deficient. This peptide formulated within the active product is able to have an immediate biological activity and to strengthen the DEJ, consequently accelerating tissue repair.

Acknowledgements

The authors would like to thank Mrs. Foussé (Laboratoires d'Anjou) for supporting this study.

References

[1] Cribier, B. and Grosshans, E. (2002) Histologie de la peau normale et lésions histopathologiques élémentaires. *Encycl*

Med Chir Dermatol, 98-085-A-10.

[2] Rousselle, P., Douglas, R.K., Ruggiero, F., *et al.* (1997) Laminin 5 Binds the NC-1 Domain of Type VII Collagen. *Journal of Cell Biology*, **138**, 719-728. http://dx.doi.org/10.1083/jcb.138.3.719

[3] Decline, F. and Rousselle, P. (2001) Keratinocyte Migration Requires Alpha2 Beta1 Integrin Mediated Interaction with the Laminin 5 Gamma 2 Chain. *Journal of Cell Science*, **114**, 811-823.

[4] Hull, M.T. and Warfel, K.A. (1983) Age-Related Changes in the Cutaneous Basal Lamina: Scanning Electron Microscopic Studies. *Journal of Investigative Dermatology*, **81**, 378-380.
http://dx.doi.org/10.1111/1523-1747.ep12519989

[5] Min, S.K., Lee, S.C., Hong, S.D., *et al.* (2010). The Effect of a Laminin-5-Derived Peptide Coated onto Chitin Microfibers on Re-Epithelialization in Early-Stage Wound Healing. *Biomaterials*, **31**, 4725-4730.
http://dx.doi.org/10.1016/j.biomaterials.2010.02.045

[6] Nguyen, B.P., Ryan, M.C., Gil, S.G. and Carter, W.G. (2000) Deposition of Laminin 5 in Epidermal Wounds Regulates Integrin Signaling and Adhesion. *Current Opinion in Cell Biology*, **12**, 554-562.
http://dx.doi.org/10.1016/S0955-0674(00)00131-9

13

Carbocysteine: A New Way for Stretch Marks Treatment

Francesco Scarci, Federico Mailland

Scientific Department, Polichem S.A., Lugano, Switzerland
Email: fscarci@polichem.com

Abstract

Background/Purpose: Although stretch marks (or striae) do not represent a medical problem, they are considered as the cause of psychological distress for women of any age that need to be treated. There are many cosmetic products or procedures claiming to improve the appearance of striae, but most of them are able to affect only striae appearance rather than physical characteristics or, even worse, they are provided with untoward effects. Our aim was to find a more efficacious and safe alternative to the existing tools. Methods: A randomized, blind observer study was conducted on 33 women to test the efficacy and safety of P-3059, a new product containing carboxymethylcysteine, Vitamin E and sweet almond oil. P-3059 was applied twice daily for 8 weeks and it was tested intra-subject in a split-body design versus an untreated area (negative control), comparing two symmetric areas with striae selected on the body/legs of each subject. The main study endpoint was the visual evaluation of striae, by means of the validated POSAS scale (consisting of two parts, OSAS and PSAS), at the end of treatment in comparison with baseline. Results: The comparison of the individual parameters of OSAS, showed significantly improved mean values for striae thickness, relief and pliability at the end of treatment (p < 0.05). The PSAS evaluation showed a statistically significant benefit in the improvement in thickness of the striae towards that of normal skin (p < 0.044). Conclusion: The new product based on carboxymethylcysteine leads to an improvement in the appearance and in the physical characteristics of striae, reducing their thickness and improving relief and pliability, as well as subjects satisfaction.

Keywords

Striae Distensae, Stretch Marks, Emollient, Carbocysteine, Sweet Almond Oil

1. Introduction

Striae distensae or stretch marks represent a common skin condition that does not induce any significant medical problem, but can cause psychological distress, due to adverse appearance and physical characteristics such as thickness and suppleness, and is undesirable to those affected [1]. Caused by pregnancy, rapid weight gain or loss, or a growth spurt in the early teens, the physiological cause is reportedly linked to hormonal changes and their consequences in the skin metabolism of the affected area [2]. The occurrence of striae affects the abdomen and the breasts of pregnant women of all races in 50% to 90% of cases [3]; in adolescents, in people overweight or in patients with excessive adrenal cortical activity, it affects thighs, hips, lower back and buttocks. Striae appear as depressed, reddish or purple lines (or in the worst cases as lesions), which later tend to gradually become white, smooth and shiny, or even wrinkled [4]. This is due to the breaks in the connective tissue. Indeed, skin distension may lead to excessive mast cell degranulation with subsequent damage to collagen and elastin [5]. Due to their physiological nature, they are considered as an aesthetic problem that can be treated with various modalities. Topical tretinoin for example, improves the appearance of striae and the improvement may persist for almost a year after discontinuation of therapy [6]. However, tretinoin may be the cause of irritation, as it indirectly increases sun sensitivity and fragility of the skin [7]. Lasers represent another option in treating striae and have minimal side effects but a moderately beneficial effect [8] [9]. Minimal pain and post treatment hyperpigmentation were the main adverse events reported in some clinical trials with lasers [10]. Abdominoplasty is a cosmetic surgery procedure used to make the abdomen thinner and more firm but it carries certain risks that may be serious or life-threatening [11]. Keratolytic and exfoliants have also been reported as useful due to their peeling effects. These products include salicylic and glycolic acid [6]. Massage with a silicone gel over a period of 6 weeks significantly increased the content of collagen in stretch marks over placebo, and decreased pliability [12]. Most of the above products may cause irritation and efficacy remains controversial [13]. There are numerous other cosmetic products that claim to improve the appearance of striae but most of these are not validated and/or only affect striae appearance rather than physical characteristics such as striae thickness and suppleness.

Thus, there is still an important medical need for topical preparations, which can be effectively and safely used for both improving the appearance of and minimizing the adverse physical characteristics of stretch marks.

The aim of this study was to assess the aesthetic efficacy and the safety profile of a new cosmetic product (P-3059), based on carboxymethylcysteine (a very safe compound commonly used in the treatment of a long-term respiratory diseases such as chronic obstructive pulmonary disease [COPD]), Vitamin E and sweet almond oil, on reducing striae on the body and legs of female subjects over a period of 8 weeks of treatment. P-3059 has the capability to decrease the rigidity of protein structures, by breaking the disulphuric bonds, resulting in an increase in the extensibility of the protein molecules.

2. Materials and Methods

A randomized, open-label, blind observer, intra-individual comparison study was performed, complying with the Declaration of Helsinki and principles of GCP, at one private clinic in Schenefeld/Hamburg in Winter 2014. The Freiburg Ethics Commission International approved the study. The subjects gave their consent to the study in writing, before entering the trial.

The study had to recruit 33 Caucasian female subjects from 18 to 65 years of age, with skin type I to III according to Fitzpatrick scale (used to classify the human skin color) and having two comparable areas with striae on the body/legs according to the Mallol score (Score 1 to 3, with 1 indicating the presence of few and thin striae and 3 the presence of many thick striae), due to either post pregnancy, weight training, weight gain or adolescent growth spurt. The main exclusion criteria included excessive loss of weight or weight gain within the last 2 months prior to and throughout the course of the study (less than 3 kg weight changes were allowed) and the presence of moles, tattoos, irritated skin, hairs etc. at the test area that could influence the investigation.

The subjects were instructed to avoid any exposure of the test area to artificial or natural UV light within the last 14 days prior to study start and for the whole study period. Moreover, they were instructed to discontinue the application of leave-on cosmetics (e.g. creams, lotions, sunscreens) in the test area within the last 5 days prior to study start and for the whole study period.

A sufficient volume of P-3059 had to be applied twice daily for 8 weeks by the subjects at home to adequately cover the whole test area (in the morning and in the evening), by means of a massage with the fingers for 5 minutes into the test area using a light pressure.

P-3059 was tested in a split-body design versus an untreated area (as negative control), choosing two comparable areas with striae to be assessed, selected on the body/legs of each subject (or one large area that could be appropriately allocated to test and control areas) by a trained clinical technician during the scheduled visit on Day 1. The test areas had to be at least 5 × 5 cm in size.

2.1. POSAS Scale

Subjects underwent an 8-week treatment, coming to the study site for the screening procedures (Day 1), after 4 weeks of treatment for a preliminary evaluation of treatment compliance and at the end of treatment for the visual evaluation of striae, performed according to the POSAS scale, in comparison with the baseline evaluation. The POSAS scale consists of two parts: the Observer Scar Assessment Scale (OSAS) and the Patient Scar Assessment Scale (PSAS). Both scales contain six items that are scored numerically on a ten-step scale with 10 indicating the worst imaginable striae or sensation [13]. Together they make up the "Total Score" of the Patient and Observer Scale; the total score for each of the scales consists of adding the scores of the six items (range 6 to 60). The lowest score, 6, reflected normal skin, whereas the highest score, 60, reflected the worst imaginable striae.

The objective assessment according to OSAS was performed by a Trained Evaluator, rating striae with regard to the following: vascularity, pigmentation, pliability, thickness, relief, surface area.

For each item of the OSAS, the following scale was used: from 1 = Normal skin to 10 = Worst striae imaginable.

To distinguish between the evaluation of vascularity (presence of vessels in striae tissue assessed by amount of redness) and pigmentation (brownish coloration of striae), a 3 mm-thick Plexiglas tool was used. The Plexiglas was pressed on the concerned areas assessing pigmentation of the striae and the surrounding skin. Then, vascularity was assessed by releasing the tool and looking at the capillary refill. For thickness, the average distance between the subcutical-dermal border and the epidermal surface of striae was considered. For the relief, the presence of surface irregularities was evaluated; for pliability the elasticity of striae was tested by wrinkling the striae between the thumb and index finger. Finally, the surface area of striae was evaluated in relation to the original affected area.

For the PSAS, the subjects were required to answer the following six questions:
a) Pain: are the striae painful?
b) Itching: are the striae itching?
c) Color (pigmentation and vascularity): is the color of the striae different from the color of your normal skin?
d) Pliability: is the stiffness of the striae different from your normal skin?
e) Thickness: is the thickness of the striae different from your normal skin?
f) Relief: are the striae more irregular than your normal skin?

The following scale was used: from 1 = No, not at all (for a and b)/No, as normal skin (from c to f) to 10 = Yes, very much (for a and b)/Yes, very different (from c to f).

2.2. Statistical Analysis

Treatments were randomly assigned to the left and right test area. The randomization was balanced 1:1, with the block size of 8 and was given according to a random vector with uniform distribution for a consecutive numbering of the subjects in this study.

Raw data for single items of OSAS and POSAS were listed by treatment and assessment time for Per Protocol (PP) population only. Separately, total scores for OSAS and POSAS, as well as differences to baseline for total scores, were calculated and listed by treatment and assessment time. Descriptive statistics (n, mean, standard deviation, standard error of the mean, median, minimum, maximum and 95% confidence limits) were given for raw data and calculated values. The mean values and differences from baseline were presented in bar charts by treatment and assessment time with 95%-confidence intervals for total scores of OSAS and POSAS separately. A significance level of 0.05 (alpha) was chosen for statistical analysis. The comparison of treatments was performed on differences from baseline separately for total scores of OSAS and PSAS using paired t-Test. Further comparison between times within each treatment group was undertaken for total scores of OSAS and PSAS with paired t-Test. Differences between times were tested by Wilcoxon test for paired samples for the individual items of OSAS and PSAS, respectively. The proportions of subjects with improvement/worsening was processed between treatments by Fisher's Exact test.

3. Results

Thirty-three subjects, with an average age of 33.1 ± 7.4 years (min age: 19; max age: 45; SEM: 1.29), were enrolled. One subject withdrew from the study and was excluded from PP population, being only included in the Safety population (SP).

The results are shown in **Table 1**.

For OSAS, the comparison of assessment times showed a significantly lower mean score for P-3059 on Day 57 compared to baseline (Day 1) (Different between times − 1.8, p = 0.009). No real changes were found for the untreated area on Day 57 compared to Day 1 for OSAS (Different between times + 0.3, N.S.). The comparison between treatments showed a significantly higher decrease in favor of P-3059 (p < 0.001).

For PSAS, a slight but not significant decrease of the mean score (Different between times − 1.3) was found for the untreated area on Day 57 compared to Day 1. A clearer decrease of the mean score was seen for P-3059 on Day 57 (Different between times − 2.2) compared to Day 1, but the level of significance was not achieved. No significant differences between treatments were found regarding PSAS.

The comparison of assessment times for the individual parameters of OSAS, showed significantly improved mean values for striae thickness, relief and pliability on Day 57 in comparison to Day 1 for P-3059 (**Table 2**).

Table 1. OSAS and PSAS—mean values ± SD and comparison between times within treatment as well as between treatments by Paired t-Test (N = 32).

| Parameter | Time | Mean values | | | p-values | |
| | | | | | Between times | |
		Untreated	P-3059	Between treatments	Untreated	P-3059
OSAS	Day 1	23.3 ± 6.5	23.8 ± 6.4	-	0.524	0.009
	Day 57	23.6 ± 6.5	22.0 ± 6.6	<0.001		
PSAS	Day 1	22.8 ± 5.7	22.8 ± 5.6	-	0.270	0.083
	Day 57	21.5 ± 6.3	20.6 ± 6.6	0.207		

OSAS and PSAS Score: 6 = normal skin to 60 = worst striae imaginable.

Table 2. Parameters of OSAS—mean values and results for the comparison of treatments and measurement time points by Wilcoxon signed-ranks test (N = 32).

| Parameter of OSAS | Time | Mean values | | | p-values | |
| | | | | | Between times | |
		Untreated	P-3059	Between treatments	Untreated	P-3059
Vascularity	Day 1	2.9 ± 1.0	3.0 ± 1.0	--	1.000	0.750
	Day 57	2.9 ± 1.0	3.0 ± 1.0	0.688		
Pigmentation	Day 1	2.8 ± 1.0	3.1 ± 1.1	--	0.625	0.531
	Day 57	2.9 ± 1.0	3.0 ±1.0	0.234		
Thickness	Day 1	4.2 ± 1.3	4.1 ± 1.3	--	1.000	0.003
	Day 57	4.2 ± 1.3	3.6 ± 1.2	0.003		
Relief	Day 1	4.1 ± 1.5	4.2 ± 1.5	--	1.000	0.034
	Day 57	4.2 ± 1.5	3.8 ± 1.5	0.038		
Pliability	Day 1	5.0 ± 1.5	5.2 ± 1.6	--	1.000	<0.001
	Day 57	5.0 ± 1.5	4.4 ± 1.6	<0.001		
Surface Area	Day 1	4.3 ± 1.4	4.3 ± 1.3	--	0.109	0.973
	Day 57	4.5 ± 1.4	4.3 ± 1.5	0.129		

Score: 1 = normal skin to 10 = worst striae imaginable.

The differences on the three parameters were significant between treatments, too. Nofurther significant differences were observed.

In **Figure 1**, the counts of subjects with improvement and worsening regarding the OSAS parameters separately by treatment are shown including percentages.

In 53% of the subjects, an improvement in skin thickness was found, an improvement in relief appeared in 44% of the subjects and an improvement in pliability was reported in 63% of the subjects treated with P-3059. In the untreated area, a negligible proportion of subject with improvement was seen for the same parameters. Fisher's Exact test between treatment groups was: $p = 0.0007$ (thickness), $p = 0.0076$ (relief), $p = 0.0435$ (pliability).

PSAS, as for OSAS, is a composite endpoint. **Table 3** presents the mean values for the scores of all PSAS parameters separately by treatment and measurement time points, the mean differences compared to baseline, and the results for the comparison of treatments and time points by Wilcoxon signed-ranks test.

The comparison of assessment times showed a significantly lower mean value in P-3059 group for the question "Is the thickness of the striae different from your normal skin" on Day 57 compared to baseline ($p < 0.044$), indicating an improvement in thickness of the striae towards that of normal skin. Furthermore, a significantly lower mean value was determined for the question "Are the striae more irregular than your normal skin" for the untreated area on Day 57 compared to baseline, indicating a worsening in irregularity of the striae. The corresponding mean value for P-3059 just missed the level of significance and no further significant differences were found for the comparison of assessment times. The comparison of treatments showed no significant differences for the parameters of PSAS. In **Figure 2**, the counts of subjects with improvement and worsening regarding the PSAS parameters separately by treatment are shown, including percentages. No significant differences between treatments were detected by Fisher's test.

Half subjects or more than half-reported improvement in striae stiffness (50%), improvement in striae thickness (56%) and improvement in striae irregularity (66%) for P-3059. For the untreated area, the improvements for the same parameters were less pronounced (34% for stiffness, 44% for thickness and 50% for irregularity).

4. Discussion

The physiopathology of striae remains unclear and a challenging issue for aesthetic medicine. The etiological mechanisms proposed relate to hormones, and structural alterations to the integument. However, it may involve

Table 3. Parameters of PSAS—mean values and results for the comparison of treatments and measurement time points by Wilcoxon signed-ranks test (N = 32).

Parameter of PSAS	Time	Mean values			p-values	
					Between times	
		Untreated	P-3059	Between treatments	Untreated	P-3059
Are the striae painful?**	Day 1	1.0 ± 0.0	1.0 ± 0.0	--	1.000	1.000
	Day 57	1.0 ± 0.0	1.0 ± 0.0	1.000		
Are the striae itching?**	Day 1	1.0 ± 0.0	1.0 ± 0.0	--	1.000	1.000
	Day 57	1.0 ± 0.0	1.0 ± 0.2	1.000		
Is the color of the striae different from the color of your normal skin?***	Day 1	5.0 ± 1.7	5.1 ± 1.8	--	0.980	0.318
	Day 57	4.9 ± 2.0	4.7 ± 2.0	0.231		
Is the stiffness of the striae different from your normal skin?***	Day 1	4.8 ± 2.0	4.7 ± 1.9	--	0.987	0.154
	Day 57	4.7 ± 1.9	4.2 ± 2.0	0.166		
Is the thickness of the striae different from your normal skin?***	Day 1	5.2 ± 2.0	5.1 ± 1.9	--	0.228	0.044
	Day 57	4.8 ± 2.0	4.5 ± 1.7	0.386		
Are the striae more irregular than your normal skin?***	Day 1	5.8 ± 1.9	5.9 ± 1.9	--	0.019	0.056
	Day 57	5.0 ± 1.8	5.1 ± 2.2	0.856		

**Score: 1 = no, not at all to 10 = yes, very much; ***Score: 1 = no, as normal skin to 10 = yes, very different.

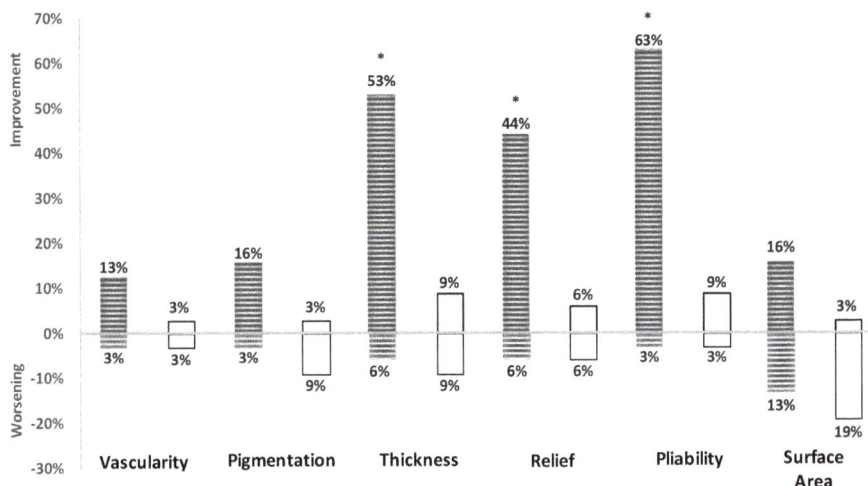

Figure 1. Counts of subjects with improvement and worsening for parameters of OSAS (N = 32) in P-3059 (shadow histogram) and in the untreated (blank histogram). Asterisks represent significant differences between treatments (Fisher's test).

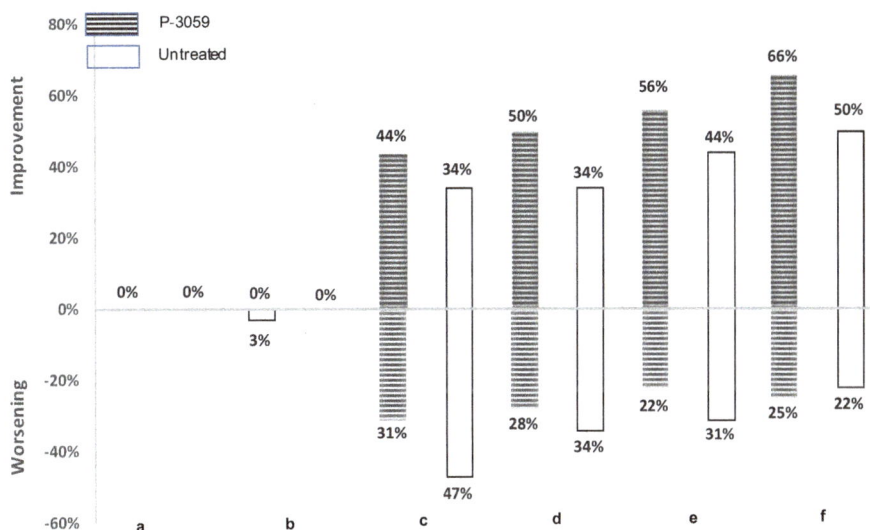

Figure 2. Counts of subjects with improvement and worsening for parameters of PSAS (N = 32), where a, b, c, d, e and f refer to pain, itching, color (pigmentation and vascularity), pliability, thickness and relief, respectively.

stretching of the skin, causing lesions in fibrilin microfibrils, which in younger spurt women are likely to be more fragile and are therefore more susceptible to rupture [14]. Nowadays, a number of therapies are available for such conditions: tretinoin, lasers, surgery and many more, are the most common treatment modalities, but they often present some disadvantages related to their efficacy or to their safety profile.

The purpose of this study was to evaluate the aesthetic efficacy of a cosmetic product, P-3059, exploiting its elasticizing and repairing properties, due to its composition based on carboxymethylcysteine, Vitamin E and sweet almond oil, on reducing striae on the body and legs of female subjects after an 8-week treatment. This was our biggest challenge, as topical treatments are in most of cases indicated in the prevention of striae occurrence instead of in the treatment of full-blown striae, where laser treatment or surgery could be more efficacious within their own limits.

Although the eligibility criteria foresaw women between 18 and 65 years old, nevertheless our population was rather homogeneous with the subjects included between 19 and 45 years old. Moreover, in order to avoid any bias in the study results, due to any rapid weight gain or loss, prior or throughout the course of the study, the weight monitoring was guaranteed during the study. Our results showed an improvement in the clinical appearance of striae treated with P-3059 on the three parameters out of six parameters in the OSAS composite endpoint that P-3059 might reasonably be expected to have an effect on. These are the three parameters where P-3059 might be expected to work. There were statistically significant improvements in striae thickness, relief and pliability following treatment with P-3059, both versus baseline and in comparison to the untreated area, as assessed objectively by a Trained Evaluator. In addition, 53% of subjects had an improvement in striae thickness, 44% an improvement in striae relief and 63% an improvement in striae pliability after treatment with P-3059. The self-assessment evaluation, done directly by the subjects, also revealed a statistical superiority of P-3059 over placebo control in the judgement of striae thickness.

Some potential limitations to this study should be mentioned: the study was randomized within subjects, but it followed an open design, which may have influenced the subject self-assessment, resulting in a study bias. However, what may have represented a limitation appeared not to be, as the Evaluator's assessment was even more favorable than the self-assessment. A second limitation may be due to the small sample size. This would explain why in some clinical parameters, besides the positive trend, there were no statistically significant differences. However, some objective parameters achieved statistical significance despite the small sample size, demonstrating the value of the trial as a preliminary study. A longer treatment period may also have improved the statistical findings.

Although POSAS score is a validated tool for striae assessment, some considerations have to be made. The observed difference between the OSAS and the PSAS score is in agreement with some recurrent findings of the literature, which tend to undervalue the influence of the subject's satisfaction, compared to trained evaluator assessment [15]. This is due to the fact that the individuals assessed their striae in a highly subjective, various, and difficult to capture way, resulting in a weak intersubjective comparability of judgments. Many factors contribute to the determination of patient's satisfaction: color, thickness and striae irregularity were the significant contributing parameters to the overall subject satisfaction as they were easier to be evaluated visually, in respect to pain, itching and stiffness, which are parameters linked to the subjects' personal perception.

Despite those limitations, the test product, P-3059, significantly improved striae according to the Observer Scar Assessment Scale. This study opens up new perspectives as carboxymethylcysteine was used to treat striae for the first time, taking advantage of the mechanism of action of P-3059. In fact, the product has the capability to decrease the rigidity of protein structures, by breaking the disulphuric bonds, resulting in an increase in the extensibility of the protein molecule. This result is achieved by acting both on ternary and quaternary structures, without affecting the primary and the secondary ones, and is therefore reversible. It seems that this action is not only efficacious in the very well-known therapy for bronchitis, to decrease sputum viscosity, but it could also be applicable in the cosmetic field to improve skin softness. Notably, unless cosmetic approaches to improved appearance of striae alone, P-3059 had the effect of improving both the appearance and distressing physical characteristics of striae, while the emollients do not.

5. Conclusion

In conclusion, the current study represents an attempt to use a product containing carboxymethylcysteine, using a validated assessment scale, to examine overall patient satisfaction in female subjects with striae in their bodies/legs. The results reported herein, showed that in the study population, the treatment with P-3059 produces a statistically significant improvement in Observer Scar Assessment Scale, with particular emphasis on improved appearance and physical characteristics of striae, such as reducing striae thickness, improving relief and pliability of striae, as well as, subject satisfaction linked to a reduction in the thickness of the striae, when compared to an untreated area. If confirmed by further, larger studies, this result could open a new way forward in the treatment of mild to moderate striae.

References

[1]   Yamaguchi, K., Suganuma, N. and Ohashi, K. (2012) Quality of Life Evaluation in Japanese Pregnant Women with Striae Gravidarum: A Cross-Sectional Study. *BMC Research Notes*, **5**, 450. http://dx.doi.org/10.1186/1756-0500-5-450

[2]   Salter, S.A. and Kimball, A.B. (2006) Striae Gravidarum. *Clinics in Dermatology*, **24**, 97-100. http://dx.doi.org/10.1016/j.clindermatol.2005.10.008

[3]   Brennan, M., Young, G. and Devane, D. (2012) Topical Preparations for Preventing Stretch Marks in Pregnancy.

Cochrane Database of Systematic Reviews, 11, Article ID: CD000066.
http://dx.doi.org/10.1002/14651858.cd000066.pub2

[4]   "Stretch Mark" (2009). Encyclopædia Britannica.

[5]   Sheu, H.M., Yu, H.S. and Chang, C.H. (1991) Mast Cell Degranulation and Elastolysis in the Early Stage of Striae Distensae. *Journal of Cutaneous Pathology*, **18**, 410-416. http://dx.doi.org/10.1111/j.1600-0560.1991.tb01376.x

[6]   Ash, K., Lord, J., Zukowski, M. and McDaniel, D.H. (1998) Comparison of Topical Therapy for Striae Alba (20% Glycolic acid/0.05% Tretinoin versus 20% Glycolic Acid/10% L-Ascorbic Acid). *Dermatologic Surgery*, **24**, 849-856. http://dx.doi.org/10.1111/j.1524-4725.1998.tb04262.x

[7]   Alldredge, B.K., Corelli, R.L., Ernst, M.E., Guglielmo, B.J., Jr., Jacobson, P.A., Kradjan, W.A. and Williams, B.R. (2013) Koda-Kimble and Young's Applied Therapeutics: The Clinical Use of Drugs. 10th Edition, Wolters Kluwer Health/Lippincott Williams & Wilkins, Baltimore.

[8]   Hernandez-Perez, E., Colombo-Charrier, E. and Valencia-Ibiett, E. (2002) Intense Pulsed Light in the Treatment of Striae Distensae. *Dermatologic Surgery*, **28**, 1124-1130.

[9]   Alexiades-Armenakas, M.R., Bernstein, L.J., Friedman, P.M. and Geronemus, R.G. (2004) The Safety and Efficacy of the 308 nm Excimer Laser in Pigment Correction of Hypopigmented Scars and Striae Alba. *Archives of Dermatology*, **140**, 955-960. http://dx.doi.org/10.1001/archderm.140.8.955

[10] Kim, B.J., Lee, D.H., Kim, M.N., Song, K.Y., Cho, W.I., Lee, C.K., *et al.* (2008) Fractional Photothermolysis for the Treatment of Striae Distensae in Asian Skin. *American Journal of Clinical Dermatology*, **9**, 33-37. http://dx.doi.org/10.2165/00128071-200809010-00003

[11] Alderman, A.K., Collins, E.D., Streu, R., Grotting, J.C., Sulkin, A.L., Neligan, P., *et al.* (2009) Benchmarking Outcomes in Plastic Surgery: National Complication Rates for Abdominoplasty and Breast Augmentation. *Plastic and Reconstructive Surgery*, **124**, 2127-2133. http://dx.doi.org/10.1097/prs.0b013e3181bf8378

[12] Ud-Din, S., McAnelly, S.L., Bowring, A., *et al.* (2013) A Double-Blind Controlled Clinical Trial Assessing the Effect of Topical Gels on Striae Distensae (Stretch Marks): A Non-Invasive Imaging, Morphological and Immunohistochemical Study. *Archives of Dermatological Research*, **305**, 603-617. http://dx.doi.org/10.1007/s00403-013-1336-7

[13] Van der Wal, M.B., Tuinebreijer, W.E., Bloemen, M.C., Verhaegen, P.D., Middelkoop, E. and van Zuijlen, P.P. (2012) Rasch Analysis of the Patient and Observer Scar Assessment Scale (POSAS) in Burn Scars. *Quality of Life Research*, **21**, 13-23. http://dx.doi.org/10.1007/s11136-011-9924-5

[14] Valente, D.S., Zanella, R.K., Doncatto, L.F. and Padoin, A.V. (2014) Incidence and Risk Factors of Striae Distensae Following Breast Augmentation Surgery: A Cohort Study. *PLoS ONE*, **9**, e97493. http://dx.doi.org/10.1371/journal.pone.0097493

[15] Consorti, F., Mancuso, R., Piccolo, A., Pretore, E. and Antonaci, A. (2013) Quality of Scar after Total Thyroidectomy: A Single Blinded Randomized Trial Comparing Octyl-Cyanoacrylate and Subcuticular Absorbable Suture. *ISRN Surgery*, **2013**, Article ID: 270953. http://dx.doi.org/10.1155/2013/270953

14

Edible Bird's Nest, an Asian Health Food Supplement, Possesses Skin Lightening Activities: Identification of N-Acetylneuraminic Acid as Active Ingredient

Gallant Kar Lun Chan, Zack Chun Fai Wong, Kelly Yin Ching Lam, Lily Kwan Wai Cheng, Laura Minglu Zhang, Huangquan Lin, Tina Tingxia Dong, Karl Wah Keung Tsim*

Division of Life Science and Center for Chinese Medicine R&D, The Hong Kong University of Science and Technology, Kowloon, Hong Kong, China
Email: *botsim@ust.hk

Abstract

Edible bird's nest (EBN; Yan Wo), or cubilose, is originated from the salivary secretion of *Aerodramus fuciphagus*. In Asia, EBN is famous for its unproven skin lightening function. Here, we aim to reveal the active ingredients of EBN responsible for skin lightening function. Three major fractions were isolated from EBN water extract by chromatography using LC-MS/MS, bioactivities of these isolated fractions were analyzed by assays of tyrosinase, melanocytes and 3D human skin model, from which, N-acetylneuraminic acid (NANA), the second isolated fraction showed an inhibition effect on tyrosinase activity in a dose-dependent manner. The IC_{50} of tyrosinase originated from mushroom and human was 16.93 mM and 0.10 mM respectively. Furthermore, only EBN with higher content of NANA (e.g. White and Red EBN), but not EBN with less NANA (e.g. Grass EBN), showed promising skin lightening function. This is the first report to reveal NANA being an active ingredient of EBN on skin lightening function.

Keywords

Cubilose, N-Acetylneuraminic Acid, Chemical Analysis, Skin Lightening, Human Skin Model

---

*Corresponding author.

1. Introduction

Edible bird's nest (EBN; Yan Wo), or named cubilose, is made of the salivary secretion of specific swiftlets (e.g. *Aerodramus fuciphagus*). EBN is an ingredient of an ancient Chinese delicacy—the EBN soup, which has been consumed for several hundred years in Asia according to the historical record. Until now, EBN is still a popular luxurious food supplement for women in the oriental population. However, the biological functions of EBN are still unclear.

There are two major problems in studying the biological functions of EBN. Firstly, the progress of mechanistic study is largely hindered by our insufficient knowledge on the bioactive ingredients of EBN. EBN consists of 40% - 60% of protein, 9% of sialic acid and trace amount of fat and minerals [1]. However, those chemical parameters are too superficial to unveil the biological functions of EBN. Secondly, there is a large variety of EBN on the market, and there is no standardized EBN for biological determinations (e.g. skincare functions). Even worse, most of the current authentication methods of EBN, including microscopic [2], proteomics [3] and *genomics* [4] approaches, all fail to differentiate different grades of EBN [5].

The free form of N-acetylneuraminic acid (NANA) could serve as a quantitative marker to grade different EBNs [6] [7]. The abundant of which increases in line with higher prices of EBN. Furthermore, NANA is known to have biological activities. NANA was proposed to be a major component for anti-influenza function of EBN [8] [9]. Moreover, NANA has proliferation effect on Caco-2 cells [10]. However, the biological functions of NANA on skin functions are unknown. Furthermore, skincare-related bioactive compounds other than protein and NANA might also be found in EBN. Thus, a full scanning of total ion chromatography was performed by LC-MS/MS, and the performances on skincare functions by different fractions were analyzed.

2. Materials and Methods

2.1. Material

NANA was purchased from Sigma-Aldrich (St. Louis, MO) as standard solution. Volume were measured accurately from the stock, diluted with fresh Milli-Q to produce a series of solution standards (1, 2, 5, 10, 15, 20 μM). Tyrosinase from mushroom (≥1000 U/mg) and recombinant human tyrosinase (Activity ≥ 95%) were purchased from Sigma-Aldrich. L-3, 4-dihydroxyphenyl-alanine (L-DOPA), vitamin C and tert- Butylhydroquinone (tBHQ) and alpha melanocyte stimulating hormone (α-MSH) were purchased from Sigma-Aldrich. All EBN samples and its adulterants were purchased in the market of Hong Kong.

2.2. Sample Preparation

For LC-MS/MS analysis, EBN samples were ground into powder (approximately 1 - 3 mm) and mixed thoroughly. Ten mg of each was weighed and extracted by 1 mL of fresh Milli-Q water under sonication for 10 min. Followed by centrifugation at 14,000 rpm for 5 min, the supernatants were filtered, and the filtrates were collected for LC-MS/MS analysis. For bioassay, one g of EBN sample, or its adulterants, was individually soaked in 100 folds of water for overnight at room temperature. The mixture was then stewed at 80°C for 6 - 9 hours until completely molten and then left to cool down to room temperature. This method of preparation is a common cooking method for the consumers, as well as a high protein extraction efficiency [11]. The extracts were kept at 4°C until further usage.

2.3. HPLC-MS/MS System

The liquid chromatograph was equipped with an Agilent 6410 Triple Quad MS/MS and a (2.1 × 100 mm) Eclipse XDB-C18 column (3.5 μm particle size). The injection volume was 2 μL. A 5-min linear gradient at flow rates of 0.4 mL/min between solvent A (Milli-Q water, 0.1% formic acid) and solvent B (Acetonitrile, 0.1% formic acid) was used. After reaching 80% B, the system returned to 100% A in 0.5 min. For column equilibration, a total cycle time of 10 min was needed. The MS was operated in negative electron spray ionization mode. A capillary voltage of 3.5 kV and a cone voltage of 10 V were applied. Source temperature was 100°C, and desolvation temperature was 325°C. Ultra-high purity nitrogen was used for cone gas (3.0 L/min), desolvation gas (10.0 L/min) and nebulising gas (35 psi). For collision induced dissociation (CID) a collision energy of 5 eV was used. Spectra from m/z 50 to m/z 1000 were recorded.

2.4. Quantification of NANA and Citric Acid

In calibration of NANA in EBN, a 5-point calibration curve having concentrations of 1, 2, 5, 10 and 20 µM was made. All calibrators were prepared in fresh Milli-Q water. Triplicate results were taken for each sample. Retention time of NANA was 0.65 - 0.69 min. A negatively single charged ion [M-H]⁻ of NANA (m/z 307.9) was selected as precursor ion for CID. The precursor ion was dissociated into two major product ions (m/z 87.0 and 170.0), and the product ion m/z 87.0 was the most abundant from NANA. Multiple reaction monitoring (MRM) was applied, the transitions m/z 307.9 → 87.0 and m/z 307.9 → 170.0 were chosen as the qualifiers, whilst the transitions m/z 307.9 → 87.0 was measured for quantification. The determination of citric acid was similar to that of NANA. The retention time of citric acid was at 1.50 min. The solution having known spiked amount of citric acid was defined as the quality control (QC) solution. Negatively single charged ion [M-H]⁺ of citric acid (m/z 191.0) was selected as precursor ion for CID. The precursor ion was dissociated into two major product ions (m/z 111.0 and 86.9), and the product ion m/z 111.0 was the most abundant from NANA. Multiple reaction monitoring was applied, the transitions m/z 191.0 → 111.0 and m/z 191.0 → 86.9 were chosen as the qualifiers, whilst the transitions m/z 191.0 → 111.0 was measured for quantification. The ethyl β-D-glucuronide (m/z 221.1) was used as the internal standard in the calibrators and QC samples, and the concentration was kept consistent at 100 ng/mL. The transitions m/z 221.1 → 84.9 and m/z 221.1 → 75.0 were chosen as the qualifiers, whilst the transitions m/z 221.1 → 84.9 was quantified as reference.

2.5. Tyrosinase Assay

The enzyme activities of mushroom and human tyrosinase were monitored by dopachrome formation at 492 nm through the oxidation of substrate (L-DOPA). The reaction medium (200 µL) contained 0.5 mM L-DOPA in 50 mM sodium phosphate buffer (pH 6.8) and (pH 7.4). Five mM of vitamin C was used as an inhibitor control. The final concentration of mushroom tyrosinase was 0.2 mg/mL. In this method, 0.1 mL of different concentrations of effectors, including EBN extracts, adulterants of EBN and NANA, were added to the reaction medium. The reaction mixtures were loaded on a 96-well plate, and the formation of dopachrome was measured in optical density at 492 nm after 20 min of incubation under dark at room temperature. Absorption was recorded using micro-plate spectrophotometer.

2.6. Melanogenesis Assay on Human and Mouse Melanocytes

B16 cells (CRL-6323™; American Type Culture Collection (ATCC), Manassas, VA) and A375 cells (CRL-1619™, ATCC) were purchased from ATCC and cultured according to the recommendations provided. B16 and A375 cells were cultured in Dulbecco's Modified Eagle's Medium (DMEM) supplemented with 10% fetal bovine albumin and Penicillin-Streptomycin (100 U/mL). Cells were sub-cultured every alternate day.

For melanogenesis assay, two hundred thousands of B16 cells and A375 cells were seeded onto each well of 6-well culture plates and incubated for 2 days, or 4 days, with or without the extracts of EBN, respectively. Five mM of vitamin C, 50 µM of tBHQ and 2% kojic acid served as positive controls. For A375 cells, α-MSH was added on day 2 as to stimulate the formation of melanin. To extract melanin from cells, the samples were dissolved in 100 mL of 1 M NaOH after washing twice with PBS. Samples were incubated at 60°C for 1 hour and mixed to solubilize the melanin. The optical density of mixed solution was detected at 405 nm, and the absorbance was converted to melanin concentration by a standard curve.

2.7. 3D Human Skin Model Assay

Twenty-four 3D human skin model constructed with keratinocytes and melanocytes in a ratio of originated from Asian skin tissue were purchased from MatTek Corporation (Lot # 21822). The model was specific for melanogenesis study (MelanoDerm™ Part # MEL-300-A). All procedures for macroscopic and microscopic analysis followed the instructions provided by the manufacturer. In brief, the testing samples (20 mM NANA and 1 mg/mL EBN extract) and positive control (2% of kojic acid) were applied either to the inner chambers of trans-well (keratinocyte side) or culture medium directly (melanocyte side). Culture medium having same concentration of tested chemicals was replaced every 2 - 3 days. The inner chamber was rinsed twice with phosphate buffer provided by the manufacturer and replaced with fresh testing samples and positive control. Macroscopic and microscopic images were captured on day 18. Macroscopic images were captured by top view

microscope (keratinocyte side), while microscopic images were captured by inverted microscope under 100×
magnification (melanocyte side).

2.8. Protein Assay and Statistical Tests

The concentration of protein was determined following the instructions of Bradford's method with a kit from
Bio-Rad Laboratories. The analysis was done on a 96-well microtiter plate. In brief, one part dye reagent con-
centrate was diluted with 4 parts of double distilled water before use. Six dilutions of BSA standard (0.05 - 0.5
mg/mL) were used for the test: Ten µL of each standard, or a sample solution, were added with 0.2 mL of diluted dye reagent into separate wells and mixed well. After 10 min incubation at room temperature, absorbance
at 595 nm was taken. The concentration of protein was determined from the standard curve. Statistical tests were
done by using student t test provided in GraphPad Prism 5.0. Statistically significant changes were classed as [*]
where $p < 0.05$, [**] where $p < 0.01$ and [***] where $p < 0.001$.

3. Results and Discussion

3.1. Fractionation of EBN by LC-MS/MS

EBNs are graded and priced according to their color, $i.e.$ Red > White > Grass. These EBNs were collected from
local market, and which were subjected to LC-MS/MS analysis. Three major fractions (named peak 1, 2 and 3)
from EBN water extracts were notified and appeared at different retention time after the separation using the full
scanning mode of LC-MS/MS chromatography (**Figure 1(a)**). Interestingly, the full scans of total ion chromatogram of different grades of EBN showed differentiable patterns. The full scan of Grass EBN showed a strong
peak 1 and a barely recognizable peak 2. The full scan of White EBN showed both notable peaks 1 and 2. While
the full scan of Red EBN showed all three distinguishable 3 peaks. After the analysis with molecular weight using MRM mode quantitation and the chemical standards, the identities of peak 2 and peak 3 were confirmed as
NANA and citric acid, respectively (**Figure 1(b)**). Peak 1 consisted of compounds with different sizes, and the
pattern of mass spectrum was similar to those spectrums of collagen-like proteins (data not shown). Having the
identities of NANA and citric acid, the amounts of them in different grades of EBN were quantified by the established MS system. The contents of protein, free NANA and citric acid for different grades of EBN were
summarized (**Supplementary Table**). The protein contents for different types of EBNs were rather similar;
however, the contents of NANA and citric acid were significantly higher in Red EBN and lower in Grass EBN.
Citric acid was not detected in Grass EBN.

For safety reason, EBN needs to be proper processed before the consumption by human [11]. As NANA and
citric acid are the most abundant soluble chemicals and therefore considered to be the targeted inhibitors. Here,
we aimed to reveal the amount of NANA and citric acid in EBN after standard processing procedures. Different
sample preparation procedures were applied onto EBN preparation to mimic the standard cooking processes.
The content of free NANA increased during the cooking processes, and an increase of ~4 folds after stewing in
different types of EBN (**Supplementary Figure 1(a)**). The increase could be an outcome of the release of conjugated NANA as the free form after extensive cooking. In contrast, the content of citric acid dropped by 90%
after the processing (**Supplementary Figure 1(b)**), suggesting the free salt form of citric acid within EBN. Thus,
the cooking EBN could result in different amounts of NANA and citric acid.

3.2. Skin Lightening Effect of EBN

Tyrosinase inhibition assay is a commonly used method in screening skin lightening agents [12]-[15]. The activity of tyrosinase (mushroom) was calculated on the formation of dopachrome from L-DOPA against time: the
concentration of dopachrome was obtained by absorbance at 492 nm (**Figure 2(a)**). The inhibition of mushroom
tyrosinase was determined in different EBN water extracts. Vitamin C was used as a positive control. White and
Red EBNs inhibited the activity of tyrosinase by about 50% (**Figure 2(b)**). In contrast, Grass EBN reduced the
tyrosinase activity of only ~10%. No inhibitory functions on tyrosinase for all common EBN adulterants, e.g.
agar, fungi and pig skin. In order to search for ingredient corresponding for tyrosinase inhibition, the protein-
depleted fraction of EBN water extract was tested. In different types of EBN, the inhibiting activity was
enriched in the protein-depleted fraction (**Figure 2(c)**), which suggested the role of water soluble small chemicals in such function.

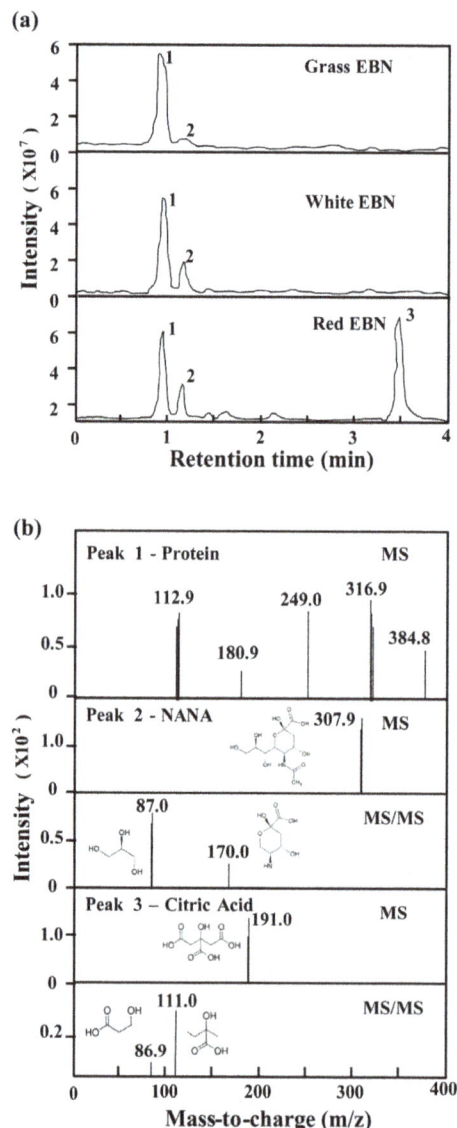

Figure 1. Screening of major ingredients from EBN by LC-MS/MS. (a) Full scan of total ion chromatography of different water extracts of different grades of EBNs. Three outstanding peaks with the highest abundance were recorded along with the retention time. (b) Mass spectrums of the outstanding peaks from the full scan were obtained. From which, peak 1 were identified as protein-like molecules while peak 2 and peak 3 were identified as NANA (m/z 307.9 → 87.0 and m/z 307.9 → 170.0) and citric acid (m/z 191.0 → 111.0 and m/z 191.0 → 86.9) respectively. NANA and citric acid standards were applied for the identification. $n = 4$.

3.3. NANA Shows Skin Lightening

The skin lightening effect by NANA becomes the focus of study here. Having tyrosinase assay, NANA inhibited both mushroom and human tyrosinases in a dose-dependent manner (**Figure 3(a)**). The IC_{50} of NANA on mushroom tyrosinase and human tyrosinase was 16.93 mM, and 0.10 mM, respectively (**Figure 3(a)**). The original Km for mushroom and human tyrosinase on L-DOPA were 1.491 mM and 0.545 mM, respectively; and Vmax were 0.394 μM/min and 0.308 μM/min, respectively. Observed from Lineweaver-Burk plot, the values of Km and Vmax of tyrosinase were altered in the presence of NANA: the changes were in a dose-dependent manner (**Figure 3(b)**). By adding 10 mM NANA to the mushroom enzyme, the Km increased from 1.491 to 1.818 mM, while the Vmax decreased from 0.394 to 0.287 μM/min. In human tyrosinase, the effect of NANA did not

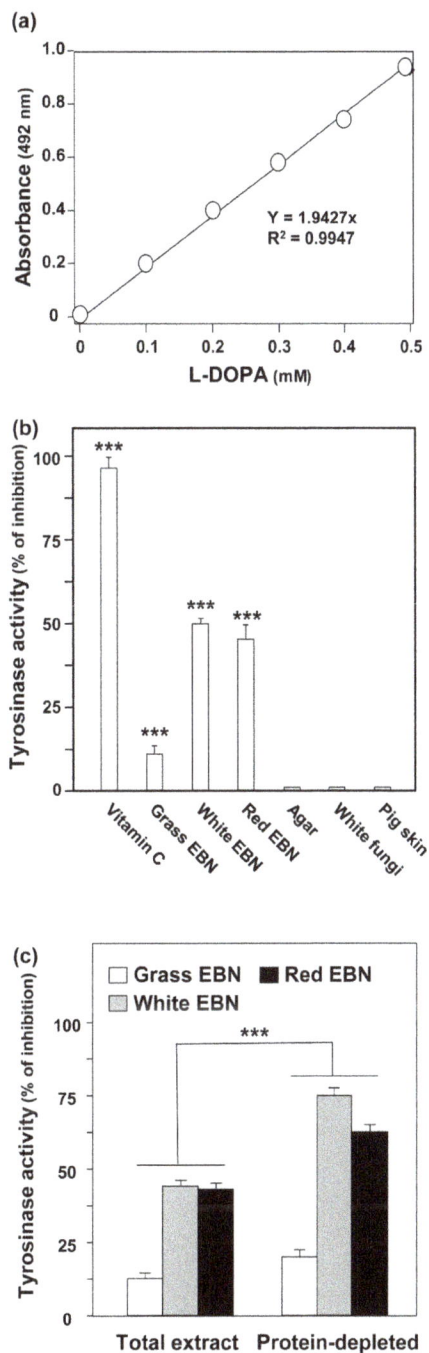

Figure 2. EBNs inhibit the activity of tyrosinase. (a) Different concentrations of L-DOPA were added to testing reagent containing mushroom tyrosinase (5000 U/mL) and incubated for 1 hour. Absorbance readings were taken at 492 nm. (b) The dopachrome formed by oxidation of 0.5 mM of L-DOPA incubated for 20 min with 0.2 mg/mL mushroom tyrosinase, served as blank control. Vitamin C (5 mM) served as a positive control. The dopachrome concentration, after treatment of different EBNs or adulterants (all at 10 mg/mL water extract), was determined. (c) Protein was depleted from the water extracts of different EBNs by precipitation using acetonitrile. The percentage of inhibition on tyrosinase activities before and after protein depletion was recorded. One mg/mL extract was added. The percentage of inhibition on tyrosinase activities was presented as Mean ± SD ($n = 3$). ***$p < 0.001$ versus reference group.

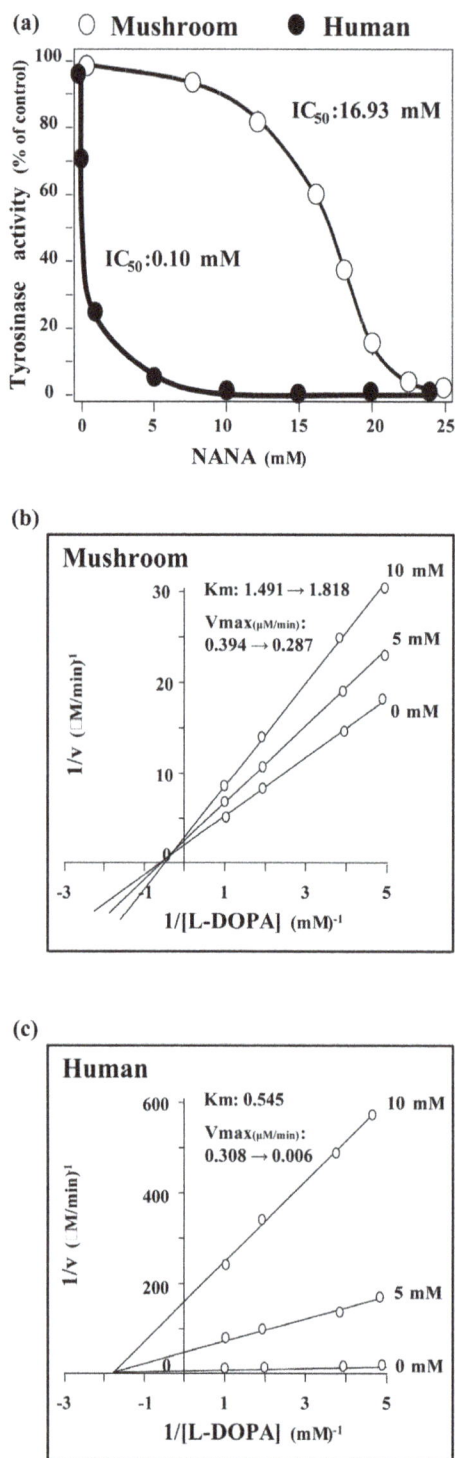

Figure 3. NANA inhibits tyrosinase (a) The reaction rate of mushroom and human tyrosinase was defined as 100% activity (*i.e.* 29.75 μM/min and 147.20 nM/min, respectively) with the substrate of 0.5 mM of L-DOPA. The inhibition effects of NANA from 0 mM to 25 mM on the mushroom and human tyrosinase activity were shown. The reaction velocity was calculated by the concentration of dopachrome, measured by spectrometer at 492 nm against time in min. Lineweaver-Burk plot of different concentrations of NANA on (b) mushroom tyrosinase and (c) human tyrosinase. Values are Mean ± SD (*n* = 3).

change the Km value, while the Vmax decreased from 0.308 to 0.006 μM/min (**Figure 3(c)**). Referring to the Lineweaver-Burk plot, the inhibition mechanism of NANA on mushroom tyrosinase was classified as mixed type I inhibition, whilst the inhibition mechanism of NANA on human tyrosinase was classified as non-competitive inhibition. Enzymatic parameters of other known tyrosinase inhibitors were compared (**Table 1**). The enzymatic parameters of inhibition by NANA were comparable to those existing known inhibitors.

In cultured B16 mouse melanoma cells, the color of culture medium was turned into dark brown after 48 hours of culture (**Figure 4(a)**). This phenomenon was due to formation and release of melanin-rich melanosome from B16 melanoma [16]. For A375 human melanoma, after stimulated by α-MSH, culture medium was also turned into dark brown after 48 hours of culture (**Figure 4(c)**) Vitamin C, tBHQ and 2% kojic acid, served as positive control, successfully abolished the formation of melanin, and hence the medium color remained unchanged, *i.e.* inhibition of melanin formation (**Figure 4(a)** and **Figure 4(c)**). The melanin concentration extracted from the treated B16 mouse melanoma and A375 human melanoma also agreed with these observations. The melanin concentration of cultured B16 and A375 were significantly lower than the blank control after incubation with NANA and White or Red EBN extract; however, the abolishing effect was not found by the extract of Grass EBN (**Figure 4(b)** and **Figure 4(d)**).

In 3D human skin model, treatment of 2% kojic acid successfully lightened the apparent intensity of skin color (**Figure 5(a)**) and reduced the density of melanocytes (**Figure 5(b)**). Similar inhibitory results were obtained by NANA and the extract of White EBN (**Figure 5(a)**, **Figure 5(b)**). No significant differences in inhibition effects between treatments on the sides of keratinocyte and melanocyte. Thus, kojic acid, NANA and EBN extracts were all suggested to be permeable through the 3D human skin model (**Figure 5(a)**, **Figure 5(b)**).

4. Conclusions

EBN has been consumed for several hundred years in China and other Southeast Asian countries. In the descriptions of ancient Chinese literatures, EBN was often used to treat respiratory disorder. The most famous record about EBN usage, as the form of "bird's nest congee", can be found in "Dream of the Red Chamber", or called that as "The Story of the Stone", a masterpiece of Chinese literature written in 18th century and is generally acknowledged to be the pinnacle of Chinese fiction. Until now, EBN is a popular food supplement for skin lightening. The trend of EBN consumption is growing [17] but stopped by the safety incident of nitrite in 2011 [11]. Although EBN has a long historical consumption record and strong belief in its skincare functions by the general public in Asia is reported, no scientific evidence has shown any relationship between EBN and skin healthiness. Here, we demonstrated the skin lightening functions of different types of EBN. On top of this, we discovered that NANA was the major ingredient of EBN responsible for the skincare functions after systematic fractionation by LC-MS/MS.

From our previous finding, the content of free NANA varied with the grading of EBN [6]. Coincidently, EBN with higher grade showed stronger skin lightening. NANA should be one of the major compounds responsible for the skin lightening function of EBN. However, NANA should not be the only compound within EBN, which is responsible for skin lightening function. The IC_{50} of NANA on human tyrosinase inhibition is 0.10 mM which is coherent to our previous study on over a hundred batches of EBNs. The maximum content of free NANA was around 1000 ppm (*i.e.* about 3 mM). Certainly, the inhibition of EBN on tyrosinase activity may also involve the

Table 1. Comparison of NANA and other skin lightening agents.

Skin lightening agent	IC_{50}[a]	Inhibitory mechanism[b]
Hydroquinone[c]	0.037 mM	Competitive
Arbutin	24.0 mM	Competitive
Gallic acid	4.50 mM	Unknown
Kojic acid	0.030 mM	Unknown
NANA (Sialic acid)	0.100 mM	Non-competitive

[a]IC_{50} value was calculated by GraphPad 5.0 after plotting the activity of mushroom tyrosinase against the concentration of different inhibitors, were presented ($n = 3$). [b]The inhibitory mechanism of different inhibitors on tyrosinase was deducted by Lineweaver-Burk plot and calculated by GraphPad 5.0. [c]Hydroquinone was banned by FDA in 2006 for its potential carcinogenicity.

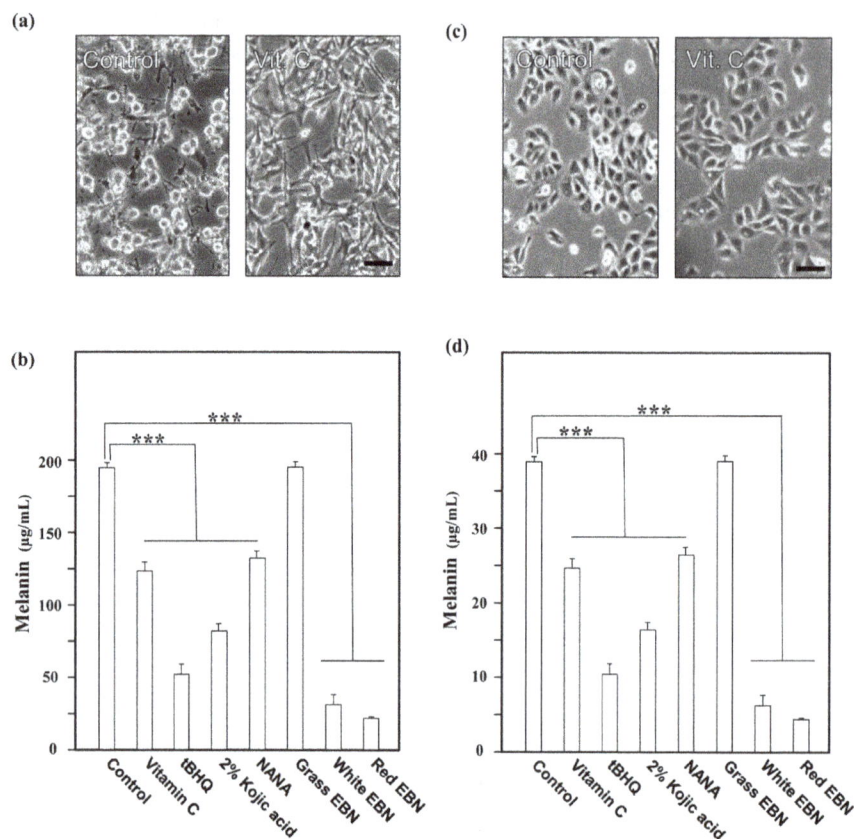

Figure 4. NANA and EBN inhibit melanin formation in cultured B16 and A375 cells. (a) B16 murine melanoma and (c) A375 human melanoma cells were seeded on 6-well plate and cultured in DMEM supplemented with 10% fetal bovine serum. On the following day, B16 cells were exposed to vitamin C (5 mM), as a positive control. For A375 human melanoma, 10 nM of α-MSH was applied to all samples to stimulate melanogenesis on day 2. Microscopic views of different wells were captured after 48 hours of incubation. Images were captured from intact B16 cells to observe the release of melanosomes. Scale bar = 100 μm. (b) Melanin from B16 cells and (d) A375 cells with or without the treatment of vitamin C (5 mM), or tBHQ (50 μM), or 2% kojic acid, or NANA (20 mM), or EBN extracts (1 mg/mL), were extracted and measured by spectrometer at 405 nm. Melanin concentrations were converted from the absorbance of 405 nm using melanin standard curve. The content of melanin were presented as Mean $\pm$ SD (n = 3). One-way ANOVA was performed on the data set by GraphPad 5.0. Statistical significant differences were indicated. ***$P < 0.001$ versus reference group.

conjugated form of NANA, and/or there are other active ingredients within EBN that perform skin lightening function synergistically with NANA.

NANA was reported to play functional roles in physiological developments in human. NANA is usually the terminal residue of cellular glycocalyx and plays important role for cellular recognition. Moreover, NANA is a major component for brain development. Disorder of NANA regulation results in retardation of brain development [18] [19]. Furthermore, NANA was reported for its functions in anti-viral [8], transformation of lymphocyte [20], growth of CaCo-2 cells [10], development of human adipose-derived stem cells [21] and proliferation of corneal keratinocytes [22]. However, no report had been found on the skincare function of NANA. In the past several years, 2% hydroquinone was accepted as a golden standard for skin lightening [23]. However, the drug was banned by FDA in 2006 because of its potential carcinogenicity. A derivative of hydroquinone with the addition of glycoside, named arbutin, was then developed into a substitute. However, the low skin lightening efficiency of arbutin had always been complained. Subsequently, the development of new skin lightening agents is an urgent need in the cosmetic market. New agents like gallic acid from gallnut and kojic acid from the by-products

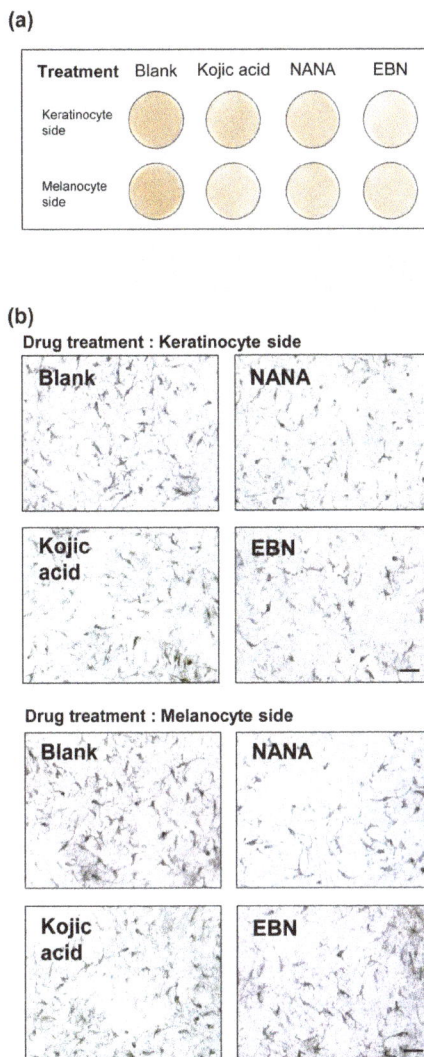

Figure 5. NANA and EBN inhibit melanin formation in 3D human skin model Blank control, 20 mM NANA, 1 mg/mL EBN extract and 2% of kojic acid (positive control) were applied either to the inner chambers of trans-well containing the 3D human skin model (keratinocyte side) or culture medium directly (melanocyte side). Macroscopic and microscopic images were captured on day 18 after treatment. (a) Macroscopic images were captured by the top view (keratinocyte side), (b) while microscopic images were captured by inverted microscope under 100× magnification (melanocyte side). Scale bar = 100 μm, $n = 3$.

of Japanese rice wine (*i.e.* Sake) were developed for their skin lightening functions [24]. However, the mechanisms of tyrosinase inhibition of gallic acid and kojic acid is still under investigation. Here, we discovered that NANA could be a potential new skin lightening agent. Firstly, NANA is derived from natural source. Secondly, the skin lightening efficiency of NANA is comparable to known skin lightening agents. Lastly, the inhibition mechanism of NANA on tyrosinase activity is different from the inhibition mechanism of hydroquinone and arbutin (competitive inhibition). In addition, the chemical structure of NANA is different to other skin lightening agents, *i.e.* a phenolic ring was replaced by a glucose ring. Thus, NANA should have a high potential to be developed into a new skin lightening agent.

Acknowledgements

Supported by Hong Kong Research Grants Council Theme-based Research Scheme (T13-607/12R), ITF (UIM/

254), GRF (661110, 662911, 660411, 663012, 662713, M-HKUST604/13), TUYF12SC02, TUYF12SC03, TUYF15SC01, The Hong Kong Jockey Club Charities Trust (HKJCCT12SC01) and Foundation of The Awareness of Nature (TAON12SC01) to Karl Tsim. Zach Wong received a scholarship from HKJEBN Scholarship for Health and Quality Living.

References

[1]   Marcone, M.F. (2005) Characterization of the Edible Bird's Nest the "Caviar of the East". *Food Research International*, **38**, 1125-1134. http://dx.doi.org/10.1016/j.foodres.2005.02.008

[2]   Lin, J.R., Zhou, H. and Lai, X. (2006) Application of Stereoscopy on Edible Bird's Nest Identification. *Journal of Chinese Medicinal Materials*, **29**, 219-221.

[3]   Lin, J.R., Dong, Y., Zhou, H., Lai, X.P. and Wang, P.X. (2006) Identification of Edible Bird's Nest by Electrophoresis. *World Science Technology/Modernization of Traditional Chinese Medicine*, **8**, 30-32.

[4]   Lin, J.R., Zhou, H., Lai, X.P., Hou, Y., Xian, X.M., Chen, J.N., Wang, P.X., Zhou, L. and Dong, Y. (2009) Genetic Identification of Edible Birds' Nest Based on Mitochondrial DNA Sequences. *Food Research International*, **42**, 1053-1061. http://dx.doi.org/10.1016/j.foodres.2009.04.014

[5]   Chan, G.K. (2013) The Quality Assurance of Edible Bird's Nest: Removal of Nitrite Contamination and Identification of an Indicative Chemical Marker. Ph.D. Thesis, The Hong Kong University of Science and Technology, Hong Kong.

[6]   Chan, G.K., Zheng, K.Y., Zhu, K.Y., Dong, T.T. and Tsim, K.W. (2013) Determination of Free N-Acetylneuraminic Acid in Edible Bird Nest: A Development of Chemical Marker for Quality Control. *Journal of Ethnobiology and Traditional Medicine*, **120**, 620-628.

[7]   Yang, M., Cheung, S.H., Li, S.C. and Cheung, H.Y. (2014) Establishment of a Holistic and Scientific Protocol for the Authentication and Quality Assurance of Edible Bird's Nest. *Food Chemistry*, **151**, 271-278. http://dx.doi.org/10.1016/j.foodchem.2013.11.007

[8]   Guo, C.T., Takahashi, T., Bukawa, W., Takahashi, N., Yagi, H., Kato, K., Hidari, K.I., Miyamoto, D., Suzuki, T. and Suzuki, Y. (2006) Edible Bird's Nest Extract Inhibits Influenza Virus Infection. *Antiviral Research*, **70**, 140-146. http://dx.doi.org/10.1016/j.antiviral.2006.02.005

[9]   Yagi, H., Yasukawa, N., Yu, S.Y., Guo, C.T., Takahashi, N., Takahashi, T., Bukawa, W., Suzuki, T., Khoo, K.H., Suzuki, Y. and Kato, K. (2008) The Expression of Sialylated High-Antennary N-Glycans in Edible Bird's Nest. *Carbohydrate Research*, **343**, 1373-1377. http://dx.doi.org/10.1016/j.carres.2008.03.031

[10] Rashed, A.A. and Nazaimoon, W.M. (2010) Effect of Edible Bird's Nest on Caco-2 Cell Proliferation. *Journal of Food Technology*, **8**, 126-130. http://dx.doi.org/10.3923/jftech.2010.126.130

[11] Chan, G.K., Zhu, K.Y., Chou, D.J., Guo, A.J., Lau, D.T., Dong, T.T. and Tsim, K.W. (2013) Surveillance of Nitrite Level on Edible Bird's Nest in Hong Kong: Evaluation of Removal Method and Proposed Origin of Contamination. *Food Control*, **34**, 637-644. http://dx.doi.org/10.1016/j.foodcont.2013.06.010

[12] Chen, Q.X., Song, K.K., Qiu, L., Liu, X.D., Huang, H. and Guo, H.Y. (2005) Inhibitory Effects on Mushroom Tyrosinase by *p*-Alkoxybenzoic acids. *Food Chemistry*, **91**, 269-274. http://dx.doi.org/10.1016/j.foodchem.2004.01.078

[13] Iwata, M., Corn, T., Iwata, S., Everett, M.A. and Fuller, B.B. (1990) The Relationship between Tyrosinase Activity and Skin Color in Human Foreskins. *Journal of Investigative Dermatology*, **85**, 9-15. http://dx.doi.org/10.1111/1523-1747.ep12872677

[14] Jeon, S.H., Kim, K.H., Koh, J.U. and Kong, K.H. (2005) Inhibitory Effects on L-Dopa Oxidation of Tyrosinase by Skin-Whitening Agents. *Bulletin of the Korean Chemical Society*, **26**, 1135-1137. http://dx.doi.org/10.5012/bkcs.2005.26.7.1135

[15] Moon, J.Y., Yim, E.Y., Song, G., Lee, N.H. and Hyun, C.G. (2010) Screening of Elastase and Tyrosinase Inhibitory Activity from Jeju Island Plants. *EurAsian Journal of Biological Sciences*, **4**, 41-53. http://dx.doi.org/10.5053/ejobios.2010.4.0.6

[16] Kasraee, B., Hügin, A., Tran, C., Sorg, O. and Saura, J.H. (2004) Methimazole Is an Inhibitor of Melanin Synthesis in Cultured B16 Melanocytes. *Journal of Investigative Dermatology*, **122**, 1338-1341. http://dx.doi.org/10.1111/j.0022-202X.2004.22509.x

[17] Leung, C.Y. (2004) Three Billions Market Competition for Edible Bird's Nest Shops. *Economic Digest*, **1197**, 68-69.

[18] Ham, M., Prinsen, B.H., Huijmans, J.G., Abeling, N.G., Dorland, B., Berger, R., Koning, T.J. and Sain-van Der Velden, M.G. (2007) Quantification of Free and Total Sialic Acid Excretion by LC-MS/MS. *Journal of Chromatography B*, **848**, 251-257. http://dx.doi.org/10.1016/j.jchromb.2006.10.066

[19] Sillanaukee, P., Pönniö, M. and Jääskeläinen, I.P. (1999) Occurrence of Sialic Acids in Healthy Humans and Different Disorders. *European Journal of Clinical Investigation*, **29**, 413-425.

http://dx.doi.org/10.1046/j.1365-2362.1999.00485.x

[20] Hou, Y., Xian, X., Lin, J., Lai, X. and Chen, J. (2010) The Effects of Edible Birds' Nest (*Aerodramus*) on Con A-Induced Rats' Lymphocytes Transformation. *China Modern Medicine*, **17**, 9-11.

[21] Roh, K.B., Lee, J., Kim, Y.S., Park, J., Kim, J.H., Lee, J. and Park, D. (2011) Mechanisms of Edible Bird's Nest Extract-Induced Proliferation of Human Adipose-Derived Stem Cells. *Evidence-Based Complementary Alternative Medicine*, **2012**, Article ID: 797520. http://dx.doi.org/10.1155/2012/797520

[22] Fadhilah, Z.A., Chua, K.H., Ng, S.L., Elvy, S.M., Lee, T.H. and Norzana, A.G. (2011) Effects of Edible Bird's Nest (EBN) on Cultured Rabbit Corneal Keratinocytes. *BMC Complementary and Alternative Medicine*, **11**, 1-11.

[23] Makino, E.T., Mehta, R.C., Banga, A., Jain, P., Sigler, M.L. and Sonti, S. (2013) Evaluation of a Hydroquinone-Free Skin Brightening Product Using *in Vitro* Inhibition of Melanogenesis and Clinical Reduction of Ultraviolet-Induced Hyperpigmentation. *Journal of Drugs in Dermatology*, **12**, s16-s20.

[24] Kumar, K.J., Vani, M.G., Wang, S.Y., Liao, J.W., Hsu, L.S., Yang, H.L. and Hseu, Y.C. (2013) *In Vitro* and *in Vivo* Studies Disclosed the Depigmenting Effects of Gallic Acid: A Novel Skin Lightening Agent for Hyperpigmentary Skin Diseases. *BioFactors*, **39**, 259-270. http://dx.doi.org/10.1002/biof.1064

Supplementary

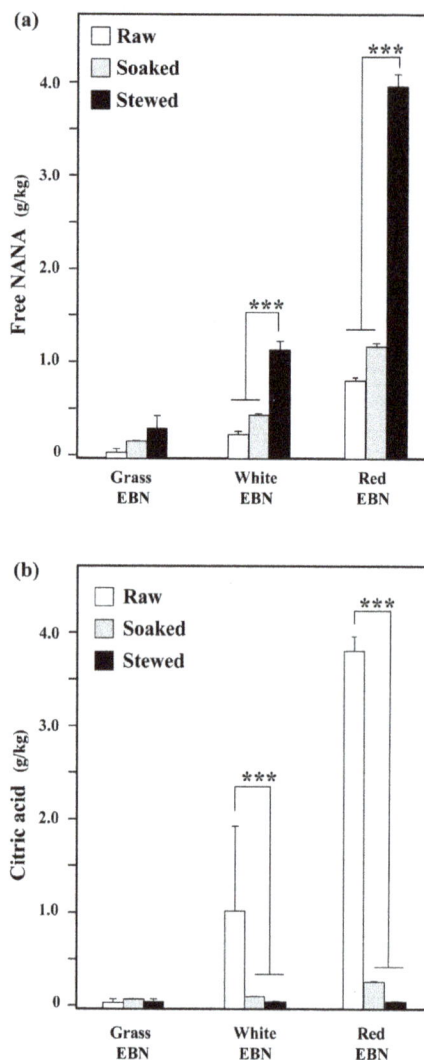

Supplementary Figure 1. The contents of NANA and citric acid during cooking. Twelve batches purchased EBN were processed by standard procedure. For Grass and White EBN, EBNs were soaked in 100 folds of water (w/v) for 3 hours and stewed in 30 folds of water for 0.5 hour. For Red EBN, EBN were soaked for 15 hours and stewed in 30 folds of water for 2.5 hours. The content of free NANA (A) and citric acid (B) on Grass EBN, White EBN and Red EBN during different stages of processing were determined. The free NANA and citric acidin g/kg of dry material was presented as Mean + SD (n = 3). ***P < 0.001 versus reference group.

Supplementary Table. The contents of protein, free NANA and citric acid of different grades of EBN.

EBN Type[a]	Protein[b] (g/kg)		Free NANA[c] (mg/kg)		Citric acid[d] (g/kg)	
	Range	Medium	Range	Medium	Range	Medium
Grass EBN	314.52 - 558.81	507.11	51.35 - 130.03	54.31	0.00	0.00
White EBN	507.28 - 695.04	680.53	96.57 - 691.23	170.46	0.00 - 2.04	1.00
Red EBN	459.27 - 504.00	477.32	310.26 - 910.81	802.51	1.05 - 4.03	3.24

[a]Twelve batches of EBN were randomly purchased from local market of Hong Kong, at least three batches for each type of EBN. The original production countries included Indonesia, Malaysia, Vietnam, Thailand and Philippines. [b]Protein content of EBN was measured by Bradford's method after completely solubilized by stewing. [c]Free NANA content was measured by calculating the peak area in LC-MS/MS chromatogram with free NANA standard. [d]Citric acid content was measured by calculating the peak area in LC-MS/MS chromatogram with citric acid standard. All contents were presented as per kilogram of crude EBN, the contents of each items were presented (n = 3).

15

The Effect of Novel Low Energy Pulsed Light Combined with Galvanic Energy for Home-Use Hair Removal of Dark Skin

Michael H. Gold[1], Hela Goren[2]

[1]Tennessee Clinical Research Center, Nashville, USA
[2]Home Skinovation Ltd., Yokneam, Israel
Email: Rgoren4@gmail.com

Abstract

Background and Objectives: Permanent reduction of unwanted hair on skin types V and VI is the most challenging procedure among all hair removal technologies based on selective absorption of light or laser. The objective of this study is to evaluate the safety and efficacy of a low energy pulsed-light device combined with galvanic energy, intended for home-use hair removal on dark skin. Materials and Methods: Fifteen women with skin types V and VI and dark terminal hair in axillaarea self-administrated 6 treatments at 2 week intervals, using a hand-held IPL combined with galvanicenergy device, using HPL (Home Pulsed Light) technology. Hair count and photographs were performed pre-treatment and 1 and 3 months after the last sixth treatment. Adverse events and subject satisfaction scores were recorded. Results: All patients showed a positive clinical response to treatment, with reduction of unwanted hair. Hair counts were significantly reduced by 57.3% 1 month following last treatment and by 44.5% 3 months following last treatment. No adverse events were recorded. Subject satisfaction scores of the device usability and the treatment outcome were high. Conclusions: Low energy pulsed light combined with galvanic energy may be applied safely and effectively for at-home hair removal for people with dark skin types V and VI.

Keywords

Hair Removal, Dark Skin, Home-Use, IPL, Galvanic Energy

1. Introduction

Long-term removal of unwanted hair is the most popular skin treatment worldwide. Over the past decade, various light and laser sources have been advocated for use in the office setting with long term results [1]-[3]. Selective photothermolysis was established as the mechanism of action of optical sources of light and laser for the selective destruction of hair follicles [4] [5]. However, efficacy and safety of these technologies presented a challenge when dark skin was treated [6]. The disadvantages of in-office based hair removal methods called for the establishment of home-use devices of laser and light sources that enable people to enjoy permanent hair reduction in the comfort of their own home [7]-[11]. The challenge of treating dark skin safely and effectively at home environment still exists, as low fluence light source has to be deployed to protect the dark skin without affecting efficacy of the long-term hair removal. In an attempt to increase absorption of light in the hair melanin, continuous galvanic current has been added. The galvaniccurrent applied that may be as low as 200 µA is widely used in cosmetic treatments for a few decades [12]. Such a low direct electrical current is hardly perceptible and may affect temporarily several skin structures, including pore dilation. Dilation of the pores at the skin surface exposes a bigger portion of the hair shaft to the optical energy, thus increasing the absorption and enabling a low fluence to be efficacious. The combination of radiofrequency electrical current and intense pulsed light (IPL) energy has been previously reported for in-office system [13]. The current study is the first attempt to combine the electrical and optical energies in a home-use device in an attempt to treat dark skin safely and effectively.

2. Materials and Methods

2.1. Device and Technology

The Infinity Device is a small hair removal home-use device, employing the technology of electrical Home Pulsed Light (eHPL™) (Home Skinovation, Yokneam, Israel). It is a portable hand-held device with spot size of 1×3 cm, combining low energy IPL (475 - 1200 nm; 3 - 5 J/cm^2) and 200 µA galvanic energy (**Figure 1**). IPL may be applied in the rate of 1 pulse every 1 - 2 sec in 5 different levels according to individual skin response, following a test spot. The electrical current is a continuous direct current that depends on full contact with the skin. Failure to have this contact results in automatic inactivation of the galvanic energy by a built-in safety mechanism. This mechanism also inactivates IPL if full contact with the skin is not achieved.

2.2. Subjects

Seventeen females, 21 - 60 years old with Fitzpatrick skin type VI who had black hair in their axillae and met the inclusion and exclusion criteria were recruited to the study. Subjects were retained by in office recruitment of existing patients who would be a candidate for hair removal through an IRB (Investigational Review Board) approval study. Fifteen subjects have completed the study. All subjects signed an informed consent form.

2.3. Acceptance Criteria

Inclusion criteria included healthy females between 21 - 60 years of age with skin type VI, having unwanted

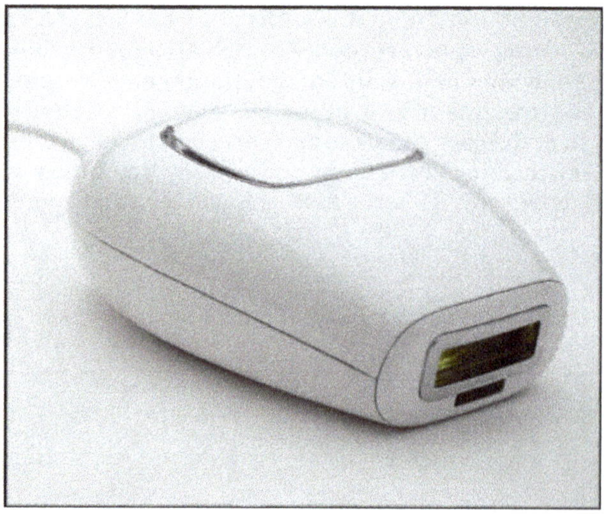

Figure 1. The Infinity Device.

black hair in their axillae and willingness to follow the study protocol. Exclusion criteria included pregnancy and lactating throughout the study period, concurrent severe diseases and history of malignancy, diseases that may be stimulated by light, such as epilepsy and lupus, scarring, inflammation or infection of the area to be treated, history of skin disorders such as keloids and abnormal wound healing, a pacemaker or internal defibrillator device, poorly controlled endocrine disorders as diabetes or PCO, history of bleeding coagulopathies or constant use of anticoagulants, previous photo-epilation hair removal or waxing and plucking in the treatment area during the last three months, history of known photosensitization or the use of a medication known to induce photosensitization; tanned skin in the treatment area within four weeks of the study, and presence of tattoo in the treatment area.

2.4. Study Design

Subjects were given the Infinity device and the instructions for use and were asked to perform the first self-treatment in the investigator's clinic in the supervision of a qualified trainer who determined the fluence used for each individual following a test spot procedure. Baseline measurements included demographic data, laboratory tests to rule out pregnancy, and initial photography and hair counts in both axillae. Subjects conducted 5 more sessions of self-treatment (total 6) at home at 2 weeks intervals. Follow-up sessions were held in the investigator's clinic 1, and 3 months following the last treatment. At each follow-up session the treated area was photographed and hair count conducted in a similar way to baseline. Photographs were taken with Nikon D100 camera with 60-mm micro lens. Hair count was done on a predetermined 2×2 cm (4 cm^2) area, using a small sticker. These stickers have a central cut out area that is a reproducible 2×2 cm in size. The axillae with the stickers were also photographed to ensure count in the same area. Furthermore, a transparency sheet was placed over each axilla of the subject, and anatomic locations (such as nevi, freckles, tags, scars) were marked to facilitate reproducibility of count area in the various visits. The duration of the entire study for each subject was up to 7 months.

2.5. Treatment Procedure

Hair was shaved and treatment was performed by applying light pressure on the treatment area with the Infinity device, to achieve complete contact with the skin and pressing the trigger button. The applicator was then moved to the next spot without overlap and with full coverage of the treated area. Post-treatment care included the application of cold Aloe Vera cream and a moisturizer cream and the patients were instructed to protect the treated areas from sun exposure and tanning throughout the whole study. After each treatment subjects were instructed to evaluateany adverse event and attend the clinic for its assessment. At each follow-up session subjects were asked to rate their satisfaction level in a scale of four: 0—Not satisfied; 1—Slightly satisfied; 2—Satisfied; 3—Very satisfied.

2.6. Statistics

Sample size was 30 treatment sites of 15 subjects. Hair count p values were performed using paired t-test analysis. Values < 0.001 were regarded statistically significant.

3. Results

All 15 subjects who enrolled and completed the study were females with an average age of 42 years, with skin type VI that were treated on both axillae for unwanted black hair. Energy levels used (out of 5 levels) were 1 - 3 with a mean value of 2.3.

Results of the clinical study and demographic data are given in **Table 1**. The Results show that the mean hair count per at baseline was 53.4 ± 3.9. At the 1 month follow-up visit, the mean hair count significantly decreased to 22.8 (SD = 4.4), by 57.3% (p < 0.001). At the 3 month follow-up visit, the mean hair count was decreased to a lesser degree 29.7 (SD = 4.8) which was still significantly lower than baseline count in 44.5% (p < 0.001).

The graphic presentation of hair count and percent hair reduction distribution is given in **Figure 2**.

Representative photographic illustrations of hair reduction in the two follow-up sessions as compared with baseline photographs are presented in **Figure 3**. Results of hair reduction on three axillae of three different patients with skin type VI are comparing baseline to 3 month follow-up (**Figure 4**). Both, hair count results and

Table 1. Hair count and percent hair reduction distribution at baseline and at 2 follow-up sessions, 1 and 3 months post 6 treatments.

Subject ID	Axilla	Age	Energy Level	Hair Count per 2 cm^2 Mean ± SD			Response
				Baseline	1 Month	3 Months	
1	Left	50	2	47	30	37	Slight erythema
1	Right		2	49	28	34	Slight erythema
2	Left	28	1	49	19	23	None
2	Right		1	49	21	25	None
3	Left	44	3	55	17	27	Slight erythema
3	Right		3	53	21	24	Slight erythema
4	Left	25	3	51	18	27	Perifollicular edema
4	Right		3	55	28	30	Perifollicular edema
5	Left	59	2	49	26	37	None
5	Right		3	47	21	37	None
6	Left	45	2	48	25	27	Perifollicular edema
6	Right		2	54	26	29	Perifollicular edema
7	Left	33	2	50	21	33	None
7	Right		2	57	19	31	None
8	Left	42	1	56	28	28	None
8	Right		2	57	30	35	None
9	Left	21	2	59	27	34	Perifollicular erythema
9	Right		2	53	27	30	Perifollicular edema
10	Left	54	3	53	25	31	Perifollicular erythema
10	Right		3	55	27	30	Perifollicular erythema
11	Left	55	3	47	17	25	None
11	Right		3	50	17	23	None
12	Left	60	1	55	19	30	None
12	Right		1	58	20	23	None
13	Left	28	2	59	29	37	None
13	Right		2	59	25	32	None
14	Left	32	3	51	17	25	None
14	Right		3	50	19	22	None
15	Left	49	3	57	25	34	Perifollicular edema
15	Right		3	56	21	35	Perifollicular edema
Mean Hair Count		42.1	2.3	53.4	22.8	29.7	
SD				3.93	4.37	4.78	
Mean % Hair Reduction					57.3%	44.5%	
p-Value					2.3502E−24	5.64221E−20	

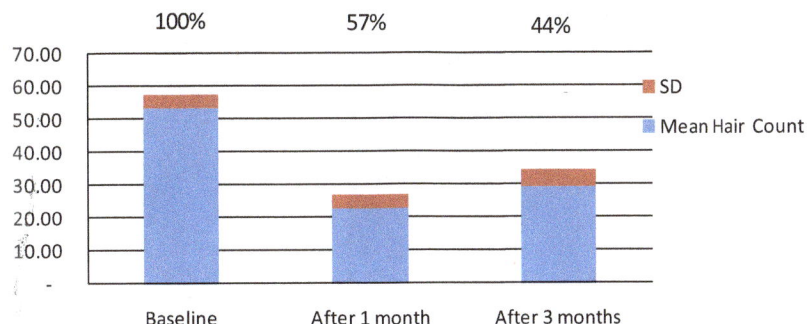

Figure 2. Graphic distribution of hair count and percent hair reduction at baseline and at 2 follow-up sessions, 1 and 3 months post 6 treatments.

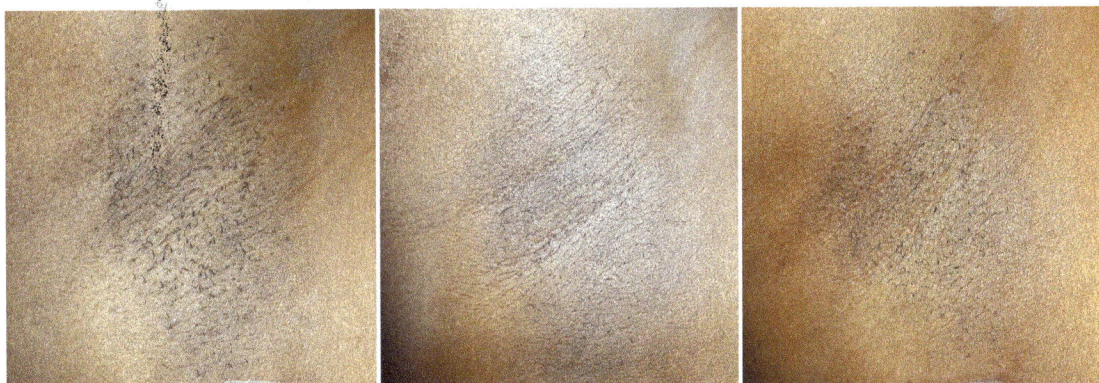

Figure 3. Photographic illustration of hair reduction in axillae of subject 1 at baseline (left), at 1 month follow-up session (center), and 3 months post last treatment (right).

photographs indicate that percent hair reduction after 3 month is smaller than after 1 month.

Subject Satisfaction Score is presented in **Table 2**. Satisfaction included subjects' impression from the results and from the usability of the device. All subjects rated the usability that reflects ease of use as "very satisfied". Regarding treatment outcome, eight subjects scored their satisfaction as "very satisfied" at the two follow-up sessions. Six subjects rated their satisfaction as "satisfied" after 1 month and 5 of them changed their rating to "very satisfied at the 3 months follow-up sessions. One subject started at "slightly satisfied" at the 1 month follow-up and changed to "satisfied" after 3 months. Altogether, satisfaction rate of both usability of the device and hair reduction outcome is very high (2.5 - 3.0). All subjects expressed their will to purchase the device following the study for home-use treatments and recommend to their friends.

No adverse events were noted during the study. Slightedema in the perifollicular sites was experienced by 33.3% of the subjects and resolved within 2 hours. This was a desirable and expected response of treatment endpoint.

4. Discussion

The current study demonstrated 57.3% hair reduction 1 month after 6 sessions every other week that was reduced to 44.5% after 3 months and was also demonstrated in the photographs (**Figure 2**, **Figure 3**). These results indicate that a maintenance session may be required after ~2 months following the treatment regime.

Long-term hair removal performed in-office by optical technologies of lasers and IPL have presented an average efficacy of 60% - 80% following a multi-session treatment [3] and with follow-up periods of 1 - 2 years [1] [12]. Home-use devices based on IPL technology proved to be efficacious on body areas [7] [10] and on the face [8] in a similar efficacy as in office-based IPL systems by using lower fluence but more frequent sessions. Thus, 83% hair reduction was demonstrated on the face after 1 month and 78% after 3 months following 6 sessions every other week [7]. Percent hair reduction on the body was lower and reached 78% after 1 month and 72% after 3 months following 6 sessions [8]. In another study [10] average percent hair reduction observed on body

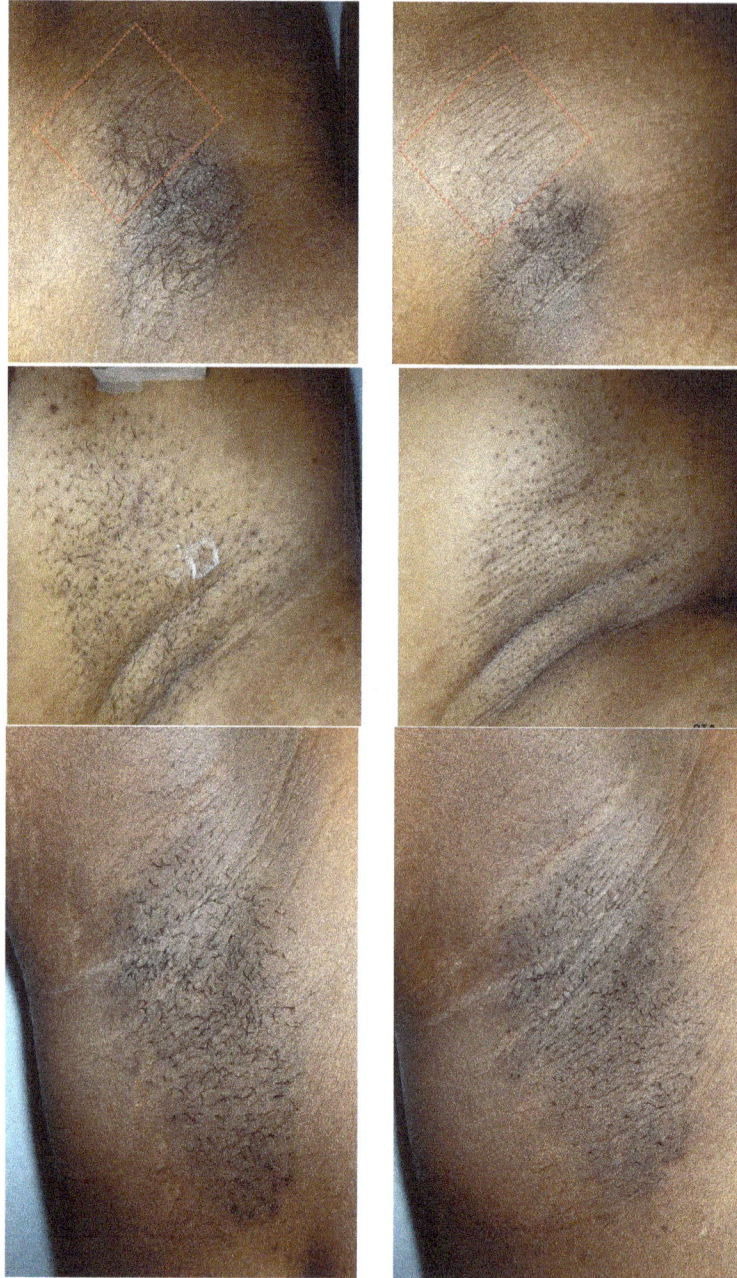

Figure 4. Photographic illustration of hair reduction in axillae of 3 subjects at baseline (Left) and 3 months post last treatment (Right). Top to bottom: subjects 3R, 10R, and 11R.

areas after 3 months following 3 treatments was 64%. The three studies were conducted on light skin types, up to Fitzpatrick skin type IV.

In an attempt to adjust the home-use hair removal device to dark skin type (V-VI), lower fluence was applied to the dark skin to ensure safety (energy levels 1 - 3), but efficacy was increased by the simultaneous addition of galvanic energy. Nevertheless, as expected, percent hair reduction was lower than on lighter skin, using a similar device. As the studies described above were conducted with a similar IPL device [7]-[9] on light skin, it is important to note that using lower level energy on dark skin types may require more treatment sessions. Therefore, to achieve similar efficacy to results on lighter skin, it is expected that treatment of darker skin types may require up to 12 treatments every other week.

Table 2. Subject satisfaction scores.

Subject ID	1 Month FU		3 Month FU	
	Usability	Outcome	Usability	Outcome
1	3	2	3	2
2	3	3	3	3
3	3	3	3	3
4	3	2	3	3
5	3	2	3	3
6	3	1	3	2
7	3	3	3	3
8	3	3	3	3
9	3	3	3	3
10	3	2	3	3
11	3	2	3	3
12	3	3	3	3
13	3	3	3	3
14	3	2	3	3
15	3	3	3	3
Mean	**3.0**	**2.5**	**3.0**	**2.9**

O = Not Satisfied; 1 = Slightly Satisfied; 2 = Satisfied; 3 = Very Satisfied.

Despite the lower efficacy achieved by the Infinity home-use device on dark skin, when compared to light skin, subject satisfaction was very high. All subjects found the device ergonomic and easy to use. Most of the subjects were very satisfied with the treatments outcome in hair reduction.

In another study [9], a similar home-use device was used for only 3 sessions bi-monthly. As a result, lower percent hair reduction (40.4%) was noted in the axillae 1 month after last treatment and it was reduced to 37.8% at 6 months follow-up. The skin types treated on axillae were II-III. According to this study, it may be worthwhile to check the percent hair reduction of the current study after 6 months.

No adverse events were recorded, like all IPL hair removal home-use devices that were reported to be safe. Some of the devices, however, had impaired efficacy due to safety [10]. In the current study efficacy was not affected, as the low optical energy was compensated by the galvanic energy used in the Infinity device. The galvanic energy which is applied in a continuous wave enables better absorption of the IPL pulses in the hair shaft by widening the skin pores [11]. As a result, less optical energy is needed to destroy the hair follicle, without creating damage to the surrounding dark skin.

5. Conclusion

Low-fluence pulsed light combined with galvanic energy, using the novel technology of eHPL™ may be applied safely and effectively for at home hair removal for subjects with dark skin type of V-VI. All patients (100%) showed a reduction in hair removal at 1 and 3 months, with zero adverse effects.

References

[1]　Gold, M.H., Bell, M.W., Foster, T.D. and Street, S. (1999) One Year Follow-Up Using an Intense Pulsed Light Source for Long Term Hair Removal. *Journal of Cutaneous Laser Therapy*, **1**, 167-171.
http://dx.doi.org/10.1080/14628839950516823

[2]　Dierickx, C.C. (2002) Hair Removal by Lasers and Intense Pulsed Light Sources. *Dermatologic Clinics*, **20**, 135-146.
http://dx.doi.org/10.1016/S0733-8635(03)00052-4

[3]   Gold, M.H. (2007) Lasers and Light Sources for the Removal of Unwanted Hair. *Clinical Dermatology*, **25**, 443-453.
        http://dx.doi.org/10.1016/j.clindermatol.2007.05.017

[4]   Anderson, R.R. and Parish, J.A. (1983) Selective Photothermolysis: Precise Microsurgery by Selective Absorption of
        Pulse Radiation. *Science*, **20**, 524. http://dx.doi.org/10.1126/science.6836297

[5]   Grossman, M.C., Dierickx, C.C., Farineli, W., Flotte, T. and Anderson, R.R. (1996) Damage to Hair Follicles by Nor-
        mal Mode Ruby Laser Pulses. *Journal of American Academy of Dermatology*, **35**, 889-894.
        http://dx.doi.org/10.1016/S0190-9622(96)90111-5

[6]   Johnson, F. and Dovale, M. (1999) Intense Pulsed Light Treatment of Hirsutism: Case Reports of Skin Phototypes V
        and VI. *Journal of Cuteneous laser Therapy*, **1**, 233-237

[7]   Gold, M.H., Foster, A. and Biron, J.A. (2010) Low-Energy Intense Pulsed Light for Hair Removal at Home. *The
        Journal of Clinical and Aesthetic Dermatology*, **3**, 48-53.

[8]   Gold, M.H., Biron, A.B. and Thompson, B. (2015) Clinical Evaluation of a Novel Intense Pulsed Light Source for Fa-
        cial Skin Hair Removal for Home Use. *The Journal of Clinical and Aesthetic Dermatology*, **8**, 30-35.

[9]   Alster, T.S. and Tanzi, E.L. (2009) Effect of a Novel Low-Energy Pulsed-Light Device for Home-Use Hair Removal.
        Dermatologic Surgery, **35**, 483-489. http://dx.doi.org/10.1111/j.1524-4725.2009.01089.x

[10]   Mulholland, R.S. (2009) Silk'n™—A Novel Device Using Home Pulsed Light™ for Hair Removal at Home. *Journal
        of Cosmetic and laser Therapy*, **11**, 106-109. http://dx.doi.org/10.1080/14764170902902806

[11]   Town, G. and Ash, C. (2010) Are Home-Use Intense Pulsed Light (IPL) Devices Safe? *Lasers in Medical Science*, **25**,
        773-780. http://dx.doi.org/10.1007/s10103-010-0809-6

[12]   Nordmann, L. (2010) Professional Beauty Therapy—The Official Guide to Level 3. 4th Edition, Cengage Learning
        EMEA, 231-237.

[13]   Sadick, N.S. and Shaoul, J. (2004) Hair Removal Using a Combination of Conducted Radiofrequency and Optical
        Energies—An 18-Month Follow-Up. *Journal of Cosmetics and Laser Therapy*, **6**, 21-26.
        http://dx.doi.org/10.1080/14764170410029013

Therapeutic Role of Isotretinoin in the Management of Recurrent Aphthous Stomatitis (Single-Blind Controlled Therapeutic Study)

Khalifa E. Sharquie[1]*, Raad M. Helmi[2], Adil A. Noaimi[1], Mohand A. A. Kadhom[3], Raafa K. Al-Hayani[4]

[1]Scientific Council of Dermatology and Venereology-Iraqi and Arab Board for Medical Specializations, Department of Dermatology and Venereology, College of Medicine, University of Baghdad, Baghdad, Iraq
[2]Department of Oral Medicine, College of Dentistry, Al-Mustansiriya University, Baghdad, Iraq
[3]School of Dentistry, Faculty of Medical Science, University of Duhok, Duhok, Iraq
[4]Department of Dermatology and Venereology, Baghdad Teaching Hospital, Baghdad, Iraq
Email: *ksharquie@ymail.com, dr_raadhelmi@yahoo.com, adilnoaimi@yahoo.com, dr_mohandduhuk@yahoo.com, raafahayani@yahoo.com

Abstract

Background: Recurrent aphthous ulcer (RAS) is a common oral disease where its etiopathogenesis is not well elucidated. There was no effective curative therapy for this disease. Isotretinoin has been recently used in the treatment of Behcet's disease. Objectives: To evaluate the efficacy and safety of isotretinoin in treating RAS and the long term remission of RAS. Patients and Methods: This single-blind controlled therapeutic study conducted in Department of Dermatology-Baghdad Teaching Hospital during February 2011-January 2012. Thirty patients with typical RAS were included in this work. Detailed history and full examination were done for all patients. They were given isotretinoin 20 mg orally once daily for three months to be seen on Day 14 firstly and then monthly to be assessed using the oral clinical manifestation index (OCMI). After isotretinoin was stopped three months later, patients were given placebo therapy for another 3 months. Results: The results of 30 treated patients were as follows: 17 (56.67%) males and 13 (43.33%) females with male to female ratio was 1.3:1. Their ages ranged from 12 - 60 (35.33 ± 12.06) years. The OCMI before isotretinoin therapy ranged from 7 - 17 (13.13 ± 2.55), while after therapy the mean started to decline to a lower level within the first 14 days (P = 0.103), and continued to decline significantly until the end of the first month of therapy (P = 0.023). Then the OCMI declined very significantly until the end of fourth month of therapy (P < 0.001). After that the mean started to

increase until the end of the 5 months (with placebo) but it remained statistically significant compared with the baseline of mean of OCMI before treatment (P = 0.046). Then it continued to increase to become not significant at the end of 6 months of therapy (P = 0.107). Conclusion: Isotretinoin is an effective therapeutic and prophylactic promising remedy in treatment of RAS.

Keywords

Recurrent Aphthous Stomatitis, Isotretinoin, Iraq

1. Introduction

Recurrent aphthous stomatitis (RAS) is a common oral problem that is encountered in a round (10% - 25% of the population [1]. There are many varieties of RAS like minor, major and herpetiform. Minor ulcers (80%) are less than one centimeter in diameter, usually heal within 2 weeks, and don't leave scars. Major ulcers (10%) usually one centimeter or more in diameter, take more than minor ulcers to heal, and may leave scars, while Herpetiform ulcers (10%) are clusters of dozens of smaller ulcers [2].

The etiology of this disease is not well elucidated [3], but there are many factors which are implicated in the etiopathogenesis like infection as herpes [4], *Streptococcus sanguis* [5] and cytomegalovirus infection [6] [7]. Other factors include immunological [8]-[11] genetics nutritional deficiency like vitamin B12 and folate deficiencies [11], trauma gastrointestinal diseases [1], hematological deficiencies [12]-[14], hormonal factors and allergies to food [1].

RAS in many cases is mild that does not need therapy but still there are other cases which are severe enough to interfere with life activities and need medical interference. Accordingly, there are many topical and systemic therapies that have been used like chlorhexidine [15], lidocainesolution [16], sucralfate suspension [16], topical honey [17], 5% lactic acid [18], nigella sativa [19], novel dexamucobasemyrtle [20], myrtle [21], colchicines, pentoxifylline [22], steroids [1] [16] thalidomide [23], BCG vaccine [24], and Etanercept [25] are used to control the symptoms. Recently an Iraqi study showed that oral zinc sulfate had an effective therapeutic and prophylactic role in management of RAS [26].

Isotretinoin is a synthetic vitamin A derivative that has been widely used to treat many dermatological diseases like acne vulgaris, ichthyosis and Darier's disease [27] through its multiple effects like increasing turnover and differentiation of epithelial cells, immunomodulator action, anti-inflammatory effect [28], inhibition of Toll like receptors 2 (TLR2) [29], and antiestrogen effect [30] Most recently, Isotretinoin had been used in treatment of Behcet's disease and was found to be effective in all the mucocutaneous manifestations including pathergy test [31].

So, the aim of the present work is to evaluate the effectiveness of isotretinoin in the treatment of RAS.

2. Patients and Methods

This single-blind controlled therapeutic study in which thirty patients with RAS who attended who attended Behcet's disease clinic Department of Dermatology-Baghdad Teaching Hospital, Medical City; Baghdad; Iraq; were enrolled in this work during the period February 2011-January 2012.

Detailed history was taken regarding: age, gender, occupation. History of the disease, recurrence rate, duration, symptoms associated with the ulceration, interference with the swallowing, drinking or eating and aggravating factors including food type, stress and trauma were evaluated. Also, the search about their general health, previous medical history, drug history, cigarette smoking and history of the same condition or other illness in the family were carried out. All patients were subjected to full examination detecting the shape, size, number and site of the lesions.

Investigations were done for all patients like Pathergy test using 24 gauge needle, HLA typing for HLAB51, B5 and HLAB27, complete blood picture, ESR, CRP, renal function test, liver function test to exclude Behcet's disease and other internal causes of oral ulcerations. All patients were examined by ophthalmologists in the same hospital to exclude findings suggestive for Behcet's disease.

The diagnosis of RAS was based on history, clinical examination and exclusion of other causes of oral ulceration.

Inclusion criteria were patients stopped their treatment three months before the start of the study, most cases had at least one attack per month.

Also, patients were selected only those who we trust their follow up during the course of therapy. While exclusion criteria were pregnant and nursing mothers, patients with lipid problems and cardiovascular diseases.

Formal consent was taken from each patient after full explanation about: the goal of the present study before using the remedy, the nature of the disease, course its complications, the methods of treatment, duration, cost, side effects of therapies and duration of follow up, prognosis. After full explanation regarding isotretinoin including: method of application, duration of therapy, side effects and follow up concentrating on documentation of any apparent oral ulceration, its size, location, number and associated symptoms. Patients were instructed not to stop study treatment during the study, and to consult for any cutaneous or systemic side effects that might develop. Also, the ethical approval was performed by the scientific committee of the Scientific Council of Dermatology & Venereology Iraqi Board for Medical Specializations.

Also, because of its teratogenic effect, this drug should not be used in ladies should not become pregnant for 2 months after stopping it. Patients were instructed to use isotretinoin capsules (Retane capsules from Asia Company, Syria) orally once daily for three months to be seen on day fourteen first and then on each month to be assessed by the oral clinical manifestation index (OCMI) which is the summation of multiple scoring numbers of the clinical status of the conditions of RAS (**Table 1**). Then, isotretinoin capsules were stopped and placebo therapy in a form of glucose capsules was given for further 3 months.

Table 1. Oral clinical manifestation index (OCMI) type score.

Type	Score
Minor ulcer	1
Major ulcer	2
Herpetiform ulcer	3
Number of ulcers/attack	
1 - 3	1
4 - 6	2
7 - 9	3
9 - 12	4
More than 12	5
Duration of the attack	
1 - 4 days	1
5 - 8 days	2
9 - 12 days	3
More than 12 days	4
Frequency (attack/date)	
0 - 2 weeks	5
3 - 4 weeks	4
5 - 6 weeks	3
7 - 8 weeks	2
More than 8 weeks	1
Associated symptoms	
Uncomfortable	1
Painful but not interfere with eating or swallowing	2
Interfere with solid feeding	3
Interfere with liquid feeding	4

The data were analyzed, and the student test was used to compare the means of OCMI before therapy and at Day 14, one month, two months, three months, four months, five months and six months of therapy.

The response was estimated by calculating the reduction in the means of OCMI at Day 14, one month, two months, three months, four months, five months and six months of therapy from the baseline of mean of OCMI before treatment. P value of less than 0.05 was considered to be statistically significant.

3. Results

Thirty patients were included in this study; 17 males (56.7%) and 13 females (43.3%), with male to female ratio was 1.3:1. Their ages ranged between 12 - 60 years with a mean ± SD of 35.4 ± 11.97872 years.

OCMI before treatment was ranged from 7 - 17 with mean ± SD of (13.133 ± 2.556). OCMI was started to decrease after two weeks of therapy but the decrease was statistically not significant (P > 0.05). After one month, this decrease was statistically significant (P = 0.023) and continued to decrease. At the end of three months, the decrease was statistically highly significant (P < 0.001). Although Isotretinoin was stopped, the effect continued till the end of fifth month and was also statistically significant (P = 0.046). Also at the end of the six months there was a slight continued effect although was not statistically significant (P > 0.05).

After placebo treatment, patients showed no improvement but the effect of Isotretinoin continued with gradual increase in the mean of OCMI until reached a level which was almost comparable to baseline data (**Table 2**).

4. Discussion

RAS is a major health problem but its etiopathogenesis is not well elucidated [3].

There are many therapies have been used to treat RAS but none of them is curable [29] and there is a high relapse rate when these therapies are stopped. Still some patients might get remission either as a result of therapy or spontaneously [26].

Dapsone and oral zinc sulfate have been used successfully in treatment of RAS through double blind therapeutic study and both of them showed effective therapeutic and prophylactic actions in controlling the disease [26].

The present work using oral Isotretinoin showed a new effective therapy in controlling RAS. The effect of this drug started after 14 days and became statistically significant after one month (P = 0.023) then the OCMI continued to decrease and became highly significant at the end of three months of therapy (P < 0.001). When the treatment was stopped and placebo started at the end of three months, the effectiveness of Isotretinoin continued and remained highly significant (P < 0.001) at the end of four months and significant at the end of fifth month (P = 0.046).

This could be explained as retinoids in general are stored in fatty tissue for longer time after stopping the therapy [32]-[34]. Acitretin could be also tried in treatment of oral aphthosis and probably might has a similar effect to isotretinoin and preferably might have longer prophylactic effect as it may stay in the body for about 2 years after stopping therapy [35].

These results are closely similar and comparable to the effectiveness of isotretinoin in controlling the oral manifestations in patient with Behcet's disease [31].

Accordingly, Isotretinoin had a prophylactic action in addition to its therapeutic effect. These results are very comparable to the results of dapsone and oral zinc sulfate although isotretinoin was less effective than zinc sulfate and dapsone (**Table 3**).

Table 2. Effects of the drug on OCMI.

		Isotretinoin therapy					Placebo therapy	
	Before therapy	Day 14	One month	Two months	Three months	Four months	Five months	Six months
Mean	13.133	10.567	7.6	5.5667	4.0667	5.9333	8.2	10.667
SD	2.556	3.9277	4.9522	5.3219	4.2421	4.7119	4.3263	3.8714
P-value		0.103 NS	0.023 S	P < 0.001 HS	P < 0.001 HS	P < 0.001 HS	0.046 S	0.107 NS

Table 3. Comparison between effects of zinc sulfate, dapsone and isotretinoin OCMI score.

OCMI score	Zinc sulfate	Reduction in mean	Dapsone	Reduction in mean	Isotretinoin	Reduction in mean	P-value
At day 0	11.93		10.87		13.133		
At 2 weeks	6.07	5.86	3.73	7.14	10.567	2.566	0.034 S
At one month	1.73	10.2	4.40	6.47	7.6	5.533	0.039 S
At 2 months	2.80	9.13	4.27	6.6	5.5667	7.566	0.089 NS
At 3 months	0.93	11	2.80	8.07	4.0667	9.066	0.048

The mechanism of action of isotretinoin in controlling RAS is difficult to be explained but it might work through its multiple actions like increasing differentiation of epithelial cells, antiinflammatory effect, immuno-modulator effect [28], Tolllike receptors 2 (TLR2) [29] and antiestrogenic effect [30].

The present study showed that isotretinoin is an effective therapy but unfortunately it might be associated with side effects like dryness of the lip, mucosa, skin and eye [32]. Also because of its teratogenic effect [32], this drug should not be used in pregnant and ladies should not become pregnant for 2 months after stopping it. But when the patient gets better, the dose of therapy could be minimized to reduce these side effects. Hence isotretinoin could be used either alone in cases failed to respond to other therapies or as a combined therapy with others like dapsone and zinc sulfate especially in difficult refractory cases.

5. Conclusion

To the best of our knowledge, this is the first study that has been carried out using isotretinoin in treatment of RAS. Isotretinoin is an effective new therapy for RAS either alone in cases failed to respond to other therapies or as a combined therapy with other drugs. Other retinoids like acitretin will be tried in management of oral aphthosis and Behcet disease by further studies which will be published.

Disclosure

This study was an independent study and not funded by any drug companies.

References

[1] Cawson, R.A., Odell, E.W. and Porter, S.R. (2002) Cawson's Essentials of Oral Pathology and Oral Medicine. 7th Edition, Churchill Livingstone, New York.

[2] Natah, S.S., Konttinen, Y.T., Enattah, N.S., Ashammakhi, N., Sharkey, K.A. and Hayrinen Immonen, R. (2004) Recurrent Aphthou Ulcers Today: A Review of the Growing Knowledge. *International Journal of Oral and Maxillofacial Surgery*, **33**, 221-234. http://dx.doi.org/10.1006/ijom.2002.0446

[3] Rivera Hidalgo, F., Shulman, J.D. and Beach, M.M. (2004) The Association of Tobacco and Other Factors with Recurrent Aphthous Stomatitis in an US Adult Population. *Oral Diseases*, **10**, 335-345. http://dx.doi.org/10.1111/j.1601-0825.2004.01049.x

[4] Katz, J., Chaushu, G. and Peretz, B. (2001) Recurrent Oral Ulcerations Associated with Recurrent Herpes Labialis—Two Distinct Entities? *Community Dentistry and Oral Epidemiology*, **29**, 260-263. http://dx.doi.org/10.1034/j.1600-0528.2001.290404.x

[5] Sun, A., Chia, J.S. and Chiang, C.P. (2002) Increased Proliferative Response of Peripheral Blood Mononuclear Cells and T Cells to *Streptococcus mutans* and Glucosyltransferase D Antigens in the Exacerbation Stage of Recurrent Aphthous Ulcerations. *Journal of the Formosan Medical Association*, **101**, 560-566.

[6] Fawaz, A. (2003) Cytological Cytogenetic and Biochemical Analysis of Behcet's Disease and Recurrent Aphthous Stomatitis. A Thesis Submitted to the College of Dentistry University of Baghdad in Partial Fulfillment of the Requirements for the Degree of Doctor of Philosophy in Oral Medicine, 44-55.

[7] Pedersen, A. and Horsleth, A. (1993) Recurrent Aphthous Ulceration: A Possible Clinical Manifestation of Reaction of Varicella Zoster of Cytomegalovirus Infection. *Journal of Oral Pathology & Medicine*, **22**, 64-68.

[8]   Jurge, S., Kuffer, R., Scully, C. and Porter, S.R. (2006) Mucosal Disease Series. Number VI. Recurrent Aphthous Sto-matitis. *Oral Diseases*, **12**, 1-21. http://dx.doi.org/10.1111/j.1601-0825.2005.01143.x

[9]   Buno, I.J., Huff, J.C. and Weston, W.L. (1998) Elevated Levels of Interferon Gamma, Tumor Necrosis Factor α, Inter-leukin 2, 4, and 5, but Not Interleukin 10, Are Present in Recurrent Aphthous Stomatitis. *Archives of Dermatology*, **134**, 827-831. http://dx.doi.org/10.1001/archderm.134.7.827

[10] Bazrafshani, M.R., Hajeer, A.H., Ollier, W.E. and Thornhill, M.H. (2002) IL1B and IL6 Gene Polymorphisms Encode Significant Risk for the Development of Recurrent Aphthous Stomatitis (RAS). *Genes & Immunity*, **3**, 302-305.

[11] Kozlak, S.T., Walsh, S.J. and Lalla, R.V. (2010) Reduced Dietary Intake of Vitamin B12 and Folate in Patients with Recurrent Aphthous Stomatitis. *Journal of Oral Pathology & Medicine*, **39**, 420-423.

[12] Jacobson, J.M., Greenspan, J.S., Spritzler, J., Ketter, N., Fahey, J.L. and Jackson, J.B. (1997) Thalidomide for the Treatment of Oral Aphthous Ulcers in Patients with Human Immunodeficiency Virus Infection. National Institutes of Allergy and Infectious Diseases AIDS Clinical Trials Group. *The New England Journal of Medicine*, **336**, 1487-1493. http://dx.doi.org/10.1056/NEJM199705223362103

[13] Demiroglu, H. and Dunder, S. (1997) Behcet's Disease and Chronic Neutropenia. *Scandinavian Journal of Rheuma-tology*, **26**, 130-132. http://dx.doi.org/10.3109/03009749709115832

[14] Burns, D.A. and Breathnach, S.M. (2004) Recurrent Aphthous Stomatitis. In: Cox, N. and Griffiths, C., Eds., *Rook's Textbook of Dermatology*, Blackwell Publishing, Oxford, 43-46. http://dx.doi.org/10.1002/9780470750520

[15] Barrons, R.W. (2001) Treatment Strategies for Recurrent Oral Aphthous Ulcers. *American Journal of Health-System Pharmacy*, **58**, 41-50.

[16] William, D.J., Timothy, G.B. and Dirk, M.E. (2006) Recurrent Aphthous Stomatitis. Andrew's Disease of the Skin: Clinical Dermatology. 10th Edition, WB Saunders Company, Philadelphia, 810-812.

[17] Sharquie, K.E. and Najim, R.A. (2001) Honey as a New Skin Tissue Preservative. *Pan Arab League of Dermatologists*, **12**, 49-54.

[18] Sharquie, K.E., Al Tammimi, S.M., Al Mashhadani, S., Hayani, R.K. and Al-Nuaimi, A.A. (2006) Lactic Acid 5 Per-cent Mouthwash Is an Effective Mode of Therapy in Treatment of Recurrent Aphthous Stomatitis. *Dermatology Online Journal*, **12**, 2.

[19] Abdoli, S., Hadi, N., Ali, A., Waiz, M. and Hayani, R. (2004) A Comparative Study in the Effect of Nigella Sativa Oil, Eugenol and Betamethasone in the Treatment of Recurrent Oral Ulcerations. *Clinical and Experimental Rheumatology Journal*, **22**, 120.

[20] Al Na'mah, Z.M., Carson, R. and Thanoon, I.A. (2009) Dexamucobase: A Novel Treatment for Oral Aphthous Ulcera-tion. *Quintessence International*, **40**, 399-404.

[21] Babaee, N., Mansourian, A., Momen Heravi, F., Moghadamnia, A. and Momen Beitollahi, J. (2010) The Efficacy of a Paste Containing *Myrtus communis* (Myrtle) in the Management of Recurrent Aphthous Stomatitis: A Randomized Controlled Trial. *Clinical Oral Investigations*, **14**, 65-70. http://dx.doi.org/10.1007/s00784-009-0267-3

[22] Fontes, V., Machet, L., Huttenberger, B., Lorette, G. and Vaillant, L. (2002) Recurrent Aphthous Stomatitis: Treat-ment with Colchicines. An Open Trial of 54 Cases. *Annales de Dermatologie et de Venereologie*, **129**, 1365-1369.

[23] Scully, C. (2006) Clinical Practice. Aphthous Ulceration. *The New England Journal of Medicine*, **355**, 165-172. http://dx.doi.org/10.1056/NEJMcp054630

[24] Sharquie, K.E. and Hayani, R.K. (2005) BCG as a New Therapeutic and Prophylactic Agent in Patients with Severe Oral Aphthosis. *Clinical and Experimental Rheumatology Journal*, **23**, 914.

[25] Sfikakis, P.P., Markomichelakis, N., Alpsoy, E., *et al.* (2007) Anti-TNF Therapy in the Management of Behcet's Dis-ease: Review and Basis for Recommendations. *Rheumatology (Oxford)*, **46**, 736-741.

[26] Sharquie, K.E., Najim, R.A., Al Hayani, R.K., Al Nuaimi, A.A. and Maroof, D.M. (2008) The Therapeutic and Proph-ylactic Role of Oral Zinc Sulfate in Treatment of Recurrent Aphthous Stomatitis in Comparison with Dapsone. *Saudi Medical Journal*, **29**, 734-738.

[27] Kontaxakis, V.P., Skourides, D., Ferentinos, P., Havaki-Kontaxaki, B.J. and Papadimitriou, G.N. (2009) Isotretinoin and Psychopathology: A Review. *Annals of General Psychiatry*, **8**, 2. http://dx.doi.org/10.1186/1744-859X-8-2

[28] Chandraratna, R.A. (1998) Rational Design of Receptor-Selective Eretinoids. *Journal of the American Academy of Dermatology*, **39**, 124-128.

[29] Fathy, A., Mohamed, R.W., Ismael, N.A. and El Akhras, M.A. (2009) Expression of Toll-Like Receptor 2 on Peripher-al Blood Monocytes of Patients with Inflammatory and Noninflammatory Acne Vulgaris. *Egyptian Journal of Immu-nology*, **16**, 127-134.

[30] Czeczuga Semeniuk, E., Anchim, T., Dzieciol, J., Dabrowska, M. and Wołczyński, S. (2004) Can Transforming Growth

Factor-Beta1 and Retinoids Modify the Activity of Estradiol and Antiestrogens in MCF-7 Breast Cancer Cells? *Acta Biochimica Polonica*, **51**, 733-745.

[31] Sharquie, K.E., Helmi, R.M.A., Noaimi, A.A., Al Hayani, R.K. and Khadom, M.A.A. (2013) The Therapeutic Role of Isotretinoin in the Management of Bahçet Disease: A Single-Blind, Controlled Therapeutic Study. *Journal of Drugs in Dermatology*, **12**, e68-e73.

[32] Malvasi, A., Tinelli, A., Buia, A. and De Luca, G.F. (2009) Possible Long Term Teratogenic Effect of Isotretinoin in Pregnancy. *European Review of Medical and Phamacological Sciences*, **13**, 393-396.

[33] Sampaio, S.P.A. and Rivitti, E.A. (2001) Dermatologia. Artes Médicas, São Paulo.

[34] Soprano, D.R. and Blaner, W.S. (1994) Plasma Delivery of Retinoic Acid to Tissues in the Rat. In: Sporn, M.B., Roberts, A.B. and Goodman, D.S., Eds., *The Retinoids, Biology, Chemistry and Medicine*, 2nd Edition, Raven Press, Ltd., New York, 257-282.

[35] McNamara, P.J., Jewell, R.C., Jensen, B.K., *et al.* (1988) Food Increases the Bioavailability of Acitretin. *The Journal of Clinical Pharmacology*, **28**, 1051-1055.

17

Solid Lipid Nanoparticles (SLN) and Nanostructured Lipid Carriers (NLC): Occlusive Effect and Penetration Enhancement Ability

R. López-García, A. Ganem-Rondero*

División de Estudios de Posgrado (Tecnología Farmacéutica), Facultad de Estudios Superiores Cuautitlán, Universidad Nacional Autónoma de México, Cuautitlán Izcalli, Mexico
Email: mrosario.logar@hotmail.com, *ganemq@hotmail.com

Abstract

Objective: This work compares the occlusive effect and the penetration enhancement ability of solid lipid nanoparticles (SLN) and nanostructured lipid carriers (NLC), through *in vitro* skin. Methods: SLN and NLC were prepared by high shear homogenization and characterized by size, polydispersity index, zeta potential, morphology and physical stability. Occlusive effect was assessed by an *in vitro* test and by measuring TEWL using pig skin. Skin treated with the lipid carriers was visualized by SEM. A penetration test through skin, followed by tape stripping, was carried out using Nile red as a marker. Results: SLN (200 ± 6 nm) and NLC (192 ± 11 nm) were obtained. An occlusion factor of 36% - 39% was observed for both systems, while a reduction in TEWL of 34.3% ± 14.8% and 26.2% ± 6.5% was seen after treatment with SLN and NLC, respectively. SEM images showed a film formed by the lipid carriers, responsible for the occlusion observed. No differences were found between the occlusive effect produced by SLN and NLC in both tests. NLC allowed the penetration of a greater amount of Nile red than SLN: 4.7 ± 1.3 μg and 1.7 ± 0.4 μg, respectively. Conclusion: Both carriers form a film on the skin, providing an occlusive effect with no differences between these two systems. The penetration of a marker (Nile red) into the stratum corneum was quite higher for NLC than for SLN, suggesting an influence of the composition of these particles on their penetration enhancing ability.

Keywords

Solid Lipid Nanoparticles, Nanostructured Lipid Carriers, Occlusive Effect, Transepidermal Water Loss, Skin Penetration

---

*Corresponding author.

1. Introduction

Nanotechnology is a highly useful tool for the design of innovative solutions for many sciences including health and beauty. The understanding and handling of compounds at nanoscale have allowed the development of materials with interesting characteristics to use in cosmetic science as seen in the design of nanoparticles of different materials as carrier systems for cosmetic actives.

Solid lipid nanoparticles (SLN) were developed at the beginning of the 1990's based on the concept of solid particles, emulsions and liposomes. They are produced by exchanging the oil in an emulsion by a solid lipid, resulting in lipid nanoparticles being solid at both room and body temperature [1]. Although SLN possess several advantages, e.g., the use of physiological lipids, the avoidance of organic solvents in the preparation process, protection of sensitive molecules from the environment and controlled release characteristics, some disadvantages have been associated such as particle growth, unpredictable gelation tendency, polymorphic transitions and inherently low incorporation capacities due to the crystalline structure of the solid lipid [2]. The second generation of lipid nanoparticles, nanostructured lipid carriers (NLC) which are prepared by blending solid and liquid lipids leading to amorphous solids, arose to overcome limitations of SLN by introducing a less ordered inner structure [3].

Nanoparticles based on lipid systems are the most common type of nanoparticles studied for topical application [4]. The current focus of the SLN and NLC research is quite related towards topical and dermal application, both in pharmaceutical and cosmetic purposes. However, since NLC represent the latest innovation, several researchers preferred them over SLN as they avoid lipid recrystallization that causes expulsion of active substances as observed with SLN [5]. Nevertheless, both SLN and NLC are widely used for cosmetics, since they show many favorable features such as adhesiveness, occlusion, skin hydration, lubrication, smoothness, emolliency, skin penetration enhancement, modified release, improvement of formulation appearance providing a whitening effect and offering protection of actives against degradation [6]-[8]. These positive features of lipid nanoparticles have led to the market introduction of a number of cosmetic products including numerous actives such as coenzyme Q10, extracts, peptides, oils, fatty acids and sun blockers [9].

The effects of lipid nanoparticles on skin barrier properties have been well established. It has been reported that SLN form an invisible, occlusive film with affinity for the stratum corneum (SC), which ensures drug release for a prolonged period of time, reduces transepidermal water loss and improves skin hydration [1] [10]. Penetration enhancement ability of SLN and NLC has also been studied [11]-[13]. Moreover, even if several papers discuss the effects of SLN and NLC on skin and their performance as carrier systems, the advantages of NLC over SLN have not yet been well established [14]-[17].

The aim of this study was to evaluate and compare the performance of SLN and NLC on the skin barrier properties through the assessment of the occlusive effect they produce and their penetration enhancement ability through SC in order to determine if differences in composition modify the performance of these systems. It is expected that the results obtained contribute to the understanding of these lipid-based carriers and improving their performance as carrier systems for cosmetic actives.

2. Materials and Methods

Glyceryl dibehenate (Compritol® 888 ATO) was a gift from Lyontec (Mexico City). Caprylic capric triglycerides were purchased from Droguería Cosmopolita (Mexico City) and poloxamer 188 (Lutrol® F-68) was obtained from BASF (Germany). Methanol was purchased from J. T. Baker, and Nile Red was obtained from Sigma-Aldrich (USA). Water was obtained from a Milli-Q® system (Millipore®, Germany). Porcine skin was obtained from pig ears collected from a local slaughterhouse immediately post-mortem and and prior to steam cleaning (the procedure followed the guidelines of The Mexican Official Standard NOM—194-SSA1-2004, related to the sanitary specifications for abbatoirs). Pig ears with no injuries and with uniform coloration were selected and stored at –20˚C until required.

2.1. SLN and NLC Preparation

SLN (composed of glyceryl dibehenate) and NLC (including glyceryl dibehenate/caprylic capric triglycerides 90:10) were prepared by high shear homogenization using an Ultra Turrax® T18 Basic (IKA®, Germany). Briefly, a hot 2.5% poloxamer 188 solution (90˚C) was added to the melted lipid phase (solid lipid or lipids blend). This mixture was emulsified at 20,000 rpm for 5 min at 90˚C. The resultant emulsion was cooled down in a cold water bath (7°C) to room temperature in order to obtain nanoparticles.

2.2. SLN and NLC Characterization

Particle size, polydispersity index (PI) and zeta potential were determined by photon correlation spectroscopy using a Malvern Zetasizer® Nano-ZS90 (Malvern Instruments, USA). For size and PI, the samples were diluted with distilled water to a proper mean count rate prior to the measurements, which were performed at a 90° scattering angle at 25°C (n = 5). To measure zeta potential, samples were diluted with deionized water and the measurements were done considering viscosity, refraction index and dielectric constant of water at 25°C (n = 5). The morphology of the lipid nanoparticles was evaluated by means of scanning electron microscopy (SEM) using a JEOL JSM-25SII Scanning microscope (JEOL Tokyo, Japan). To prepare the sample, nanoparticle aqueous dispersion was left to dry over a coverslip and covered with gold.

2.3. SLN and NLC Stability

SLN and NLC formulations were stored in glass vials at 5°C, 25°C and 40°C. Particle size, PI and zeta potential were measured at 8, 15, 30, 60 and 90 days (n = 3), as previously described.

2.4. Test of *in Vitro* Occlusive Effect

Occlusive effect of SLN and NLC was determined using a modified *in vitro* occlusion test [18]. Briefly, bakers were filled with 40 mL of water and covered with Whatman® filter paper grade 42 (Sigma-Aldrich, USA). A sample of SLN or NLC (300 µL, 10% w/v lipid content) was spread on the filter surface, using water as reference, instead lipid carriers. Bakers were stored at 32°C to mimic the temperature of skin surface and weighted at 0, 6, 24 and 48 h to calculate water evaporation through the filter paper in terms of water loss. The occlusion factor F was calculated at 6, 24 and 48 h using Equation (1) [18].

$$F = \frac{R-S}{R} \times 100 \tag{1}$$

where R = reference water loss and S = sample water loss. An $F = 0$ means no occlusive effect while an $F = 100$ means maximum occlusiveness. At the end of the experiment, filter paper was observed by scanning electron microscopy (SEM), using a JSM-25-SII scanning electron microscope (JEOL, Tokyo, Japan) in order to visualize film formation.

2.5. Effect of SLN and NLC on the TEWL

Transepidermal water loss (TEWL) is the outward diffusion of water through skin [19]. Skin was excised from pig ears. Skin slides (700 µm thickness) were obtained using an Electric Dermatome (Zimmer®, USA). Impaired skin was obtained removing the SC by means of tape stripping (20 tapes). Both impaired and intact pig skin samples were mounted on the receptor compartment of a Franz cell filled with phosphate buffer solution pH 7.4 and basal TEWL value was recorded with a Tewameter® TM 210 (Courage & Khazaka, Germany). A volume of 50 µL (10% w/v) of SLN or NLC dispersion was spread on the skin surface and TEWL was measured 2 h later. The occlusive effect was determined by the reduction of the TEWL value using Equation (2):

$$\%\text{TEWL reduction} = \frac{B-T}{B} \times 100 \tag{2}$$

where B is the basal TEWL value and T is the TEWL value after lipid carrier treatment. SEM was used to visualize film formation on the skin. Pig skin was fixed, dehydrated and coated with gold previous observation under the microscope (JEOL JSM-25-SII, JEOL, Tokyo, Japan).

2.6. Penetration Test through Pig Skin

Penetration test through the SC of pig skin was carried out using SLN and NLC containing Nile red as a marker. Nile red-loaded SLN and NLC (0.005% w/w) were prepared as described before, incorporating the dye in the melted lipid phase. Skin excised from pig ears was mounted in Franz diffusion cells containing phosphate buffer pH 7.4 as receptor solution, and the surface of the skin was treated with 1 mL sample of Nile red-loaded SLN or

NLC dispersion. The Franz diffusion cells were kept in a water bath at 37°C and, after 2 h contact, the remaining formulation was removed and tape stripping was performed on the skin. Fifteen tapes (Scotch® packaging tape) of 2 × 2 cm were used, weighting each tape before and after skin application. Nile red was extracted from the tapes, stirring with a volume of methanol during 24 h. Tapes 1 to 5 were extracted individually and subsequent tapes were extracted in clusters (6 - 10 and 11 - 15). The extracts were filtered and Nile red was quantified by spectrophotometry UV/Vis (λ = 555 nm) (Varian Cary® 50 UV-Vis spectrophotometer, Australia). Penetration distance was determined from tapes weight data, using Equation (3):

$$\text{Penetration distance} = \frac{TW_f - TW_0}{SCD \times A} \tag{3}$$

where TWf is the tape weight after the stripping, TW_0 is the tape weight before the stripping, SCD is the SC density considered as 1 g cm^3 and A is the tape area.

2.7. Statistical Analysis

The statistical analysis was performed with $p < 0.05$ as level of significance (STATGRAPHICS® Centurion XVI).

3. Results and Discussion

3.1. Lipid Nanoparticle Characterization

Although high pressure homogenization (HPH) is the most used technique for lipid nanoparticle preparation [9], high shear rate homogenization is a feasible technique to prepare lipid nanoparticles at laboratory scale since it is an easy handle technique, that requires low cost equipment compared to HPH, and that allows to obtain particles of nanometric size (~200 nm) [20]. **Table 1** shows the results of SLN and NLC characterization.

No differences in particle size between SLN and NLC ($p > 0.05$) were found. SLN and NLC of similar particle size were desirable so that this variable was not a factor directly influencing the results observed on the skin (occlusive effect and penetration enhancement ability). PI indicates the width of the particle size distribution. Theoretically, monodisperse distributions are described as PI = 0, however, PI < 0.2 is considered as narrow size distribution [16]. PI > 0.2 for the lipid nanoparticles prepared could be due to the preparation method used, giving a wider size distribution compared to HPH [20]. Zeta potential is a parameter used to predict stability of colloidal suspensions throughout storage time. A zeta potential higher than ±30 mV may assure good physical stability, being optimal when zeta potential is close to ±60 mV [21]. It is well known that zeta potential depends on the nature of the particles and the medium composition. For lipid nanoparticles, the molecular arrangement of lipids in the external layer of nanoparticles and its interaction with stabilizers are determinant. For the lipid nanoparticles prepared, poloxamer 188 was used as stabilizer, and due to its non-ionic nature, this molecule does not contribute with additional charges to zeta potential. Furthermore, the lipid that composes SLN is in fact a blend of acylglycerols (**Figure 1(a)**): glyceryl tribehenate (28% - 32%), glyceryl dibehenate (52% - 54%) and glyceryl monobehenate (12% - 18%) [22], all of them being glycerol esters of long-chain-length fatty acids (C22) so that they provide neither charge nor polarity that contributes to zeta potential. On the other hand, NLC are made of the same lipid blend but including a certain amount of caprylic/capric triglyceride, which is a diacylglycerol of medium-chain-length fatty acids (**Figure 1(b)**). In this case, due to the non-esterified hydroxyl group of the glycerol and the length of the fatty acids, this molecule exhibits certain polarity that contributes to zeta potential, which explains the higher value compared to SLN. A similar result was observed by Teeranachaideekul et al. [18] for nanoparticles composed of cetyl palmitate and medium-chain-length triglycerides. The authors explain that it might be due to the accumulation of oil at the surface of NLC. Being the melting point of the solid lipid higher than that of the oil, when preparing NLC, the solid lipid recrystallizes first, holding a portion of the oil within the solid lipid matrix. Subsequently, the excess of oil remains in the outer shell of nanoparticles, then the oil contributes largely to zeta potential. Despite this difference in zeta potential between SLN and NLC, both values are under the desired ±30 mV, which may indicate physical stability issues during storage. Nevertheless, poloxamer 188 stabilizes lipid nanoparticles because of the steric effect it produces which avoids coalescence of the particles [21]. Such steric effect is possible due to the structure and conformation of poloxamer. Poloxamer 188 is a block copolymer of ethylene

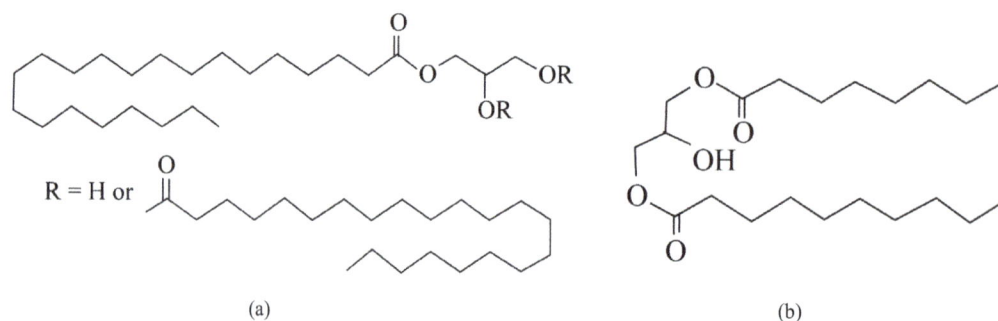

| (a) | (b) |

Figure 1. Chemical structure of (a) glyceryl dibehenate as a mix of glyceryl tribehenate (28% - 32%), glyceryl dibehenate (52% - 54%) and glyceryl monobehenate (12% - 18%); and (b) caprylic capric triglyceride.

Table 1. Particle size, PI and zeta potential of SLN and NLC prepared by high shear homogenization. Results are displayed as mean ± SD (n = 5).

	Particle size (nm)	PI	Zeta potential (mV)
SLN	200 ± 6	0.436 ± 0.022	−7.5 ± 0.6
NLC (90:10)[1]	192 ± 11	0.311 ± 0.014	−11.1 ± 0.8

[1]Glyceryl dibehenate: caprylic capric triglycerides.

oxide and propylene oxide with the formula $HO(C_2H_4O)_{80}(C_3H_6O)_{27}(C_2H_4O)_{80}H$. The polyoxyethylene segments are hydrophilic and the polyoxypropylene segment is hydrophobic [22], so this last part of the molecule is located on the lipid nanoparticle surface whereas the long hydrophilic polymer chains are oriented towards the medium. Regarding the morphology of the lipid nanoparticles, **Figure 2** shows SEM images for SLN and NLC. Both systems exhibit similar characteristics since they are assembled out of the same main lipid and were prepared under the same conditions. Particles appear as spherical or almost spherical structures of approximately 200 nm, which agrees with the results obtained from the photon correlation spectroscopy technique.

3.2. SLN and NLC Stability

Physical stability of SLN and NLC was assessed measuring particle size, PI and zeta potential to determine whether there are changes or not, depending on the storage temperature and storage time. Results showed no significant changes in either PI or zeta potential through storage time under different storage conditions (data not shown). Conversely, both storage time and temperature have effect on the particle size of the lipid carriers (**Figure 3**). For SLN, particle size increased at 90 days and 40°C, whereas NLC size increased at 90 days for both 25 and 40°C (ANOVA test showed significant differences between 40°C and the other two temperatures for SLN and between 5°C and the other two temperatures for NLC). Hence, storage at 5°C seems to preserve the particle size more effectively for both SLN and NLC up to 90 days.

3.3. Test of *in Vitro* Occlusive Effect

Results of *in vitro* occlusive effect (**Figure 4**) showed that occlusion factor (Equation (1)) took values between 35.9 and 38.9 throughout the test for SLN and NLC. Although no statistical difference was found between SLN and NLC, differences between 6 h and the other two times were found, which might be due to the formation of a film on the filter paper at the beginning of the test. When a nanoparticle suspension is applied onto the skin, lipid nanoparticles tend to fusion forming a film on the skin [23], so, it is expected that this effect occurs on the filter paper as well. The formation of this nanoparticle film was confirmed by scanning electron microscopy. **Figure 5** shows the presence and characteristics of the film formed with the lipid carriers: fibers that compose filter paper (without treatment) are shown in **Figure 5(a)**, whereas **Figure 5(b)** and **Figure 5(c)** show these fibers covered by the lipid carriers. This film is thought to be responsible for the occlusive effect observed in the test, as it acts like a barrier that avoids water vapor to escape through the filter paper. As shown, the films formed by both SLN and NLC are alike between each other. It has been demonstrated previously that the degree

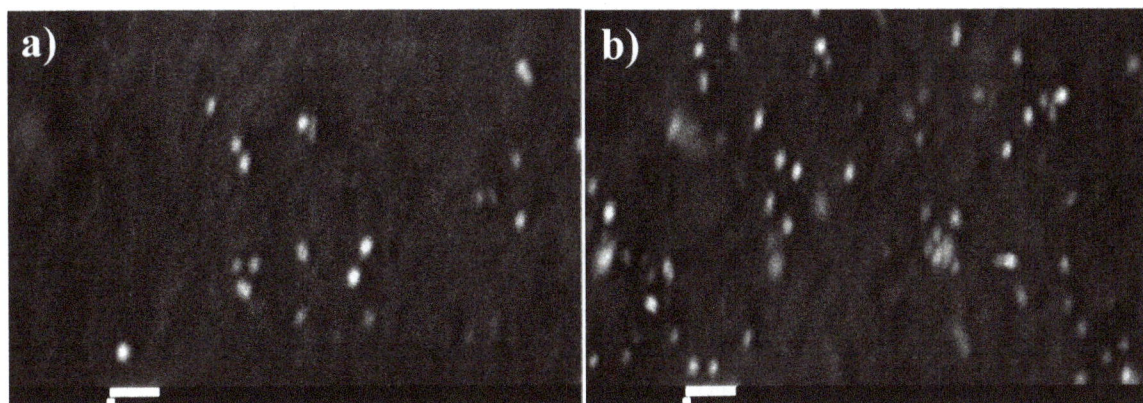

Figure 2. SEM images of a) SLN and b) NLC. The bar at the bottom equals 1 µm (10,000×).

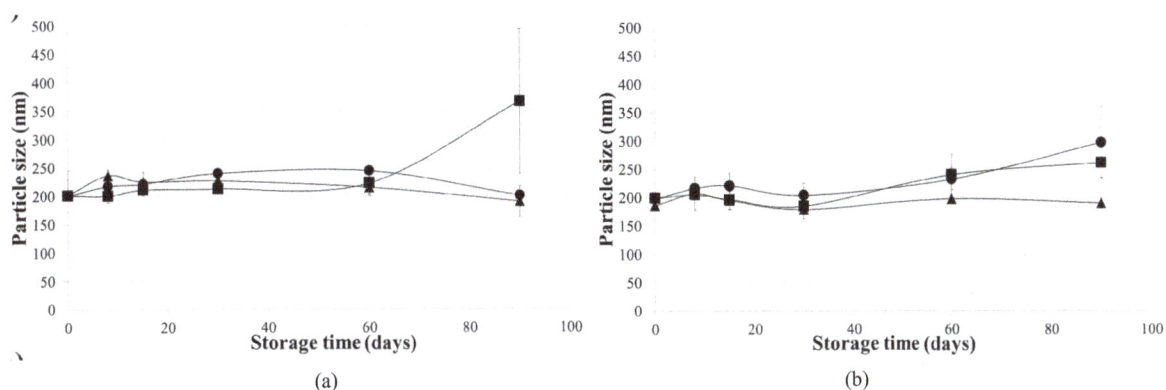

Figure 3. Lipid nanoparticle stability at different temperatures: (▲) 5˚C, (●) 25˚C, (■) 40˚C. Particle size of (a) SLN and (b) NLC plotted as a function of time (0, 8, 15, 30, 60 and 90 days). Values are plotted as mean (n = 3) and the bars correspond to SD. Significant differences were found between 40˚C and the other two temperatures for SLN and between 5˚C and the other two temperatures (NLC).

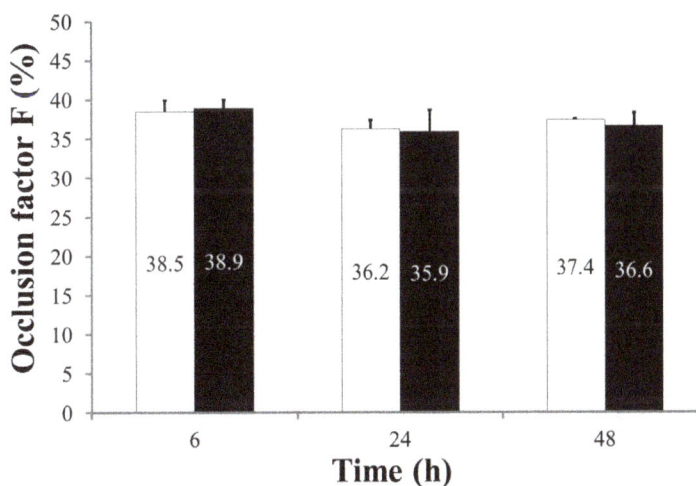

Figure 4. Occlusion factor (F) for SLN (□) and NLC (■) at 6, 24 and 48 h. Data is given as the mean value and the bars correspond to SD.

of occlusion of these films depends on the particle size [24], therefore, as the size of SLN and NLC are very close, it is clear that the inclusion of oil for preparing NLC does not have effect either on the film formation or on the occlusive effect.

3.4. Effect of SLN and NLC on the TEWL

In order to evaluate the effect of SLN and NLC on the TEWL value, reduction of this parameter as percentage (Equation (2)) is shown in **Figure 6**. A significant reduction in TEWL of intact skin was observed for SLN and NLC respectively, without statistical difference between these systems (p > 0.05). Such effect is due to the occlusive effect of lipid carriers as result of film formation on the skin. The film formed at the surface of pig skin was observed by SEM. **Figure 7(a)** shows intact skin without treatment, where the microrelief lines as well

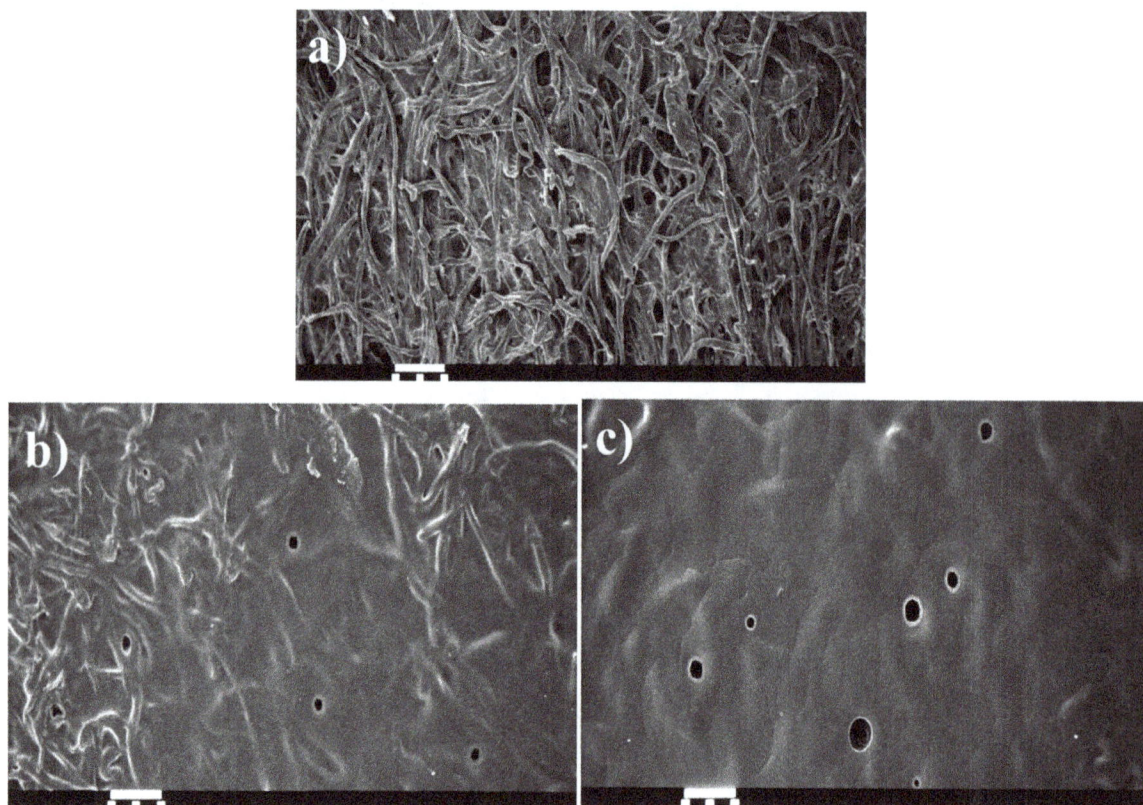

Figure 5. SEM images showing filter paper: a) without lipid nanoparticles; b) with SLN; c) with NLC. Bar at the bottom equals 100 μm (100×).

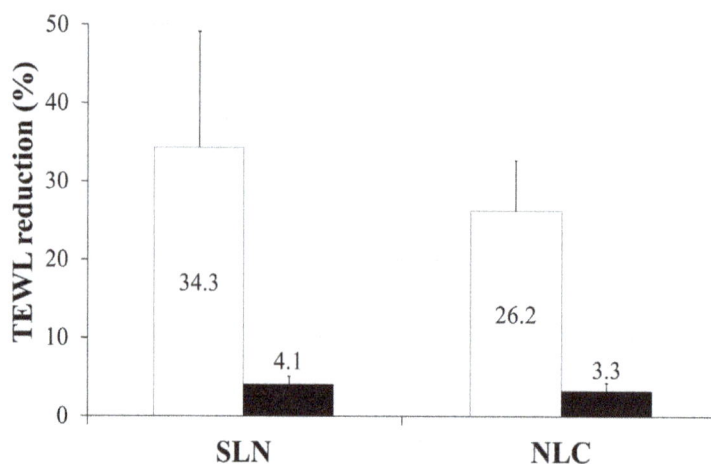

Figure 6. Reduction of the TEWL after treatment with SLN and NLC in intact (☐) and impaired skin (■). Values are plotted as mean (n = 6) and the bars correspond to SD.

as hairs are clearly seen. On the contrary, in **Figure 7(b)** and **Figure 7(c)**, which correspond to intact skin treated with SLN and NLC respectively, microrelief lines and some parts of hair remain under the film formed by the carriers. In the case of impaired skin, carriers did not have a significant effect on the TEWL ($p > 0.05$). Due to stripping of SC the high humidity on the skin surface prevents film formation, since lipid carrier suspensions applied on the skin have to lose their own humidity in order to form the film. Jenning *et al.* [25] studied water loss from SLN, by applying lipid nanoparticles on a glass surface and measuring water loss. They determined that formulation lost their own water almost completely within 1 h. In the present work, even 2 h after applying formulations, the film was not formed on the stripped-skin surface and therefore, a reduction in TEWL was not detected.

3.5. Penetration Test through Pig Skin

Tape stripping is considered a useful non-invasive technique that when coupled with other techniques, it can provide information about the transport of substances through the SC [11]. In this work, tape stripping was used to determine the amount as well as the penetration depth (Equation (3)) through the SC of Nile red included in both SLN and NLC. Lipid nanoparticles are unable to penetrate through human skin because of their size, but

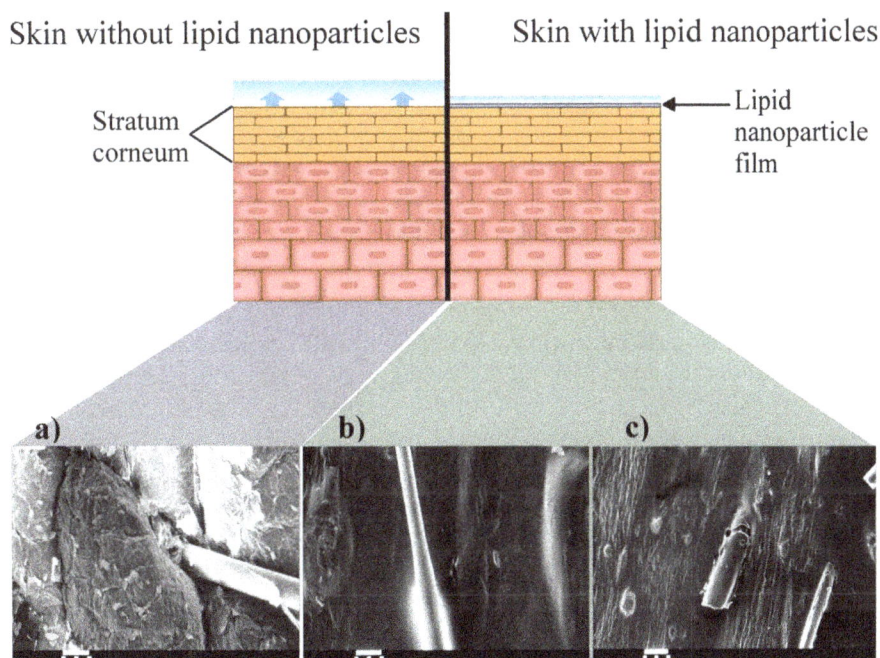

Figure 7. SEM images showing intact pig skin: a) without lipid nanoparticles; b) with SLN; c) with NLC. Bar at the bottom equals 100 μm (100×).

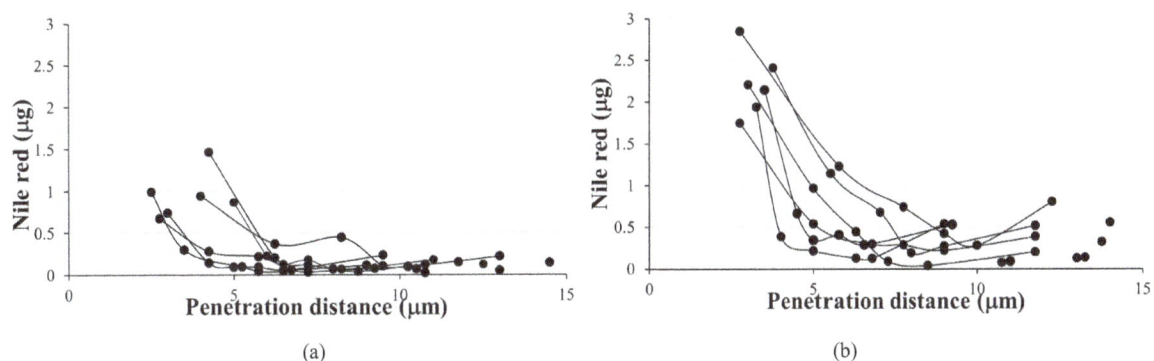

Figure 8. Penetration profile of Nile red throughout the stratum corneum. The graph shows the amount of Nile red versus penetration distance for a) SLN and b) NLC (n = 6).

they can help actives to reach deeper skin layers due to the interaction of nanoparticle lipids with the extracellular lipid matrix of the skin. **Figure 8** shows the penetration profile of Nile red included in both SLN and NLC, being NLC the system that favors the penetration of a greater amount of Nile red. At a distance of 12.2 ± 1.5 µm (SLN) and 12.6 ± 1.4 µm (NLC), the total amount of Nile red penetrated was 1.7 ± 0.4 µg and 4.7 ± 1.3 µg, respectively. This means that, even if a similar occlusive effect was found for both systems, the amount of Nile red penetrated was 2.7 fold higher for the NLC. This fact suggests that lipid nanocarrier composition affects the ability to enhance penetration of molecules through the SC, due to differences in the interaction of lipids with skin components. It has been reported that NLC have the ability to get into deeper layers of the SC. Penetration through pig skin of flufenamic acid (a model drug) included in SLN and NLC, was monitored using tape stripping. Researchers found that NLC showed the deepest skin penetration [12]. In other study, the penetration enhancement ability of lipid nanoparticles was related to the solubility parameter (SP) of lipids [26]. SP is useful to predict the release and skin penetration of any molecule by its interaction with skin lipids. Components with a SP close to that of the skin may have good miscibility with the skin lipids, and thus, can lead to greater penetration. As reported by Jensen *et al.* [26], pig skin SP is estimated in 10, thus lipids with a SP value nearby 10 are expected to exhibit a better interaction with skin lipids and so, the penetration is expected to be greater as well. In this work, SP of glyceryl behenate and caprylic/capric triglyceride was calculated upon the Fedors substituents method [27]. SP values are estimated to be 9.34 for glyceryl behenate and 10.36 for caprylic/capric triglyceride, therefore, the inclusion of this oil may improve the interaction of NLC with skin lipids as well as the penetration enhancement ability through the SC, since triglycerides are more miscible with skin lipids for having a closer value to the skin SP. Moreover, partition of Nile red within NLC contributes to explain its greater penetration. Nile red distribution within NLC was studied by fluorescence spectroscopy [28]. The authors found that the fluid lipid phase of NLC composed of glyceryl behenate and caprylic/capric triglyceride was enriched in Nile red (65% ± 8%). Hence, a better interaction with skin lipids is expected, allowing Nile red to penetrate into deeper SC layers when it is included in NLC.

4. Conclusion

The occlusive effect and penetration enhancement ability of SLN and NLC were studied in order to determine differences between these carrier systems. According to the tests performed, both SLN and NLC produced an occlusive effect of similar magnitude, which is due to the ability of lipid nanoparticles to form a film. No differences were found between film appearance and the occlusive effect degree produced by both SLN and NLC, suggesting that differences in composition did not affect those parameters. In contrast, neither occlusive effect nor film formation was observed in impaired skin, because SC removal led to an increased TEWL and so a higher humidity on the skin surface, which avoided film to form and to produce occlusion. Regarding the penetration enhancement ability of lipid carriers, Nile red included in NLC penetrated into deeper SC layers compared to dye included in SLN. Enhanced penetration is attributed to the influence of particle composition and its interaction with SC components. These findings suggest that NLC may be useful to enhance the penetration of some cosmetic ingredients into deep layers of the stratum corneum.

Acknowledgements

The authors acknowledge funding from CONACYT (129320, 271124) and PAPIIT (IN216313). The authors also thank to Mr. Rodolfo Robles Gómez for the support to obtain microscope images.

References

[1] Müller, R.H., Radteke, M. and Wissing, S.A. (2002) Solid Lipid Nanoparticles (SLN) and Nanostructured Lipid Carriers (NLC) in Cosmetic and Dermatological Preparations. *Advanced Drug Delivery Reviews*, **54**, S131-S155. http://dx.doi.org/10.1016/S0169-409X(02)00118-7

[2] Jores, K., Mehnert, W., Drechsler, M., Bunjes, H., Johann, C. and Mäder, K. (2004) Investigations on the Structure of Solid Lipid Nanoparticles (SLN) and Oil-Loaded Solid Lipid Nanoparticles by Photon Correlation Spectroscopy, Field-Flow Fractionation and Transmission Electron Microscopy. *Journal of Controlled Release*, **95**, 217-227. http://dx.doi.org/10.1016/j.jconrel.2003.11.012

[3] Teeranachaideekul, V., Müller, R.H. and Junyaprasert, V.B. (2007) Encapsulation of Ascorbyl Palmitate in Nanostructured Lipid Carriers (NLC)—Effects of Formulation Parameters on Physicochemical Stability. *International Journal of Pharmaceutics*, **340**, 198-206. http://dx.doi.org/10.1016/j.ijpharm.2007.03.022

[4]   Contri, R.V., Fiel, L.A., Pohlman, A.R., Guterres, S.S. and Beck, R.C.R. (2011) Transport of Substances and Nanoparticles across the Skin and *in Vitro* Models to Evaluate Skin Permeation and/or Penetration. In: Beck, R., Guterres, S. and Pohlman, A., Eds., *Nanocosmetics and Nanomedicines, New Approaches for Skin Care*, Springer, Berlin, 3-35. http://dx.doi.org/10.1007/978-3-642-19792-5_1

[5]   Puglia, C., Damiani, E., Offerta, A., Rizza, L., Tirendi, G.G., Tarico, M.S., Curreri, S., Bonina, F. and Perrotta, R.E. (2014) Evaluation of Nanostructured Lipid Carriers (NLC) and Nanoemulsions as Carriers for UV-Filters: Characterization, *in Vitro* Penetration and Photostability Studies. *European Journal of Pharmaceutical Sciences*, **51**, 211-217. http://dx.doi.org/10.1016/j.ejps.2013.09.023

[6]   Souto, E.B. and Müller, R.H. (2008) Cosmetic Features and Application of Lipid Nanoparticles (SLN®, NLC®). *International Journal of Cosmetic Science*, **30**, 157-165. http://dx.doi.org/10.1111/j.1468-2494.2008.00433.x

[7]   Wissing, S., Lippacher, A. and Müller, R. (2001) Investigations on the Occlusive Properties of Solid Lipid Nanoparticles (SLN). *Journal of Cosmetic Science*, **52**, 313-324.

[8]   Wissing, S. and Müller, R. (2003) The Influence of Solid Lipid Nanoparticles on Skin Hydration and Viscoelasticity— *In Vivo* Study. *European Journal of Pharmaceutics and Biopharmaceutics*, **56**, 67-72. http://dx.doi.org/10.1016/S0939-6411(03)00040-7

[9]   Pardeike, J., Hommoss, A. and Müller, R. (2009) Lipid Nanoparticles (SLN, NLC) in Cosmetic and Pharmaceutical Dermal Products. *International Journal of Pharmaceutics*, **366**, 170-184. http://dx.doi.org/10.1016/j.ijpharm.2008.10.003

[10] Müller, R., Petersen, R., Hommoss, A. and Pardeike, J. (2007) Nanostructured Lipid Carriers (NLC) in Cosmetic Dermal Products. *Advanced Drug Delivery Reviews*, **59**, 522-530. http://dx.doi.org/10.1016/j.addr.2007.04.012

[11] Iannuccelli, V., Coppi, G., Romagnolli, M., Sergi, S. and Leo, E. (2013) *In Vivo* Detection of Lipid-Based Nano- and Microparticles in the Outermost Human Stratum Corneum by EDX Analysis. *International Journal of Pharmaceutics*, **447**, 204-212. http://dx.doi.org/10.1016/j.ijpharm.2013.03.002

[12] Schwarz, J., Weixelbaum, A., Pagitsch, E., Löw, M., Resch, G. and Valenta, C. (2012) Nanocarriers for Dermal Drug Delivery: Influence of Preparation Method, Carrier Type and Rheological Properties. *International Journal of Pharmaceutics*, **437**, 83-88. http://dx.doi.org/10.1016/j.ijpharm.2012.08.003

[13] Montenegro, L., Sinico, C., Castangia, I., Carbone, C. and Puglisi, G. (2012) Idebenone-Loaded Solid Lipid Nanoparticles for Drug Delivery to the Skin: *In Vitro* Evaluation. *International Journal of Pharmaceutics*, **434**, 169-174. http://dx.doi.org/10.1016/j.ijpharm.2012.05.046

[14] Tiwari, R. and Pathak, K. (2011) Nanostructured Lipid Carrier Versus Solid Lipid Nanoparticles of Simvastatin: Comparative Analysis of Characteristics, Pharmacokinetics and Tissue Uptake. *International Journal of Pharmaceutics*, **415**, 232-243. http://dx.doi.org/10.1016/j.ijpharm.2011.05.044

[15] Kovacevic, A., Savic, S., Vuleta, G., Müller, R. and Keck, C. (2011) Polyhydroxy Surfactants for the Formulation of Lipid Nanoparticles (SLN and NLC): Effects on Size, Physical Stability and Particle Matrix Structure. *International Journal of Pharmaceutics*, **406**, 163-172. http://dx.doi.org/10.1016/j.ijpharm.2010.12.036

[16] Das, S., Kiong, W. and Tan, R. (2012) Are Nanostructured Lipid Carriers (NLCs) Better Than Solid Lipid Nanoparticles (SLNs): Development, Characterizations and Comparative Evaluations of Clotrimazole-Loaded SLNs and NLCs? *European Journal of Pharmaceutical Sciences*, **47**, 139-151. http://dx.doi.org/10.1016/j.ejps.2012.05.010

[17] Bose, S. and Michniak-Kohn, B. (2013) Preparation and Characterization of Lipid Based Nanosystems for Topical Delivery of Quercetin. *European Journal of Pharmaceutical Sciences*, **48**, 442-452. http://dx.doi.org/10.1016/j.ejps.2012.12.005

[18] Teeranachaideekul, V., Boonme, P., Souto, E.B., Müller, R.H. and Junyaprasert ,V.B. (2008) Influence of Oil Content on Physicochemical Properties and Skin Distribution of Nile Red-Loaded NLC. *Journal of Controlled Release*, **128**, 134-141. http://dx.doi.org/10.1016/j.jconrel.2008.02.011

[19] Levin, J. and Maibach, H. (2009) The Correlation between Transepidermal Water Loss and Percutaneous Absorption: An Overview. In: Barel, A., Paye, M. and Maibach, H. Eds, *Handbook of Cosmetic Science and Technology*, Informa Healthcare, NewYork, 165-171. http://dx.doi.org/10.1201/9780849359033.ch43

[20] Mehnert, W. and Mäder, K. (2001) Solid Lipid Nanoparticles: Production, Characterization and Applications. *Advanced Drug Delivery Reviews*, **47**, 165-196. http://dx.doi.org/10.1016/S0169-409X(01)00105-3

[21] Garzón, M., Vázquez, M., Villafuerte, L., García, B. and Hernández, A. (2009) Effect of Formulation Components on the Properties of Solid Lipid Nanoparticles. *Revista Mexicana De Ciencias Farmacéuticas*, **2**, 26-40.

[22] Rowe, R., Sheskey, P. and Owen, S. (2006) Handbook of Pharmaceutical Excipients. Pharmaceutical Press, London, 304-305, 535-538.

[23] Wissing, S. and Müller, R. (2001) A Novel Sunscreen System Based on Tocopherol Acetate Incorporated into Solid Lipid Nanoparticles. *International Journal of Cosmetic Science*, **23**, 233-243.

http://dx.doi.org/10.1046/j.1467-2494.2001.00087.x

[24] Wissing, S. and Müller, R. (2003) Cosmetic Applications for Solid Lipid Nanoparticles (SLN). *International Journal of Pharmaceutics*, **254**, 65-68. http://dx.doi.org/10.1016/S0378-5173(02)00684-1

[25] Jenning, V., Gysler, A., Schäfer-Korting, M. and Gohla, S. (2000) Vitamin A Loaded Solid Lipid Nanoparticles for Topical Use: Occlusive Properties and Drug Targeting to the Upper Skin. *European Journal of Pharmaceutics and Biopharmaceutics*, **49**, 211-218. http://dx.doi.org/10.1016/S0939-6411(99)00075-2

[26] Jensen, L., Petersson, K. and Nielsen, H. (2011) *In Vitro* Penetration Properties of Solid Lipid Nanoparticles in Intact and Barrier-Impaired Skin. *European Journal of Pharmaceutics and Biopharmaceutics*, **79**, 68-75. http://dx.doi.org/10.1016/j.ejpb.2011.05.012

[27] James, K.C. (1986) Solubility and Related Properties. Marcel Dekker, New York.

[28] Lombardi, S., Regehly, M., Sivaramakrishnan, R., Mehnert, W., Korting, H.C., Danker, K., Röder, B., Kramer, K.D. and Schäfer-Korting, M. (2005) Lipid Nanoparticles for Skin Penetration Enhancement—Correlation to Drug Localization within the Particle Matrix as Determined by Fluorescence and Parelectric Spectroscopy. *Journal of Controlled Release*, **110**, 151-163. http://dx.doi.org/10.1016/j.jconrel.2005.09.045

18

Infliximab Therapy in Iraqi Patients with Moderate to Severe Psoriasis

Hayder R. Al-Hamamy[1]*, Ihsan A. Al-Turfy[2], Farah S. Abdul-Reda[3]

[1]Scientific Council of Dermatology & Venereology, Iraqi Board for Medical Specializations, Baghdad, Iraq
[2]College of Medicine University of Baghdad, Baghdad, Iraq
[3]Department of Dermatology & Venereology, Baghdad Teaching Hospital, Baghdad, Iraq
Email: *hayder317@gmail.com, dr_ihssanalturfy@yahoo.com, dr.farah248@yahoo.com

Abstract

Background: Tumor necrosis factor alpha (TNF-α) is a proinflammatory cytokine which plays a critical role in the pathogenesis of psoriasis. Infliximab is an anti-TNF-α drug widely used for the treatment of psoriasis. Objectives: To assess the efficacy and safety of infliximab in Iraqi patients with moderate-to-severe psoriasis. Patients and Methods: In this therapeutic, single-center study, a total of 23 patients with moderate-to-severe psoriasis resistant to conventional treatments were enrolled to receive infusions of infliximab 5 mg/kg at weeks 0, 2, and 6, then every 8 weeks for at least 22 weeks. Psoriasis Area and Severity Index(PASI), Body Surface Area (BSA) and Dermatology Life Quality Index (DLQI) were calculated at each visit to assess the response to treatment and all side effects were recorded. Results: PASI score was reduced from a mean ± SD of 17.41 ± 8.53 before treatment to 2.44 ± 2.68 after 22 weeks. At week 22, 84% of patients achieved PASI 75, 42% achieved PASI 90 and 28% achieved complete clearance. BSA and DLQI score were reduced from a mean ± SD of 35.69 ± 22.44 and 20.04 ± 4.68 before treatment to 3.52 ± 4.94 and 3.87 ± 5.60 after 22 weeks, respectively. Pruritus, boils, infusion reactions were recorded and relapse during treatment was found in 3 patients. Conclusion: Infliximab monotherapy is highly effective in the treatment of moderate-to-severe psoriasis, with rapid onset of action and relatively low side effects.

Keywords

Psoriasis, TNF-α, Infliximab

1. Introduction

Psoriasis is a common chronic and immunomediated skin disease which typically follows a relapsing and remitting course [1]. Psoriasis affects approximately 2% - 3% of world's population [2].

---

*Corresponding author.

The proinflammatory cytokine tumor necrosis factor alpha (TNF-α) plays an important role in the pathogenesis of psoriasis [3] [4].

The TNF-α antagonist infliximab, a chimeric monoclonal IgG1 antibody, has been shown to be highly effective for the treatment of psoriasis. In addition to blocking soluble TNF-α, infliximab is also capable of binding transmembrane TNF-α, resulting in complement fixation and antibody-mediated cytolysis [5]-[7]. Given infliximab's characteristic rapid onset of action and high response rates, it is recommended when rapid disease control is required in unstable conditions such as erythrodermic or pustular psoriasis [5].

The significant reduction in quality of life and the psychosocial disability suffered by patients underline the need for prompt, effective treatment, and long-term disease control.

Therefore the present study was designed to evaluate the efficacy and safety of infliximab in Iraqi patients with moderation to severe psoriasis.

2. Patients and Methods

This phase IV, prospective, therapeutic, single centerinterventional study was carried out at the Department of Dermatology and Venereology, Baghdad Teaching Hospital, from May 2013 to July 2014. This is the largest hospital in Baghdad city with more than 1000 beds.

Formal consent was taken from each patient after full explanation about the nature of the study and an ethical approval was granted by the Scientific Council of Dermatology & Venereology-Iraqi Board for Medical Specializationson March 2013.

Adult patients with chronic moderate to severe psoriasis resistant to conventional systemic treatments were included in this study. The exclusion criteria include pregnant or lactating women, patients younger than 18 years, those with severe hepatic, renal, hematological or other systemic disorders, moderate-to-severe heart failure, immunosuppression, history or risk of serious infection, lymphoproliferative, demyelinating disease or active or latent tuberculosis and positive virology for hepatitis or HIV infection.

Psoriasis Area and Severity Index (PASI) score was calculated according to dermnet [8]. Body Surface Area (BSA) was calculated as the patient's hand, including the palm, fingers and thumb represent roughly 1% of the body's surface [9]. Dermatology Life Quality Index (DLQI) score was calculated according to Cardiff University Dermatology Department work group [10].

Depending on the above mentioned parameters for measuring severity of psoriasis, patients with moderate to severe psoriasis in the present work were defined as having PASI > 10, BSA > 10 and/or DLQI > 10.

They received intravenous infliximab infusion in a dose of 5 mg/kg to be repeated at 2, 6 and then every 8 weeks there after according to British Association of Dermatologists' guidelines for the treatment of psoriasis with biologics [11].

Clinical response was assessed by calculating PASI scores, BSA and DLQI score at baseline and at each infusion session. In patients with pustular psoriasis PASI score is not applicable so BSA was depended for evaluation. Safety was assessed by measurement of routine laboratory parameters and reporting of adverse events at all study visits.

Student t-test was used to compare the results with p values < 0.05 were considered to indicate statistical significance.

3. Results

Twenty three patients completed at least 22 weeks of treatment, 21 patients had plaque psoriasis and 2 patients had generalized pustular psoriasis. Seventeen (73.91%) were males and 6 (26.08%) were females. Their ages ranged from 20 - 62 years with a mean ± SD of 39.69 ± 10.57 years. The duration of their disease ranged from 1 - 33 years with a mean ± SD of 12.39 ± 8.19 years, 12 patients (52%) had negative family history of psoriasis and 11 (47%) had positive family history. The patients had no other diseases and they were not on any other medications. Their mean baseline PASI score ranged from 6.4 - 31.9 with a mean ± SD of 17.41 ± 8.53. Their baseline BSA% ranged from 6% - 75% with a mean ± SD of 35.69 ± 22.44. Baseline DLQI score was ranged from 13 - 28 with a mean ± SD of 20.04 ± 4.68 (see **Figures 1-3**).

3.1. PASI Score

PASI score was reduced from a mean ± SD of 17.41 ± 8.53 before treatment to 9.75 ± 6.34 at 2 weeks, to 4.26 ±

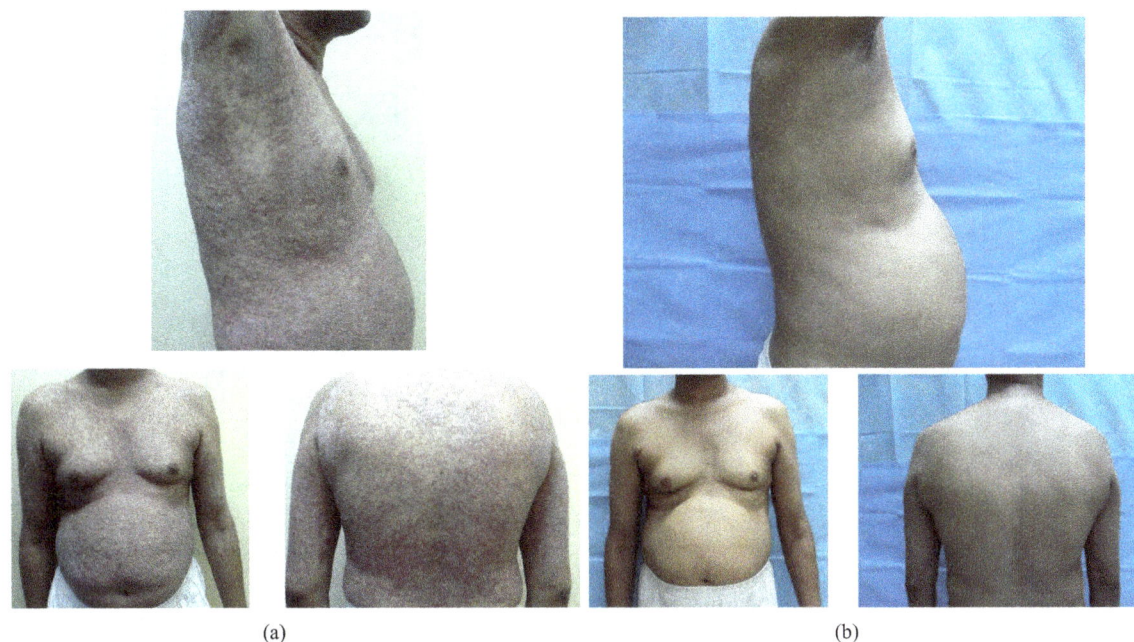

Figure 1. Forty-one year old male with generalized plaque psoriasis for 2 years. (a) Before treatment; (b) after 6 weeks of treatment.

4.01 at 6 weeks, to 3.39 ± 3.46 at 14 weeks and to 2.44 ± 2.68 at 22 weeks of treatment.

Table 1 shows comparison of PASI score at each visit with the previous visit with p-values.

The reduction in PASI score was calculated as percent of the original PASI. It was 43.99%, 75.53%, 80.52% and 85.98% after 2, 6, 14 and 22 weeks of treatment respectively.

After 14 wks of treatment, 90% of patients with plaque psoriasis achieved >50% reduction in PASI score (PASI 50), 71% of patients achieved >75% reduction (PASI 75), 33% of patients achieved >90% reduction (PASI 90) and 14% of patients achieved complete clearance (100% reduction).

At 22 wk, 88% of patients achieved PASI 50, 84% of patients achieved PASI 75, 42% of patients achieved PASI 90 and 28% of patients achieved complete clearance.

3.2. BSA Percent

BSA percent was reduced from a mean ± SD of 35.69 ± 22.44 before treatment to 25.35 ± 19.60, 11.43 ± 12.64, 4.91 ± 5.55 and 3.52 ± 4.94 at 2, 6, 14 and 22 weeks of treatment, respectively.

Table 2 shows comparison of BSA at each visit with the previous visit with p-values.

The reduction in BSA percent was 28.97%, 67.97%, 86.24% and 90.13% after 2, 6, 14 and 22 weeks of treatment respectively.

At the end of 22 weeks, the two patients with generalized pustular psoriasis achieved complete clearance.

3.3. DLQI Score

DLQI score was reduced from a mean ± SD of 20.04 ± 4.68 before treatment to 14.00 ± 6.95, 7.96 ± 5.91, 4.52 ± 4.82 and 3.87 ± 5.60 at 2, 6, 14 and 22 weeks of treatment, respectively.

Table 3 shows comparison of DLQI score at each visit with the previous visit with p-values.

The reduction in DLQI score was 30.13%, 60.27%, 77.44% and 80.68% after 2, 6, 14 and 22 weeks of treatment respectively.

3.4. Side Effects

The following side effects were noticed during the period of study.

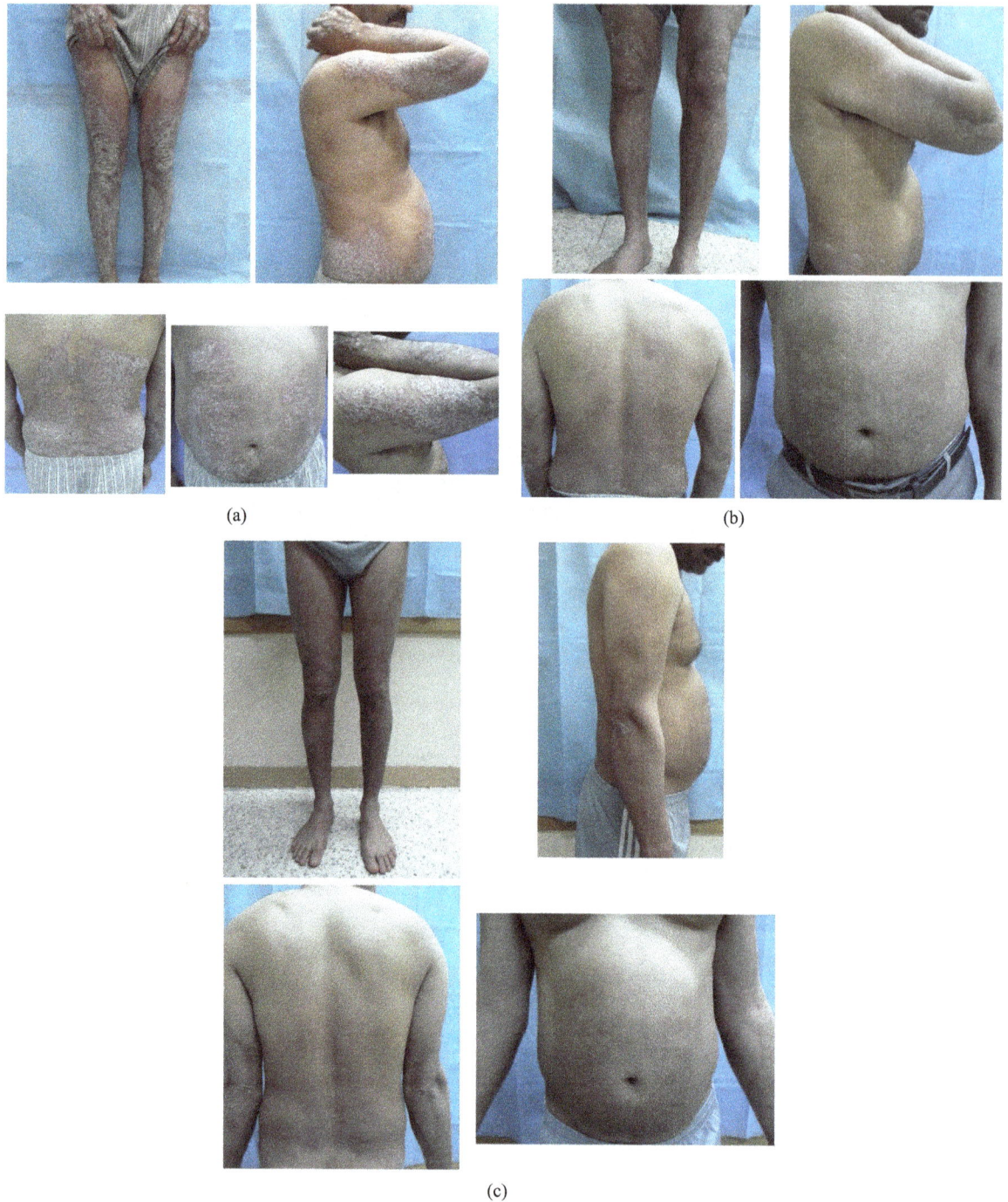

Figure 2. Thirty-nine year old male with generalized plaque psoriasis for 20 years. (a) Before treatment; (b) after 14 weeks of treatment; (c) after 30 weeks of treatment.

Pruritus was recorded in 2 patients, boils were reported in 1 patient, both were disappeared with continuation of treatment. Alopecia are at a developed in one patient. Four patients had infusion reaction, only in one patient the treatment was stopped. One patient developed new onset psoriatic arthritis and methotrexate was added for this patient.

In 2 patients tuberculin skin test became positive, the treatment was suspended and INH was instituted.

Three patients had relapse during treatment. For the first patient acitretin was added to infliximab and for the second one methotrexate was added. For the third patient infliximab was discontinued because his PASI score

Table 1. PASI score (mean ± SD) at different weeks with p-values.

	Weeks	PASI score Mean ± SD	p-value
*Pair 1	0 2	17.41 ± 8.53 9.75 ± 6.34	<0.000001
Pair 2	2 6	9.75 ± 6.34 4.26 ± 4.01	<0.0001
Pair 3	6 14	4.26 ± 4.01 3.39 ± 3.46	<0.1236 **(N.S)
Pair 4	14 22	3.39 ± 3.46 2.44 ± 2.68	<0.0214

*Pair1, 2, 3 and 4 compare the results of treatment at subsequent visits. **(N.S) not significant.

Table 2. BSA (mean ± SD) at different weeks with p-values.

	Weeks	BSA% Mean ± SD	p-value
*Pair 1	0 2	35.69 ± 22.44 25.35 ± 19.60	<0.00005
Pair 2	2 6	25.35 ± 19.60 11.43 ± 12.64	<0.0003
Pair 3	6 14	11.43 ± 12.64 4.91 ± 5.55	<0.005
Pair 4	14 22	4.91 ± 5.55 3.52 ± 4.94	<0.1105 **(N.S)

*Pair 1, 2, 3 and 4 compare the results of treatment at subsequent visits. **(N.S) not significant.

Table 3. DLQI score (mean ± SD) at different weeks with p-values.

	Weeks	DLQI score Mean ± SD	p-value
*Pair 1	0 2	20.04 ± 4.68 14.00 ± 6.95	<0.0000001
Pair 2	2 6	14.00 ± 6.95 7.96 ± 5.91	<0.000001
Pair 3	6 14	7.96 ± 5.91 4.52 ± 4.82	<0.001
Pair 4	14 22	4.52 ± 4.82 3.87 ± 5.60	<0.2072 **(N.S)

*Pair 1, 2, 3 and 4 compare the results of treatment at subsequent visits. **(N.S) not significant.

became more than the baseline.

4. Discussion

Biologics are relatively new modalities for treatment of psoriasis [12]. They target different steps in the immunological reactions. [7] Infliximab was approved for the treatment of moderate to severe psoriasis by FDA at 2006 [13].

In Iraq, there is only one center in which infliximab is administrated for the treatment of psoriasis (Medical City Teaching Hospital) and all the data of the patients are presented in this work.

In the present study, PASI score, BSA and DLQI score were significantly improved with the treatment and this improvement begun at the second week of therapy with infliximab.

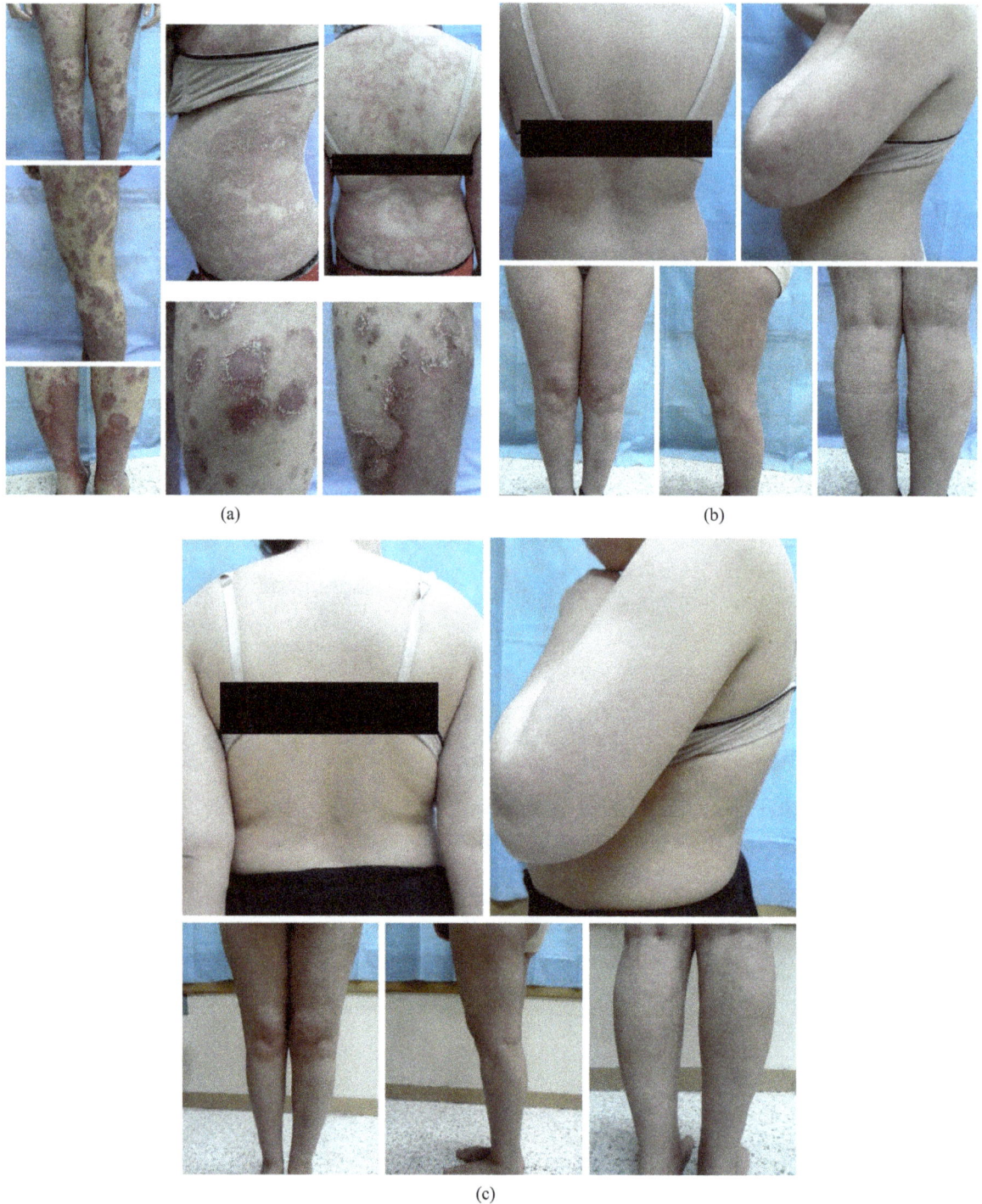

(a)

(b)

(c)

Figure 3. Thirty year old female with generalized pustular psoriasis for 5 years. (a) Before treatment; (b) after 14 weeks of treatment; (c) after 30 weeks of treatment.

On comparing our results with other studies on infliximab, Reich *et al.*, [14] found that at week 24 of treatment, 82% of patients achieved PASI 75 and 58% achieved PASI 90, while in our study 84% of patients achieved PASI 75, 42% achieved PASI 90 and 28% achieved complete clearance after 22 weeks of treatment.

Smith *et al.*, [15] reported that at week 10, 95% of patients achieved PASI 50% and 77% achieved PASI 75 while in the present study, at week 14, 90% of patients achieved PASI 50, 71% achieved PASI 75, 33%

achieved PASI 90% and 14% of patients achieved complete clearance.

Several workers studied the effect of infliximab on DLQI score in psoriatic patients. Feldman *et al.*, on 2005 [16] showed that DLQI score reduced from a mean ± SD of 13.2 ± 7.0 at baseline to 2.8 ± 5.0 at week 10 with a mean percentage improvement of 79.4%, while in the present work DLQI score was reduced from a mean ± SD of 20.04 ± 4.68 at baseline to 4.52 ± 4.82 with a mean percentage improvement of 77.4% at 14 weeks of treatment. All these results are comparable to the results of the present study.

Regarding side effects, the following were reported in different studies: infusion reactions, upper respiratory tract infection, headache, arthralgia, pharyngitis and neoplasms including squamous cell carcinoma and basal cell carcinoma.

In the present study, pruritus, boils, alopecia areata, tuberculin skin test conversion to positive, infusion reactions and new onset psoriatic arthritis were recorded as side effects.

Limitations of the present study include lack of control and small number of patients (23 patients) and this is because it is a single center study. Other limitation include relatively short period of treatment (22 weeks) and this is because infliximab is a new drug in our department. Infliximab is given by infusion and this require a trained nursing staff and beds which are occupied for at least 2 hrs and since the infusion is only given at the morning, few patients can be treated each day.

5. Conclusion

In conclusion, infliximab monotherapy seems to be an effective treatment for psoriasis with rapid onset of action and side effects were relatively mild and did not affect the life of the patients.

Disclosure

This study was an independent study and not funded by any drug companies.

References

[1] Christophers, E. (2001) Psoriasis—Epidemiology and Clinicalspectrum. *Clinical and Experimental Dermatology*, **26**, 314-320. http://dx.doi.org/10.1046/j.1365-2230.2001.00832.x

[2] Naldi, L.N. (2004) Epidemiology of Psoriasis. *Current Drug Target-Inflammation & Allergy*, **3**, 121-128. http://dx.doi.org/10.2174/1568010043343958

[3] Gottlieb, A.B. (2003) Clinical Research Helps Elucidate the Role of Tumor Necrosisfactor-α in the Pathogenesis of T1-Mediated Immune Disorders: Use Oftargeted Immunotherapeutics as Pathogenic Probes. *Lupus*, **12**, 190-194. http://dx.doi.org/10.1191/0961203303lu354xx

[4] Krueger, J.G. (2002) The Immunologic Basis for the Treatment of Psoriasis with Newbiologic Agents. *Journal of the American Academy of Dermatology*, **46**, 1-23. http://dx.doi.org/10.1067/mjd.2002.120568

[5] Ali, A. and Ibrahim, A. (2013) Biologic Systemic Therapy for Moderate-to-Severe Psoriasis: A Review. *Journal of Taibah University Medical Sciences*, **8**, 142-150. http://dx.doi.org/10.1016/j.jtumed.2013.09.001

[6] Stephen, K.R. and Joel, M.G. (2012) Immunobiologicals, Cytokines, and Growth Factors in Dermatology. In: Wolf, K., Goldsmith, L.A., Katz, S.I., Gilchrest, B.A., Paller, A.S. and Leffell, D.J., Eds., *Fitz Patrick's Dermatology in General Medicine*, 8th Edition, McGraw Hill, New York, 2: 234: 2814-2826.

[7] Breathnach, S.M., Smith, C.H., Chalmers, R.J. and Hay, R.J. (2010) Systemic Therapy. In: Burns, T., Breathnach, S., Cox, N. and Griffiths, C., Eds., *Rook's Textbook of Dermatology*, 8th Edition, Wiley-Blackwell Publishing Company, Singapore, 4: 74.4.

[8] Severity and Extent of Psoriasis (Psoriasis Area and Severity Index). http://www.dermnetnz.org/scaly/pasi.html

[9] Krueger, G.G. (2000) Two Considerations for Patients with Psoriasis and Their Clinicians: What Defines Mild, Moderate, and Severe Psoriasis? What Constitutes a Clinically Significant Improvement When Treating Psoriasis? *Journal of the American Academy of Dermatology*, **43**, 281-285. http://dx.doi.org/10.1067/mjd.2000.106374

[10] Quality of Life. Dermatology Life Quality Index. http://www.dermatology.org.uk/quality/dlqi/quality-dlqi.html

[11] Smith, C.H., Anstey, A.V., Barker, J.N., Burden, A.D., Chalmers, R.J. and Chandler, D.A. (2009) British Association of Dermatologists Guidelines for Biological Intervention for Psoriasis 2009. *British Journal of Dermatology*, **161**, 987-1019. http://dx.doi.org/10.1111/j.1365-2133.2009.09505.x

[12] Mathur, M., Kedia, S.K. and Chimire, R.B.K. (2011) An Intravenous Biological Therapy for Psoriasis: Infliximab. *Journal of College of Medical Sciences-Nepal*, **7**, 69-72.

[13] Jeniffer, S. and Robert, E. (2008) Infliximab for the Treatment of Plaque Psoriasis. *Biologics*, **2**, 115-124.

[14] Reich, K. (2005) Infliximab Induction and Maintenance Therapy Formoderate-to-Severe Psoriasis: A Phase III, Multi-centre, Double-Blind Trial. *Lancet*, **366**, 1367-1374. http://dx.doi.org/10.1016/S0140-6736(05)67566-6

[15] Smith, C.H., Jackson, K., Bashir, S.J., Perez, A., Chew, A.L., Powell, A.M., Wain, M. and Barker, J. (2006) Infliximab for Severe, Treatment-Resistant Psoriasis: A Prospective, Open-Label Study. *British Journal of Dermatology*, **155**, 160-169. http://dx.doi.org/10.1111/j.1365-2133.2006.07316.x

[16] Feldman, S.R., Gordon, K.B. and Bala, M. (2005) Infliximab Treatment Results in Significant Improvement in the Quality of Life of Patients with Severe Psoriasis: A Double-Blind Placebo-Controlled Trial. *British Journal of Dermatology*, **152**, 954-960. http://dx.doi.org/10.1111/j.1365-2133.2005.06510.x

19

Safety and Efficacy of a Thermally Regulated Radiofrequency Home-Device for Rhytide and Laxity Treatment

Judith Hellman[1], Hela Goren[2], R. Stephen Mulholland[3]*

[1]New York, USA
[2]Yokneam, Israel
[3]Private Plastic Surgery Practice, Toronto, Canada
Email: *info@spamedica.com

Abstract

The growth of the medical aesthetic industry is tremendous, and not surprisingly, has been followed by the introduction of new novel technologies for home use. This study focuses on the Silk'n Home Skin Tightening (HST), a home use device that uses a thermally regulated radiofrequency (RF) delivery technology. This technology allows the end point dermal temperatures to be sustained safely for a prolonged period of time, optimizing the non-ablative dermal collagen, elastin and ground substance production. Enhancement of the clinical results of rhytides and laxity improvement are noted. In this study, the HST protocol and technology innovation is outlined. The results of a blinded, independent assessment of photographs before and 1 month after 20 biweekly sessions demonstrated that 96% of patients achieved an average improvement of 1.6 grades (32%) in their Fitzpatrick wrinkling and elastosis scale, with no significant complications.

Keywords

Radiofrequency, Wrinkle Reduction, Skin Tightening, HST

1. Introduction

Patient demand for non-surgical, non-invasive and no-downtime wrinkle and laxity reduction procedures has grown dramatically over the past decade. This increased demand has fuelled the growth of new technologies that deliver these non-invasive and non-ablative, anti-aging outcomes. The disadvantages of in-office based treat-

---
*Corresponding author.

ments are availability, inconvenience of travel to the clinic for multiple sessions, cost of the treatments, discomfort with the high fluence devices, and risks of pigmentation issues and scars. Using a small low energy home-use system can alleviate these disadvantages.

The non-ablative rhytide reduction technologies can be divided into a) laser and infrared (IR) devices with single spot size or laser/IR "stampers", and b) radiofrequency (RF) or RF/IR combination with single spot size and "stamping" technologies, both yielding high peak thermal end points. The early prototypes for the "stamping" laser devices included the CoolTouch 1320 nm laser, the Titan for the pure IR "stampers", and Thermage for the "RF stamping" technology. Each of these aforementioned devices had considerable success by heating the dermis to non-ablative temperatures of 45°C - 50°C, while protecting the epidermis from overheating by direct cooling systems or specific pulse configurations. The non-ablative heating resulted in a thermally mediated, micro-inflammatory production of collagen, elastin and ground substances, with a moderate improvement in rhytides and laxity. Due to the short pulse durations and short exposure time of the dermis to the non-ablative temperatures, multiple pass and multiple session protocols evolved. However, the high peak temperatures and short pulse durations of these "stampers" led to a high and often unacceptable level of patient discomfort and clinically inconsistent rhytide improvement outcomes.

In attempt to overcome these limitations of the early generation non-ablative skin heating devices, there evolved a class of continuous radio frequency (RF) thermal skin heaters that necessitated moving the applicator around on the skin surface, while the RF heated the epidermal-dermal tissues. These "moving" RF heating systems include Accent (Alma Lasers), Exilis (Aesthetic Precision) and Venus Freeze (Venus Concept) and have grown in popularity to dominate the market, as they sustain the dermal matrix to elevated thermal temperatures for prolonged periods of time, leading to more consistent rhytide and laxity results. There are several monopolar, bipolar and multipolar RF devices in the market, however, this current generation of "moving" RF applicators does not have thermal feedback control and can lead to "thermal spikes", patient discomfort and compromised outcomes or patient compliance issues.

This paper introduces novel technology advancement and "moving" RF soft tissue heating application, which is called the Silk'n HST by HomeSkinovations Ltd., Yokneam, Israel. It introduces for the first time, an RF device that senses skin temperatures and controls the deliverd RF energy, allowing a prolonged, sustained, safe and efficacious dermal heating.

The effects of dermal heating are well recognized to include immediate effects on collagen structure with stimulation of neocollagenesis [1]. These changes can help reduce the appearance of fine wrinkles and enhance skin tightening. RF energy has been used in medicine for several decades. It heats tissue through intermolecular motion, molecular friction and the induction of rotational movement in water molecules. During the course of treating wrinkles and laxity, the treatment creates enough thermal effect to induce collagen, elastin and ground substance remodeling with no ablative thermal damage of the epidermis or dermis, nor thermal reduction of the subcutaneous adipose tissue.

This study was performed in order to evaluate the efficacy and safety of the HST home-use device, based on an innovative, noninvasive highly thermally regulated RF heating technology, intended for the reduction of rhytides and for skin tightening

2. Materials and Methods

2.1. Study Design

This study is a multicenter study, performed in 3 clinics in USA and Canada. Fifty patients were treated on 3 facial areas—2 cheeks and forehead; altogether 150 treatment sites. Twenty bi-weekly treatment sessions during 10 weeks were conducted at home, following 1st session of instruction in the clinics. Follow up session was 1 month after the last treatment.

2.2. Device Description

The HST device consists of two side electrodes and one central electrode (**Figure 1**). RF current alternates between the side electrodes and the central electrode pins, confined to the dermis and superficial subdermal layer. There is an impedance sensor and a skin surface thermal sensor built into the applicator. Addition of these sensors allows for an innovative and valuable thermal treatment, allowing the skin to be treated at the desired ther-

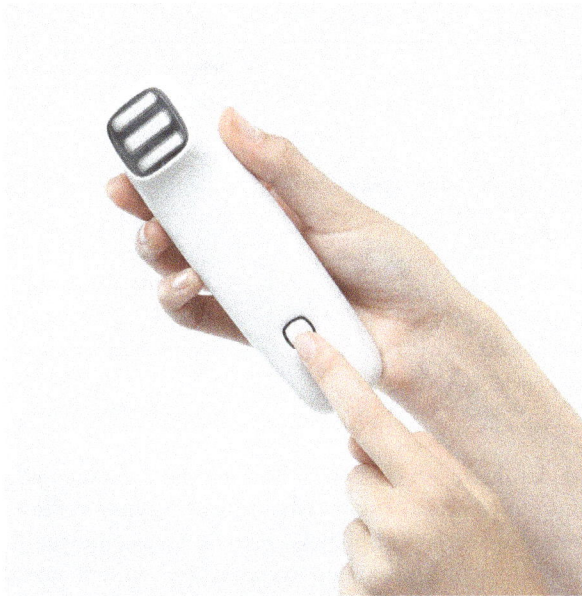

Figure 1. The HST home-device.

mal end point for prolonged periods of time, minimizing "hot spots" and patient discomfort, optimizing dermal matrix response, wrinkle reduction, and laxity improvement. There are 5 power levels that are chosen by the operator according to comfort. Levels 3 - 5 are emitting 5 watts, 10 watts, and 15 watts RF, respectively. In addition there is heating via a red spectrum LED. When the epidermal temperature reaches the end point temperature (41°C - 43°C in levels 3 -5, respectively), the device senses this temperature and the RF energy is inactivated. Once the temperature falls below the end point temperature, the RF is turned back on again. This cycle will continue as long as the operator wishes to maintain this soft tissue thermal end point. Thus, temperature end point is achieved quickly, well controlled and safely sustained. Additional safety features include the ability of the impedance sensors to detect when the dermal temperature is rising too quickly and the dermal impendence drops suddenly, resulting in the RF energy to be shut-off automatically. Conversely, if the electrodes stray off the skin, the impedance rises too high and the RF is shut-off (limiting RF arching or poor contact discomfort).

2.3. Subjects

53 subjects (44 females and 9 males) were enrolled in the study. Of all 53 subjects, 50 subjects (94%) completed the study course and received all 20 treatments and attended the 1 month follow-up visit. Three subjects withdrew from the study because they were not compliant with the treatment protocol. Subjects' age was between 36 - 77 (average 55.5 ± 10.8) with Fitzpatrick skin type I to VI (**Table 1**). Subjects were enrolled in the study after meeting all inclusion/exclusion criteria and providing a signed Informed Consent Form. Subjects' wrinkle and rhytide appearance were classified according to Fitzpatrick wrinkling and elastosis scale (**Table 2**) before and after treatment. Enrolled subjects were classified as having mild or moderate wrinkling and elastosis score according to Fitzpatrick scale. Exclusion criteria included scarring, inflammation or infection of the area to be treated, history of skin disorders, keloids, abnormal wound healing, pregnancy or lactating, subjects with current or history of malignancy, implants or a pacemaker device, Botox/HA/collagen/fat injections or other augmentation methods with bio-material in the last six months, poorly controlled endocrine disorders as diabetes or thyroid dysfunction, severe concurrent conditions such as cardiac disorders, epilepsy, uncontrolled hypertension and liver and kidney disorders, patients with history of diseases stimulated by heat, such as recurrent Herpes Simplex in the treated area, facial resurfacing, deep chemical peeling within the last 3 months, or history of bleeding coagulopathies.

2.4. Treatment Protocol

The first session took place in the clinics and the subjects were trained and performed the first treatment at the

Table 1. Subject demographic.

Age	Gender	Skin type
55.5 ± 10.8	8 males 42 females	3.3 ± 1.3

Table 2. Fitzpatrick wrinkling and elastosis scale [2].

Class	Wrinkling	Score	
I	Fine wrinkles	1 - 3	**Mild**: fine texture changes with subtly accentuated skin lines.
II	Fine to moderate depth wrinkles Moderate number of lines	4- 6	**Moderate**: distinct popular elastosis (individual papules with yellow translucency) and dyschromia.
III	Fine to deep wrinkles, numerous lines With or without redundant skin folds	7 - 9	**Severe:** multipapular and confluent elastosis (thickened, yellow and pallid) approaching with cutis rhomboidalis.

investigators' offices under the supervision of trained nurses. Treatment power level (5 - 15 W) was adjusted to each patient according to tolerance and skin response. All patients could tolerate 15 W at level 5. Prior to initiating the study, the treated areas were photographed in a standardized method, using high-resolution digital photography in order to allow comparison and assessment of wrinkle and laxity improvement at study conclusion.

All subsequent treatments were performed at home by the patients. They were instructed to call the clinic for any query that they may have or for any change in response that could be classified as an adverse event. Subjects came to the clinics after 10 bi-weekly sessions to evaluate the interim results and the treatment technique.

The treatment area was cleaned thoroughly with skin cleanser to remove any makeup, perfume, oils or other cosmetics. The face was divided into 3 treatment zones as shown in **Figure 2**, including the two zones of cheek-jaw line-lower eyelid and the brow-temporal zone, and the forehead. A thin layer of water based gel was applied on the intended treatment area. The treatment technique calls for complete contact with the skin and constant slow circular movements, figure of eights, or in lines throughout the treatment zone. Each zone was treated for 10 minutes, in areas that were sensitive or boney the treatment time could be decreased to seven minutes. The treatment area was monitored thoroughly during the treatment and assessed for any potential adverse events.

Immediately after each treatment the treated area was visually assessed for skin responses and moisturizer was applied. In addition, patients were asked to rate the pain level they felt during treatment, on a 10-point linear analog pain scale.

2.5. Safety Measures

The safety of the procedure was evaluated by monitoring the occurrence of potential procedure-related side effects. (e.g. blisters, prolonged discoloration, edema, erythema, hypopigmentation, hyperpigmentation, scars and textural changes).

2.6. Efficacy Measures

The study's efficacy end point was evaluated by comparing standardized pre- and post-treatment photographs that were assessed and graded by a blinded independent physician, who is not the study investigator, in each of the 3 clinics. Assessment was based on Fitzpatrick wrinkling and elastosis scale. Any wrinkle score improvement (downgrade score) following treatment, relative to pre-treatment wrinkle (baseline) score, was considered a "success". Subjects were considered a "success" if they gain at least one degree of facial wrinkle reduction (based on Fitzpatrick scale) following 20 treatments. Study success was declared if at least 90% of study participants were scored a rhytide improvement success.

2.7. Statistical Analyses

Descriptive statistics including mean, standard deviation, and 95% confidence interval were used to describe treatment efficacy (determined by pre and post Fitzpatrick wrinkling and elastosis score). The mean differences of Fitzpatrick Score before treatment and at follow up session were analyzed by a paired-sampled t-test. All statistical data analyses were performed using statistical software (SAS version 9.1).

3. Results

No unexpected adverse side effects were detected or reported during the study, including Fitzpatrick dark skin types V and VI. All patients participating in the study reported no significant pain during the treatment.

Photographic analysis of pre-and post treatment of the digital images was conducted by a blinded independent physician on each treatment site separately (left cheek, right cheek, and forehead) (**Figure 3**). Analysis of the 150 treatment facial sites revealed average improvement in 1.6 (STDV 0.7) Fitzpatrick score in almost all subjects (96% of 150 treatment sites). 15 treatment sites (10%) improved in 3 Fitzpatrick grades, 72 (48%) treatment sites improved in 2 Fitzpatrick grades, 57 treatment sites (38%) improved in 1 Fitzpatrick grade and only 6 treatment sites (4%) did not show any improvement. Most subjects (94%) were satisfied with treatment results.

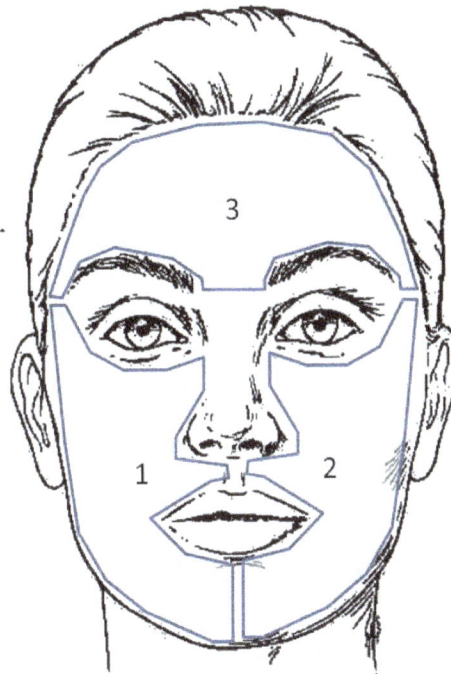

Figure 2. Treatment zones.

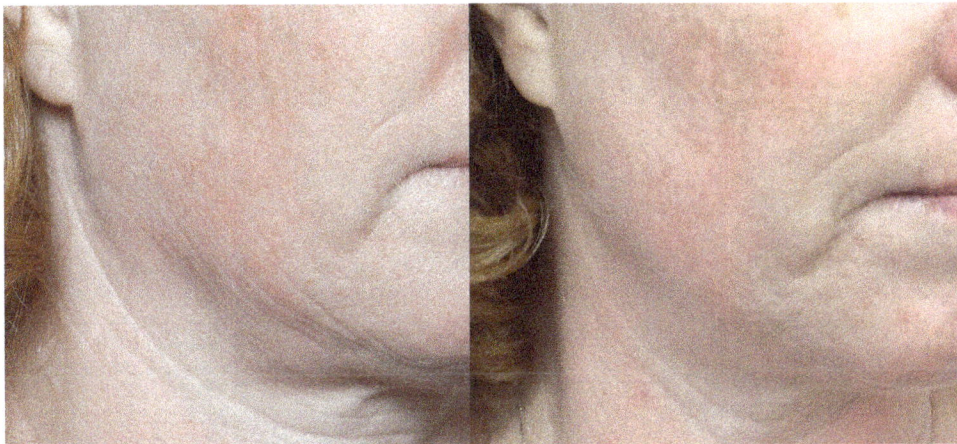

Figure 3. Before and after of lift in the cheek area.

3.1. Treatment Safety Assessment

Post treatment slight erythema was detected in all subjects. The erythema disappeared within one hour without any intervention. In some subjects, post treatment edema (hyperemia) was detected. The edema was resolved within 24 hours, and no treatment was needed. It should be noted that edema and erythema are common transient response following RF treatments and represent a desirable effect.

3.2. Treatment Efficacy Assessment

Most patients (94%) were satisfied from treatment results.

Statistical comparison (using paired t-test) was conducted among the pre treatment Fitzpatrick score (baseline) to Fitzpatrick score obtained at 1 month follow-up. The statistical analysis was conducted by SAS. Score differences were found to be statistically significant while comparing baseline scores to the scores obtained at 1 month follow-up (p < 0.001), indicating treatment efficacy. **Table 3** and **Figure 4** represent averages (±STDV) of Fitzpatrick scores given by the blinded independent physician at baseline and at 1 month follow-up. There was no significant correlation between rhytide reduction and skin type; all skin types showed improvement. The results are summarized in **Table 3**.

4. Discussion and Conclusions

The HST home-device, with its thermal control innovation allows the operator to sustain the desired dermal temperatures with exquisite control and comfort, optimizing both the patient experience and non-ablative dermal enhancement. The combination of built in impedance sensors, limiting both high and low values, allows the RF to be cut-off when the dermal temperature is rising too quickly (low impedance cut-off) or when there is poor electrode contact (high impedance cut-off), making the treatment very safe. In addition, the thermal sensor and automatic feedback loop allows the operator and system to tightly regulate the dermal temperature and sustain the thermal end point.

The data reported in this study demonstrate that the HST home-device offers a safe and effective in-home noninvasive technique to improve the appearance of age-related wrinkles and elastosis.

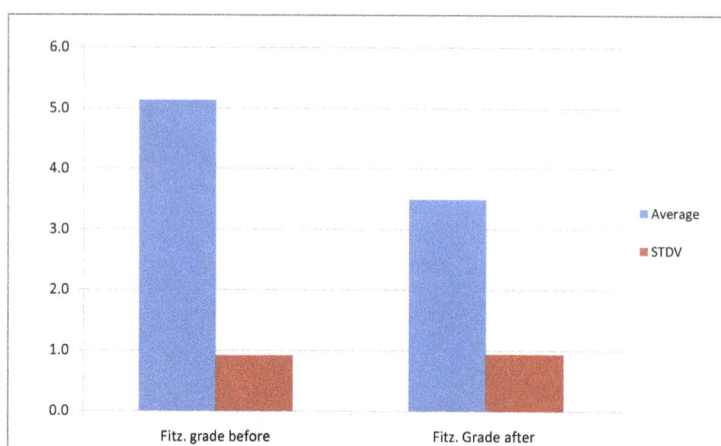

Figure 4. Average (±STDV) of Fitzpatrick scores before and 1 month after the last treatment.

Table 3. Average (±STDV) of Fitzpatrick scores at baseline and 1 month follow-up (following 20 treatments), and grade reduction, comparing to baseline with statistical results of the comparison.

Score time	Average score	Grade reduction (comparing to baseline)	Grade reduction in %	Statistical (t-test) results of the comparison
Baseline	5.1 (±0.9)			
1 month follow-up	3.5 (±0.9)	1.6 (±0.7)	31.9 (±0.1)	p < 0.001

The clinical results of nonablative RF anti wrinkle effects were first reported in the periorbital area [3]. Fitzpatrick and his colleagues demonstrated clinical improvement in periorbital rhytides in 80% of subjects. In contrast, in 24 patients who underwent a single RF treatment to improve the upper third of the face, only 36% of the patients' self-assessment reported improvement [4].

In this study, statistical analysis has revealed improvement (downgrade of average 1.6 score according to the Fitzpatrick scale) in almost all subjects. Analysis of study results has revealed statistical significance while comparing baseline score to the scores obtained at 1 month follow-up, following 20 bi-weekly treatments, indicating treatment efficacy. These results may indicate that the treatments have initiated collagen remodeling process that continues after treatment session has been completed. Study success criteria are defined as: at least 90% of study subjects are considered success. Therefore, it concludes that study success criteria are met.

In a similar device, it has been reported that the use of a RF device is associated with significant pain, and in a small but significant number of cases subcutaneous fat atrophy develops [5]. No subcutaneous fat atrophy is detected externally. All subjects participating in this study have reported no pain during treatment, although the procedure is performed without using any anesthetic agents. Furthermore, no subject considers the procedure intolerable at any stage.

The HST home-device deploys RF power of only 7.5% of the density emitted by RF devices currently on the market: up to 4.5 J/cm^2. This low energy can't cause complications and therefore is very safe to the user's skin. As a result, the potential risk is minimal.

The results of this study clearly indicate that the HST innovative RF application offers in-home noninvasive, effective, safe and virtually painless wrinkle reduction and skin laxity treatment.

The HST can also be used to treat rhytide and laxity on non-facial skin, such as the neck, back of hands, navel area, or knees. Further studies may demonstrate this versatility.

References

[1] Sadick, N. and Sorhaindo, L. (2005) The Radiofrequency Frontier: A Review of Radiofrequency and Combined Radiofrequency Pulsed Light Technology in Aesthetic Medicine. *Facial Plastic Surgery*, **21**, 131-138. http://dx.doi.org/10.1055/s-2005-872414

[2] Goldman, P. and Fitzpatrick, E. (1999) Cutaneous Laser Surgery—The Art and Science of Selective Photothermolysis. Mosby, St. Louis, 377.

[3] Fitzpatrick, R., Geronemus, R., Goldberg, D., *et al.* (2003) Multicenter Study of Noninvasive, Radiofrequency for Periorbital Tissue Tightening. *Lasers in Surgery and Medicine*, **33**, 232-242. http://dx.doi.org/10.1002/lsm.10225

[4] Bassichis, B.A., Dayan, S. and Thomas, J.R. (2004) Use of Nonablative Radiofrequency Device to Rejuvenate the upper One-Third of the Face. *Otolaryngology—Head and Neck Surgery*, **130**, 397-406. http://dx.doi.org/10.1016/j.otohns.2003.09.034

[5] Biessman, B.S. (2005) Radiofrequency Devices. Monopolar vs Bipolar vs Radiofrequency plus Laser; Indications; Treatment Approaches; Novel Applications; Results. In: Arndt, K.A., Dover, J.S. and Anderson, R.R., Eds., *Controversies and Conversations in Laser and Cosmetic Surgery*, Symposium Proceedings, Denver, CO.

20

Assessment of Using Cosmetics Containing Hydroquinone among Sudanese Women

H. M. Osman[1*], M. E. Shayoub[2], Munzir M. E. Ahmed[3], E. M. Babiker[4]

[1]Department of Biochemistry, Faculty of Pharmacy, University of National Ribat, Khartoum, Sudan
[2]Department of Pharmaceutics, Faculty of Pharmacy, University of Khartoum, Khartoum, Sudan
[3]Department of Biochemistry, Faculty of Medicine, AL-Gadarif University, Gadarif, Sudan
[4]Department of Zoology, Faculty of Sciences, University of Khartoum, Khartoum, Sudan
Email: [*]hisham1212ribat@yahoo.com, profshayoub51@gmail.com, munzirhmd@hotmail.com, embabiker@uofk.edu

Abstract

Many countries in the world wide banned hydroquinone in cosmetics skin lightening but it is still used in most of Africa countries, including Sudan. Few studies were carried out on the side effect of hydroquinone on Sudanese women. Therefore, the present study was carried out in Khartoum state in April to May/2014 to assess the awareness of Sudanese women about using hydroquinone and its probable risks. The results revealed that, highly using cosmetics containing hydroquinone by women aged between 20 - 29 years (78.3%) as well as by those classified as single (69.6%). The results also showed that the highest percentage of women was using it during evening (81.2%) and a high percentage of them was using it for skin lightening (65.2%), followed by elimination acne (20.3%) and about 10.1% for both skin lightening and elimination of acne and very little (4.3%) for freckle elimination. Moreover, the results showed a very high percentage of women (94.2%) used the chemical without being prescribed by doctors and about (85.5%) of them didn't know its nature and risks on human health. Consequently, (50.7%) of women have had sides effects, (44.9 %) used more than one and (44.1%) used it regularly. In addition, the results revealed that a wide range of products of this chemical was available in local market with amalico (34.8%) being highly used. The study can conclude that the awareness of Sudanese women about this compound was poor and needs to be raised by health authorities.

Keywords

Cosmetics, Side Effects, Hydroquinone, Skin Lightening

---

[*]Corresponding author.

1. Introduction

Cosmetics (colloquially known as makeup) are care substances used to enhance the appearance or odor of the human body. They are generally mixtures of chemical compounds, some being derived from natural sources but many are synthetic compounds [1].

Of these synthetic chemical products, hydroquinone-containing products are currently used for cosmetic purposes. Hydroquinone is an aromatic compound derived from phenol. It is a crystalline powder. It is well-known for its antioxidant properties and is widely used as a stabilizer in the coating industry. Hydroquinone pure substance may cause severe damages to human health: it is an eye irritant and a possible skin sensitizer and it is harmful if swallowed. It is suspected to cause genetic defects and cancer [2]. Hydroquinone is also very toxic to aquatic life. The pure substance is used in a large number of industrial and professional applications. Hydroquinone is benzene-1,4-diol belonging to the aromatic organic phenol compounds having the chemical formula $C_6H_4(OH)_2$. It is one of the most effective inhibitors of melanogenesis and is widely used for the treatment of melanosis and other related disorders of hyper-pigmentation. Hydroquinone is also used in many skin bleaching creams and lotions [3].

Some concerns about hydroquinone safety on skin have been expressed; the previous study found when hydroquinone comes to topical application indicates negative reactions which are minor or other is due to using extremely high concentrations of it [4]. Moreover, the World Health Organization [5] reported that the long term use of this chemical would lead to liver and kidneys failure. In addition to this, skin cancer risk probably may develop as melanin synthesis responsible for its protection against ultraviolet radiation would be inhibited by this chemical.

The present work is aimed to assess awareness of Sudanese women about the risks of hydroquinone and its side effects.

2. Materials and Methods

Data were collected in Khartoum city during April and May of 2014 via questionnaire format designed to elicit the picture of using hydroquinone by different age groups of Sudanese women as this chemical is abundant in cosmetic places and easy to buy in low prices from local market. The format included information about the age, Job and social status of participant as well as time of using, duration and dosage of cosmetic. Participants involved in the study were 69 volunteered women where prior consent from each was ensured and those did not use hydroquinone-containing cosmetic was rejected. Data collected was analyzed and presented following conventional descriptive statistical methods.

3. Results

The results of percentage of those using the cosmetic according to age distribution of participants, their marital status and the time they applied the creams during the day are shown in **Table 1**.

The results revealed that cosmetics were highly used by women aged between 20 and 29 years (78.3%) followed by the other two groups having nearly equal percentages; 11.6% for those aged between 30 and 39 years and 10.1% for those aged 40 - 50 years. According to marital status, the increasing prevalence of using cosmetics was in this order; 69.6%, 26.1% and 4.3% for the single, married and divorced women, respectively while regarding the time of the day it was in this order; 81.2%, 15.9 and 2.9% during evening, afternoon and in the morning, respectively.

The results regarding distribution of the prevalence of using cosmetics among women according to their occupation and duration of use as well as purpose of using the cream are shown in **Table 2**.

The results showed that a high prevalence of use was confined to students (56.5%), followed equally by employee (17.4%) and housewife (17.4%) while 8.6% was shown by unclassified women. For the duration of using cosmetics, the distribution of prevalence was in this sequence; (39.1%), 36.23%, 17.4% and 7.2% for extending using it for months, weeks, years, and only days, respectively. In the meantime, the results showed a high percentages of women (65.2%) was using cosmetics containing hydroquinone (65.2%) for skin lightening followed by 20.3% to eliminate acne, 10.1% for skin lightening plus to eliminate acne and 4.3% to eliminate freckles only.

The results of percentage of women aware by saying (Yes or No) regarding different aspects related to cosmetics are shown in **Table 3**. The results showed a high percentage of women (94.2%) received the cream over

Table 1. Distribution of prevalence of using cosmetic according to age group, marital status and dose during a day.

	Prevalence (%)			Total
Age group	20 - 29 years 54 (78.3%)	30 - 39 years 8 (11.6%)	40 - 50 years 7 (10.1%)	69 (100%)
Marital status	Single 48 (69.6%)	Married 18 (26.1%)	Divorced 3 (4.3%)	69 (100%)
dose during a day	Morning 11 (15.9%)	Afternoon 2 (2.9%)	Evening 56 (81.2%)	69 (100%)

Table 2. Distribution of prevalence of using cosmetic according to occupation, duration and purpose of using hydroquinone.

	Prevalence (%)				Total
Occupation	Students 39 (56.5%)	Employee 12 (17.4%)	Housewife 12 (17.4%)	Other 6 (8.6%)	69 (100%)
Duration	One week 5 (7.2%)	Weeks 25 (36.2%)	Months 27 (39.1%)	Years 12 (17.4%)	69 (100%)
Purpose	Elimination of acne 14 (20.3%)	Elimination of freckles 3 (4.3%)	Skin lightening 45 (65.2%)	Skin lightening + elimination of acne 7 (10.1%)	69 (100%)

Table 3. Percentage of (yes/no) answers of participants to questions regarding prescription, nature and risk, side effects, regularity of use and if more than one type of hydroquinone was used.

Enquiry	Yes	No	Total
If had been prescribed	4 (5.8%)	65 (94.2%)	69 (100%)
If aware of it nature and risk	10 (14.5%)	59(85.5%)	69 (100%)
If side effects being induced	34 (49.3%)	35 (%50.7)	69 (100%)
If more than one type being used	38 (55.1%)	31 (44.9%)	69 (100%)
If being used regularly	23 (33.3%)	46 (66.7%)	69 (100%)

the counter without a prescription by medical doctor and (85.5%) did not know its nature and risks on human health. Moreover, (50.7%) admitted to have side effects awareness and (44.9 %) used more than one type of cosmetics and (33.3%) used it regularly.

However, the consequences of using cosmetics informed by women are shown in **Table 4**. Of these women 50.7% showed no signs or symptoms due to this cosmetics while those showing signs were in this increasing order: redness (17.4%), pigmentations (13.0), redness plus grain (7.2%), grain (7.2%) and exfoliation (4.3%).

On the other hand, the percentages of different cosmetics containing hydroquinone that were used by women of this study are shown in **Table 5**. According to the increased percentage of use, the arrangement of these chemicals will be as follows: amalico (34.8%), lucocid (14.5%), tritospot (11.6%), avalone (7.2%), skinsucces (7.2%), baby face (5.8%), suffix (4.3%) , Divacream (4.3%), pure hydroquinone (2.9%), oranvate (1.4%), eldoquin forte (1.4%), melanofree (1.4%), civiiclemon (1.4%) and orange (1.4%).

4. Discussion

Although, a considerable number of Sudanese women are using hydroquinone to brighten their skin but only 69 participants agreed to take part in this study. This lack of cooperation of some cosmetics users probably based on their personal experience that the information given would not be used for the purpose of study or some of them might feel shy to give this information. However, despite the fact that the sample size of this study was not as large as usually would be preferred in such a kind of study, but still could give insight as to the awareness of subjects towards using cosmetics containing hydroquinone. It was evident that, a considerable proportion of Sudanese women, particularly, young unmarried students indulged in these chemicals and their time at the even-

Table 4. Number and percentage (%) of women showing different symptoms induced by hydroquinone.

Symptoms	No	Percent (%)
No signs	35	50.7
Redness	12	17.4
Grain	5	7.2
Exfoliation	3	4.3
Pigmentations	9	13.0
Redness + grain	5	7.2
Total	69	100

Table 5. Percentage of distribution of using different hydroquinone by Sudanese women.

The compound used	Frequency	Percent (%)
Amalico	24	34.8
Avalone	5	7.2
Baby face	4	5.8
Tritospot	8	11.6
Suffix	3	4.3
Oranvate	1	1.4
Lucocid	10	14.5
Eldoquin forte	1	1.4
Divacream	3	4.3
Skinsucces	5	7.2
pure hydroquinone	2	2.9
Melanofree	1	1.4
Civiiclemon	1	1.4
Orange	1	1.4
Total	69	100

ings as most of the Sudanese remained at home until the next day. Perhaps, the slightly high percentage of women who used chemicals for months rather than those for days or weeks or years might be due to achieving by lasting this duration the most preferred purpose of using the chemical which was the skin lightening.

The results of this study, unfortunately, revealed that the subjects were unaware of the hazards that might develop by exposing their skin to these chemicals. This claim can be strengthened by the fact that a high percentage of women (94.2%) neither consulted a medical doctor nor appreciating the hazards of these chemicals (85.5%). Moreover, they were using a wide range of cosmetics containing hydroquinone and perhaps ignored the appearance of the side effects which might lead to serious skin problems.

In this context, it had been reported that hydroquinone when applied at levels higher than the recommended could result in thinning of the skin, irreversible white patches where the melanin producing cells would have been destroyed and could act as an eye, nose, skin and mucous membrane, gastro-intestinal and respiratory irritant [6]. Also, increase in skin temperature could result in an increased flow rate of these compounds [7], hence that might lead to exposing skin to side effects as a result of these difficult environmental conditions. Other than these, hydroquinone was reported unsafe for use because of increasing the risk of developing skin cancers from sun exposure since it makes one's skin more sensitive to the sun's damaging ultraviolet rays. Therefore, it had been banned in some countries like France because of fears of cancer risk [8]. Together with this, hydroquinone was found to be responsible for incurred nephropathy and renal cell proliferation [5].

It is obvious that most synthetic agents were aimed to rate limiting enzyme of melanogenesis tyrosinase, and to bring about alternative hypopigmenting mechanisms [9] but on application they were abused and the customers were not complying with instructions enclosed with product package. It had been noticed that on applying a small amount of this medicine to an area of unbroken skin, this area of application must be checked within 24 hours for any serious side effects. If there was any itching, redness, puffy or blistering, the use of product should be stopped and the doctor to be contacted but with just mild redness the treatment with the product may continue.

The problem with Sudanese women was that their regular use of hydroquinone for cosmetic purposes. This regularity in using perhaps was enhanced as these products were available almost in most local markets and sold in small fractions so as to be bought with low prices. Added to this, the chemicals were brought out from their origin containers without any consideration to optimal storage conditions and that might lead to changing these chemical to harmful compounds especially when heated by the very hot weather in Sudan. Moreover, in some instances the containers did not carry labeling and this may lead to bad handling. The expected hazards of such bad handling could be inspired from previous reports advising that these products must be placed at optimal room temperature, away from light and moisture [6].

5. Conclusion

The present study concluded that the awareness of customers of hydroquinone should be raised via health education and its handling should be banned except for those with authenticated license.

References

[1] Gunter, S., SvenGohla, J., Whaltrand, K., Uwe Schonrock, H., Schmidt, L., Annegret, K., Xenia, P., Wolfgang, P., Hellmut, I. and Walter, D. (2005) Skin Cosmetics, in Ullmann's Encyclopedia of Industrial Chemistry. Willey VCH, Weinheim, 280-285.

[2] Priyanka, M., Ketki, D. and Hyacinth, H. (2013) Cytotoxic Effects of Benzene Metabolites on Human Sperm Function: An *in Vitro* Study. *ISRN Toxicology*, **2013**, Article ID: 397524, 6pp.

[3] Karamagi, E., Owino, E. and Katabira, E. (2001) Hydroquinone Neuropathy Following Use of Skin Bleaching Creams: Case Report. *East African Medical Journal*, **78**, 223-224. http://dx.doi.org/10.4314/eamj.v78i4.9069

[4] Us Food and Drug Administration (USFDA) (1992) FDA's Cosmetics Handbook Washington DC, US Department of Health and Human Services, Public Health Service. *Food and Drug Administration*, **2**, 21-23.

[5] WHO. IPCS International Programme on Chemical Safety (1996) Health and Safety. Hydroquinone, Health and Safety Guide, No. 101, Rom.

[6] Oyedeji, F., Hassan, G. and Adeleke, B. (2011) Hydroquinone and Heavy Metals Levels in Cosmetics Marketed in Nigeria. *Trends in Applied Sciences Research*, **6**, 622-639. http://dx.doi.org/10.3923/tasr.2011.622.639

[7] Vikas, B., Rajni, K., Arun, K. and Dinesh, K. (2014) A Novel Approach for Drug Delivery System. *World Journal of Pharmaceutical Research*, **3**, 318-334.

[8] Belezal, S. (2012) The Timing of Pigmentation Lightening in European. *British Journal of Dermatology*, **120**, 229-238.

[9] Lei, T., Virador, V., Vieira, W. and Hearing, V. (2002) A Melanocyte-Keratinocyte Coculture Model to Assess Regulators of Pigmentation *in Vitro*. *Analytical Biochemistry*, **305**, 260-268. http://dx.doi.org/10.1006/abio.2002.5665

Bi-Polar RF, Still the Gold Standard for Non-Invasive Fat Volume Reduction

James K. M. Chan[1], Inna Belenky[2], Monica Elman[3]*

[1]DR JAMES CLINIC, Hong Kong, China
[2]Viora Inc., Jersey City, NJ, USA
[3]Elman Medical Services Ltd., Tel Aviv, Israel
Email: *monica@elman.co.il

Abstract

Background and Objective: Non-invasive body contouring treatments is one of the fastest growing markets in the aesthetic field. The main purpose of radiofrequency (RF)-based devices for body contouring is to produce thermal stimulus which leads to skin tightening effect by dermal collagen production and decreases the volume of adipose tissue by a reduction of the adipocyte's cytosolic. The cutaneous application of RF devices in Asian patients differs in several respects from their use in Caucasians; therefore the objective of this study was to evaluate the safety and efficacy of a novel RF device used for focal fat reduction. Materials and Methods: Twenty-two Asian patients aged 24 - 51, Fitzpatrick skin types III-V, were enrolled to the study and received 6 sessions of consecutive abdomen contouring treatment with bi-polar RF device combined with a mechanical pressure. Statistical linear correlation tests and descriptive analysis were performed on the cohort. Results: All twenty-two patients treated for six treatments showed some degree of circumferential reduction with a stable weight. No adverse events were recorded during the whole period of trial. During the 3-month follow up visit, no deterioration of the body condition was detected. No statistical significant relation was found between circumference change and weight, age, height or BMI. Conclusions: The majority of the patients exhibited a substantial circumferential reduction, not at the expense of weight loss. The bi-polar RF device was found to be safe for Asian skin.

Keywords

Adipose Tissue, Asian Patients, Radiofrequency, Vacuum

1. Introduction

Non-invasive body contouring treatments is one of the fastest growing markets in the aesthetic field [1]. These

---

*Corresponding author.

treatments have grew from mechanical rollers and suction technologies, to thermal based technologies including radio-frequency (RF) energy, infrared light, high intensity focused ultrasound energy (HIFU), and for non-thermal technologies such as cryolipolysis, pulsed focused ultrasound energy, low-level laser therapy (LLLT), etc. [2]-[10]. In some devices the thermal heat is combined with mechanical pressure technology [2]-[6] [11]. The mechanical pressure stimulates the lymphatic flux which reduces edema and toxic environment.

Main purposes of RF-based devices are skin tightening and decrease the volume of adipose tissue. Skin is tightened by immediate collagen contraction, subsequent collagen production and remodeling. Reduction of the adipocyte's cytosolic volume by normal lipolysis without direct cellular destruction is also obtained due to heat generation in the tissue. The lipolysis process is a normal metabolism of the adipose tissue through stimulation of epinephrine mediated membrane bound lipase enzyme. During the lipolysis process the triglycerides (the main cytosolic volume) are converted (hydrolyzed) to glycerol and free fatty acids. These free fatty acids and glycerol egress out of the cell and are mobilized and metabolized according to body's needs [2].

The cutaneous application of RF devices in Asian patients differs in several respects from their use in Caucasians [12]. But, since RF energy is color-blind technology, the response of the Asian population to the body contouring treatments is assumed to be similar to the Caucasian Population. The objective of this study was to evaluate the safety and efficacy of a novel RF-based device used for focal fat reduction.

2. Materials and Methods

2.1. Patient's Specifications

Twenty-two Asian patients from Hong Kong (16 females and 6 males) aged 24 - 51 (average 39.59 years, SD 7.14 years), Fitzpatrick skin types III-V (according to 6 types Fitzpatrick phototyping scale), were enrolled to the study after informed consent was obtained. The patients selected according to the following inclusion criteria: 1) no contraindication for the RF-based treatment; 2) age below 18 years old; 3) BMI 18.5 - 39.9; 4) realistic treatment expectations.

The height range of patients deployed between 152 - 180 cm (average 166.27 cm, SD 7.92 cm) with initial body weight of 49 - 114.5 Kg (average 63.36 Kg, SD 14.63 Kg) and calculated BMI (Body Mass Index) of 18 - 36 (average 22.78, SD 4.06). Seventeen patients were in range of "normal" (healthy weight), one patient was in the "underweight" category, with BMI = 18.0 (patient No. 21), three patients were in "overweight" category (patient No. 1, 17 and 19) and one patient was in "obese class I" (moderately obese) category (patient No. 18) (**Table 1**).

All patients, except patients No. 18 and 21, had maintained a stable weight (weight fractionations were limited to ±2 Kg) during the whole period of the trial (**Table 1**). Patients presented similar focal fat accumulation on the abdomen area. No patient had undergone any previous treatments and/or medications for fat volume reduction.

2.2. Treatment Device and Treatment Regime

2.2.1. RF-Based Device

All twenty two patients were treated with bi-polar RF device (Viora Inc., Jersey City, NJ, USA) combined with a mechanical pressure. The system integrates CORE™ technology, which allows independent heating depth control with three distinguished frequencies of RF energy: 0.8, 1.7 and 2.45 MHz, and an additional channel which combines all three frequencies in a single pulse [11].

2.2.2. Treatment Applicator

All patients were treated with B-Contour applicator which designed for treatment of large skin areas. This applicator emits vacuum-assisted pulsed RF power up to 50 W with a treatment spot size of 35 × 30 mm [11].

2.2.3. Treatment Area and Regime

The entire study period was hold during 6 months, including the 3 months follow-up visits. All patients kept on their normal diet and level of exercise during treatment period. The patients received 6 consecutive sessions on the abdomen area with one week interval. The treatment procedure was based on "Body Contouring Protocol" designed in three phases: I) Pre-heating phase, II) adipose tissue heating phase and III) fibroblast stimulation

Table 1. Patient characteristics.

Patient No.	Age	Sex*	BMI	Weight Fluctuations (Kg)	Fitzpatrick Skin Type
1	38	F	29.7	0.0	IV
2	50	M	24.6	0.1	V
3	38	F	24.8	0.0	IV
4	51	F	22.7	0.0	V
5	43	F	20.1	−2.0	IV
6	38	F	21.0	−1.7	III
7	29	F	20.3	−0.8	III
8	38	F	23.4	1.9	III
9	46	F	21.2	0.5	IV
10	38	M	22.5	−0.2	V
11	24	F	20.0	−0.8	III
12	46	M	21.9	0.3	IV
13	31	F	23.3	−0.2	III
14	27	F	21.4	0.7	III
15	42	F	18.8	0.2	III
16	43	F	19.4	0.0	IV
17	43	M	26.2	0.6	III
18	46	M	36.1	−11.8	III
19	41	M	25.2	0.0	IV
20	38	F	19.2	0.6	III
21	35	F	18.0	4.6	III
22	46	F	21.6	−0.6	III

F: Female. M: Male.

phase (skin tightening finishing) [11]. The skin temperature was continuously monitored at 39°C - 42°C, using IR (infrared) thermometer (Fluke 561, Everett, WA USA).

Each treatment session lasted about 20 ± 2 minutes in accordance with protocol guidelines.

2.3. Clinical Measurements and Statistical Analysis

2.3.1. Clinical Measurements

During the enrollment visit, patient's parameters including gender, age, height, weight, BMI and circumferential measurements were recorded before each treatment and in 3-month follow-up visit.

The weight fluctuations (in Kg) were calculated as following: weight (Kg) measured one week after the last treatment session minus weight (Kg) measured in the baseline meeting. The BMI was calculated according to standard guidelines.

The circumferential measurements of the neck, arms, chest, upper abdomen, umbilicus, lower abdomen, hips, thighs and knees, were made using measuring tape, on constant points on each body part. The upper abdomen was determined as a part above the umbilicus and the lower abdomen, as part below. The "Total" circumferential measurement was calculated as a sum of all body parts circumferential measurements. The "Upper body" circumferential measurement was calculated as a sum of neck, arms, chest and upper abdomen circumferential measurements. The "Lower body" circumferential measurement was calculated as a sum of lower abdomen, hips, thighs and knees circumferential measurements.

The circumferential change (in cm) was calculated as following: circumference (cm) recorded one week after the last session minus circumference (cm) recorded in the baseline meeting.

Photography was taken in the baseline, one week after the 6th session and one week after the last treatment session if a patient had more than 6 treatment sessions.

2.3.2. Statistical Analysis

Twenty patients were enrolled to the statistical analysis. Patients No. 18 and 21 were excluded due to unstable weight during the trial. These patients were also excluded when we enrolled only patients that are in range of average value of the initial patient's weight ± 2SD.

All statistical tests were performed using the software package for statistical science (SPSS for Windows, Version 14, SPSS Inc., Chicago, IL, USA). Total 20 patients were included in statistical analysis since patients number 18 and 21 were excluded due to unstable weight fluctuations (over two kilos change).

Descriptive analysis was performed on the cohort, recording the number of valid cases for each test, minimum and maximum values measured, mean and standard deviation (SD), shown in **Table 2**.

Weight and BMI category refer to the initial weight and BMI. Weight change and waist's circumference change refer to the measurements' difference between the baselines and post six treatment sessions. Another parameter indicated is the percentage change, referring to each patient's net measurement divided by the initial factor. For example weight percentage change was calculated as the change between the patient's baseline and post six treatment sessions weight measurement divided by the patient's baseline weight measurement.

A linear correlation tests (R squared) were performed between two parameters: circumference change as dependent variable and weight percentage change, age, initial BMI or high as independent variable.

3. Results

All twenty two patients treated for six treatments by the bi-polar RF device showed some degree of total circumferential reduction from −25.0 cm up to −1.5 cm (**Table 2**). Since the calculation of total circumferential reduction was inconsistent (in some of the patients not all anatomic parts of body where measured), the umbilicus circumference change was chosen as a constant parameter for statistical analysis and comparison. The umbilicus circumference change ranged between the loss of 5 cm to no change with a mean value of −2 cm (SD = ~1.5; **Table 2**).

In contrary to the circumference change, the weight change was low (**Table 2**) with a mean value of −0.0720 Kg and mean percentage of −0.0016% (SD = 0.01499), demonstrating stable weight of the cohort.

No adverse events were recorded during the whole period of trial. The side effects were limited to local bruises, which resolved during the next 4 to 9 days post-treatment. Temporary erythema, which accepted as positive end-point, lasted up to 60 minutes post-treatment.

During the 3-month follow up visit, no rebound of the body condition was detected (data not shown).

A linear correlation tests (R squared) between umbilicus's circumference change and weight change %, did not reveille strong statistical significant relation, with R^2 of 0.07 and sig = 0.260.

Also, there was no statistical significant relation between the umbilicus's circumference change and the age ($R^2 = 0.09$, sig = 0.299), height ($R^2 = 0.17$, sig = 0.409) or initial BMI of the patient ($R^2 = 0.20$, sig = 0.443).

Table 2. Descriptive statistics.

Parameter	N	Minimum	Maximum	Mean	Std. Deviation
Age	20	24	51	39.50	7.280
Weight (Kg)	20	49.50	80.90	61.5185	9.19776
BMI	20	18.78	28.41	22.3478	2.61494
Weight change (Kg)	20	−2.00	1.86	−0.0720	0.84627
Weight change %	20	−0.04	0.03	−0.0016	0.01499
Total circumference change (cm)	20	−25.0	−1.5	−10.150	5.9096
Umbilicus's circumference change (cm)	20	−5.00	0.00	−2.0000	1.46898

4. Discussion and Conclusions

This is well known that body shape and body image are negatively impacted by unwanted local subcutaneous fat. Therefore body contouring treatments are increasingly popular cosmetic procedures. Thermal stimulus by non-invasive systems can increase physiological breakdown of triglycerides within adipocytes. Besides, recent animal and human studies showed there was macrophage infiltration and delayed adipocytes cellular death or Apoptosis after an adipose tissue was exposed to therapeutic temperature at 43°C to 45°C for 15 minutes. Consequently, shrinkage of subcutaneous fat layer was resulted [13]-[14].

Most RF-based systems aimed for body shaping and contouring report 2 - 4 cm circumferential reductions in abdominal-hip measurements, and usually happy patients [2]-[8] [15]. Therefore it is not surprisingly that in current study the majority of the patients exhibited a substantial circumferential reduction, not at the expense of weight loss.

Two of the patients (patient No. 3 and 13) did not exhibit any circumferential reduction, according to the umbilicus measurements, but did show substantial circumferential reduction of the hip and tights (lower body). Here it is interesting to speculate about concept called redistribution of the fat, due to "fat communication" hormones or peptides. That is why when abdominal subcutaneous fat is reduced or influenced, measurement of other areas like frank, thighs, arms, even neck may also be reduced subsequently. View of the aforesaid, it is quite interesting to investigate this area in more scientific framework.

The lack of statistically significant correlation between umbilicus's circumference change and weight change, portraits the independent relation between the two, leaving the impressive loss of patients waists' circumferential reduction be the solely result of the treatment's course. The thermal stimulus by RF energy to the superficial adipose tissue, enhance the natural lipolysis.

When randomly selected six of the enrolled patients received additional series of treatment sessions (more than six sessions), the circumferential reduction further accelerated (data not shown). These patients exhibited up to 3 times more circumferential reduction reduced, compared to the achieved reduction after the first six treatment sessions (see Example in **Figure 1**). For example, patient No. 2 reduced only 0.5 cm according to umbilicus's measurements after the first six treatment sessions and additional 1.5 cm after additional six sessions (total—2 cm post 12 treatment sessions). This acceleration of clinical outcomes can be contributed to enhanced metabolic rate of the adipose tissue. This type of "buildup" in circumferential reduction can be assumed when the initial blood microcirculation in the treatment area is poor. While increasing the blood flow by the thermal influence of RF energy, every consecutive treatment will lead to greater physiological response, due to increase in skin conductivity and the ability to reach higher end point temperature during the treatment [11].

Three of the patients enrolled in currents study were also treated on additional body areas, including underarms, hips and thighs with notable improvement in circumferential reduction (**Table 3**). Due to very small sample size of the additional areas, only abdomen area was chosen for statistical analysis. In addition, abdominal measurements were the most consistent, while other areas were highly variable and differentiated in measurement (some measurements were missing or taken in different locations on the body or position) which affected the variability of the patients.

Although no significant correlation was found between the circumferential measurements and initial patients parameters, it could have been interesting to check the correlation between the clinical outcomes and the patient's gender due to physiological/metabolic differences between the genders. In women, lipid changes occur more slowly within the femoral region than within the abdominal region; the adipocytes within the femoral region are

Table 3. Circumferential reduction on additional body areas.

Circumferential Reduction (cm)	Patient No. 3	Patient No. 8	Patient No. 17
Hip	−5.50	−3.00	NA
Right thigh	−2.50	NA	−2.50
Left thigh	−1.50	NA	−2.50
Right arm	NA	−1.50	NA
Left arm	NA	−1.50	NA

NA: Not Available.

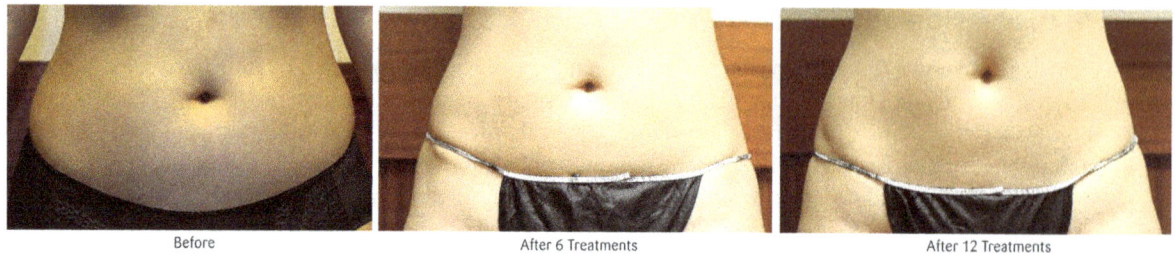

Figure 1. 38-year-old female patient, before, after 6 and 12 abdomen contouring treatments with bi-polar RF device.

larger and are influenced by female sex hormones. They are metabolically more stable and resistant to lipolysis [13]. But, since the male group in this study was relatively low (only 6 males), statistical examination of this theory was impossible.

Safety issues are main concern in performing aesthetic procedures. This non-invasive bi-polar RF-based system delivers therapeutic thermal energy selectively to subcutaneous adipose tissues without causing damages to surrounding epidermis, dermis and muscles.

Since RF energy, in contrary to light energy, produces an electrical current, epidermal melanin reminds unscathed, making the RF-based devices as a safe choice for patients of all skin types.

Facial aging are resulted from combination effects of gravity, reduced skin elasticity, rearrangement of subcutaneous volume, change in supporting bony structure and etc. There may be areas of fat accumulation such as at lower face, submental and submandibular regions, which are particularly common in aging Asians.

Recently, the safety and efficacy of the system was also evaluated on Asian patients with facial aging and local facial fat accumulation (data not shown). A group of 15 participants underwent a treatment course of 4 - 8 sessions and showed notable facial skin tightening, upward repositioning of facial volume and reduction in excessive fat accumulation at lower face and neck regions.

In conclusion, the bi-polar RF system, which is a bi-polar RF system utilizing multiple frequencies of RF together with vacuum associated mechanical pressure, is a safe and effective treatment option of non-invasive body contouring and localized fat reduction among Asian population.

References

[1] Sadick, N.S. and Mulholland, R.S. (2004) A Prospective Clinical Study to Evaluate the Efficacy and Safety of Cellulite Treatment Using the Combination of Optical and RF Energies for Subcutaneous Tissue Heating. *Journal of Cosmetic and Laser Therapy*, **6**, 187-190. http://dx.doi.org/10.1080/14764170410003039

[2] Alster, T.S. and Tanzi, E.L. (2005) Cellulite Treatment Using a Novel Combination Radiofrequency, Infrared Light, and Mechanical Tissue Manipulation Device. *Journal of Cosmetic and Laser Therapy*, **7**, 81-85. http://dx.doi.org/10.1080/14764170500190242

[3] Zachary, C.B., Mian, A. and England, L.J. (2009) Effects of Monopolar Radiofrequency on the Subcutaneous Fat Layer in an Animal Model [Abstracts]. *American Society for Laser Medicine and Surgery*, **38**, 105.

[4] Anolik, R., Chapas, A.M., Brightman, L.A. and Geronemus, R.G. (2009) Radiofrequency Devices for Body Shaping: A Review and Study of 12 Patients. *Seminars in Cutaneous Medicine and Surgery*, **28**, 236-243.

[5] Goldberg, D.J., Fazeli, A. and Berlin, A.L. (2008) Clinical, Laboratory, and MRI Analysis of Cellulite Treatment with a Unipolar Radiofrequency Device. *Dermatologic Surgery*, **34**, 204-209. http://dx.doi.org/10.1097/00042728-200802000-00009

[6] Emilia del Pino, M., Rosado, R.H., Azuela, A., Graciela Guzmán, M., Argüelles, D., *et al.* (2006) Effect of Controlled Volumetric Tissue Heating with Radiofrequency on Cellulite and the Subcutaneous Tissue of the Buttocks and Thighs. *Journal of Drugs in Dermatology*, **5**, 714-722.

[7] Kaplan, H. and Gat, A. (2009) Clinical and Histopathological Results Following TriPollar Radiofrequency Skin Treatments. *Journal of Cosmetic and Laser Therapy*, **11**, 78-84. http://dx.doi.org/10.1080/14764170902846227

[8] Teitelbaum, S.A., Burns, J.L., Kubota, J., Matsuda, H., Otto, M.J., *et al.* (2007) Noninvasive Body Contouring by focused Ultrasound: Safety and Efficacy of the Contour I Device in a Multicenter, Controlled, Clinical Study. *Plastic and Reconstructive Surgery*, **120**, 779-789. http://dx.doi.org/10.1097/01.prs.0000270840.98133.c8

[9] Shek, S.Y., Chan, N.P. and Chan, H.H. (2012) Non-Invasive Cryolipolysis for Body Contouring in Chinese—A First Commercial Experience. *Lasers in Surgery and Medicine*, **44**, 125-130. http://dx.doi.org/10.1002/lsm.21145

[10] McRae, E. and Boris, J. (2013) Independent Evaluation of Low-Level Laser Therapy at 635 nm for Non-Invasive Body Contouring of the Waist, Hips, and Thighs. *Lasers in Surgery and Medicine*, **45**, 1-7. http://dx.doi.org/10.1002/lsm.22113

[11] Belenky, I., Margulis, A., Elman, M., Bar-Yosef, U. and Paun, S.D. (2012) Exploring Channeling Optimized Radio-frequency Energy: A Review of Radiofrequency History and Applications in Esthetic Fields. *Advances in Therapy*, **29**, 249-266. http://dx.doi.org/10.1007/s12325-012-0004-1

[12] Chan, H.H.L. (2005) Effective and Safe Use of Lasers, Light Sources, and Radiofrequency Devices in the Clinical Management of Asian Patients with Selected Dermatoses. *Lasers in Surgery and Medicine*, **37**, 179-185. http://dx.doi.org/10.1002/lsm.20244

[13] Franco, W., Kothare, A., Ronan, S.J., Grekin, R.C. and McCalmont, T.H. (2010) Hyperthermic Injury to Adipocyte cells by Selective Heating of Subcutaneous Fat with A Novel Radiofrequency Device: Feasibility Studies. *Lasers in Surgery and Medicine*, **42**, 361-370. http://dx.doi.org/10.1002/lsm.20925

[14] Weiss, R., Weiss, M., Beasley, K., Vrba, J. and Bernardy, J. (2013) Operator Independent Focused High Frequency ISM Band for Fat Reduction: Porcine model. *Lasers in Surgery and Medicine*, **45**, 235-239. http://dx.doi.org/10.1002/lsm.22134

[15] Brightman, L., Weiss, E., Chapas, A.M., Karen, J., Hale, E., *et al.* (2009) Improvement in Arm and Post-Partum Abdominal and Flank Subcutaneous Fat Deposits and Skin Laxity Using a Bipolar Radiofrequency, Infrared, Vacuum and Mechanical Massage Device. *Lasers in Surgery and Medicine*, **41**, 791-798. http://dx.doi.org/10.1002/lsm.20872

22

Clinical and Biochemical Evaluation of Facial Acanthosis Nigricans

Khalifa E. Sharquie[1,2*], Adil A. Noaimi[1,2], Halla G. Mahmood[3], Sameerah M. Al-Ogaily[4]

[1]Department of Dermatology, College of Medicine, University of Baghdad, Baghdad, Iraq
[2]Arab Board for Dermatology & Venereology, Baghdad Teaching Hospital, Medical City, Baghdad, Iraq
[3]Department of Clinical Biochemistry, College of Medicine, University of Baghdad, Baghdad, Iraq
[4]Department of Dermatology, Baghdad Teaching Hospital, Medical City, Baghdad, Iraq
Email: [*]ksharquie@ymail.com, adilnoaimi@yahoo.com, halla_ghazi@yahoo.com,
drsameraalokailimahde@yahoo.com

Abstract

Background: Acanthosis nigricans is a well known cause of facial melanosis in Iraqi males and usually it is a part of ordinary acanthosis nigricans. It is commonly associated with many metabolic derangements. Objectives: To evaluate cases of acanthosis nigricans of the face for all metabolic disturbances including fasting blood sugar, fasting serum insulin, total cholesterol, triglyceride, growth hormone and serum leptin. Patients and Methods: Twenty seven cases of acanthosis nigricans of the face were included in this case descriptive, clinical and biochemical study. This was conducted in Department of Dermatology-Baghdad Teaching Hospital and Department of Clinical Biochemistry, College of Medicine, Baghdad, Iraq during the period from November 2012-August 2014. It consisted of 26 males and one female, their ages ranged from 16 - 58 (39 ± 4.9) years. The diagnosis was established by clinical and histopathological evaluation. Sharquie's ANSI scoring of acanthosis nigricans of face was carried out for all patients, also body mass index was assessed. Biochemical evaluation was carried out for all patients including total cholesterol, triglyceride, fasting blood sugar and insulin, insulin resistance, growth hormone and leptin enzyme immunoassay. Twenty seven healthy control non obese individuals with comparable ages and gender were assessed for all tests. Results: Biochemical results showed that fasting blood glucose, fasting serum insulin, insulin resistance, fasting serum triglyceride, total cholesterol, growth hormone and serum leptin were statistically significantly high in patients with acanthosis nigricans of the face in comparison with control individuals and all were positively correlated with the scoring of acanthosis nigricans of the face apart from high density lipoprotein was negatively correlated. Conclusion: Acanthosis nigricans of the face is a good marker for the associated metabolic diseases and these metabolic changes were statistically significantly correlated with the severity of acanthosis nigricans.

---

[*]Corresponding author.

Keywords

Acanthosis Nigricans, Face, Sharquie's Ansi Scoring, Facial Melanosis, Biochemical Changes

1. Introduction

Acanthosis nigricansis (AN) a skin disease characterized by hyperpigmented, thickened, verrucous plaques with a velvety texture typically symmetrical in distribution. It usually involves intertriginous areas including: neck, axillae, groin, antecupital and popliteal fossae, knuckles and umbilicus; occasionally it involves the mucosa such as oral, esophageal, pharyngeal, laryngeal, conjunctival, and anogenital mucosa [1]. The earliest changes in acanthosis nigricans of the face are usually dryness, pigmentation and roughness of the skin, which in affected area is gray-brown or black [1]. The hyperpigmentation is later accompanied by hypertrophy, increased skin marking, and velvety texture. The most commonly involved locations are the forehead, temples, nasolabial folds and cheeks [2]. Facial melanosis although is commonly caused by acanthosis nigricans of the face among adult males [3] but unfortunately was not reported and documented in the medical literatures until *Sharquie et al.* 2014, 2015 published their work. This study showed that acanthosis nigricans of the face has the same clinical and histopathological features of acanthosis of neck and axillae mainly pigmentation of the skin, thickening with or without velvety appearance and acanthosis with or without papillomatosis together with epidermal and dermal melanosis [2].

Acanthosis nigricans has a variety of causes but the likely common mechanism is stimulation of tyrosine kinase growth factor receptor signaling pathways in epidermis [4]. In insulin resistance syndromes, high levels of circulating insulin directly or indirectly activate the insulin-like growth factor 1 receptor (IGF1R) [5]. Insulin resistance due to obesity underlies the hyperinsulinaemia in obesity-associated acanthosis nigricans [6] [7]. An elevated fasting blood insulin level confirms the presence of hyperinsulinaemia underling the diagnosis of atypical acanthosis nigricans [8]. In malignant acanthosis nigricans, tumor deriver growth factors, in particular transforming growth factor-α, acting through the epidermal growth factor receptor (EGFR) is presumed, although anti-insulin receptor antibodies have also been implicated [9].

The metabolic disorder parameters like fasting blood sugar, fasting serum insulin, total cholesterol, triglyceride, serum growth hormone and serum leptin were not evaluated before. So the aim of present work is to assess these metabolic markers and to be correlated with the severity of acanthosis nigricans of the face.

2. Patients and Methods

This case descriptive, clinical and biochemical study was conducted in the Department of Dermatology-Baghdad Teaching Hospital and Department of Clinical Biochemistry, College of Medicine, Baghdad, Iraq during the period from November 2012 to August 2014. Twenty seven patients were enrolled in this study 26 males and 1 female. The nature and aim of this study were explained for each patient. Formal consent was taken from them before this study and photographs were taken. Also, the ethical approval was given by the Scientific Council of Dermatology & Venereology-Iraqi Board for Medical Specializations.

Clinical and histopathological study of acanthosis nigricans of the face of these patients were already published [2].

Body mass index for all patients were calculated in addition the atherogenic co-efficiency, atherogenic index plasma and cardiac risk ratio were assessed.

Color photographs for all patients were performed by 8 megapixels camera of mobile Samsung Galaxy Note II, in the same place and distance with fixed illumination.

Sharquie's ANSI scoring [2] was carried out for all patients regarding the followings:

Score 1 = Light brown;

Score 2 = Brown;

Score 3 = Dark brown;

Score 4 = Black.

1) Texture: Scoring from 0 - 3

Score 0 = No thickening;

Score 1 = Mild thickening;

Score 2 = Moderate thickening;

Score 3 = Severe thickening.

2) Percentage of the total area involved, this was measured by using transparent square paper. By this method the acanthosis nigricanc and the total surface areas were measured accurately by square centimeters, then the percentage of the acanthosis nigricansarea relative to the total area of the same region was measured and scoring was done as follows:

a) Forehead:

Score 1 = 1% - 25%;

Score 2 ≥ 25% - 50%;

Score 3 ≥ 50% - 75%;

Score 4 ≥ 75%.

b) Cheek:

Score 1 = 1% - 25%;

Score 2 ≥ 25% - 50%;

Score 3 ≥ 50% - 75%;

Score 4 ≥ 75%.

c) Nasolabial folds:

Score 1 = 1% - 25%;

Score 2 ≥ 25% - 50;

Score 3 ≥ 50% - 75%;

Score 4 ≥ 75%.

d) Temporal area:

Score 1 = 1% - 25%;

Score 2 ≥ 25% - 50%;

Score 3 ≥ 50% - 75%;

Score 4 ≥ 75%.

The scoring for each area were done separately including: forehead, right temporal, left temporal, right cheek, left cheek, right nasolabial fold and left nasolabial fold for all patients.

The **ANSI score** was calculated by the following equation:

$$\text{ANSI} = \left(\text{DF} + \text{TF} + \text{AF}\right) + \left(\text{DTR} + \text{TTR} + \text{ATR}\right) + \left(\text{DTL} + \text{TTL} + \text{ATL}\right) + \left(\text{DCR} + \text{TCR} + \text{ACR}\right)$$
$$+ \left(\text{DCL} + \text{TCL} + \text{ACL}\right) + \left(\text{DNR} + \text{TNR} + \text{ANR}\right) + \left(\text{DNL} + \text{TNL} + \text{ANL}\right).$$

where D is darkness, T is thickness, A is area, F is forehead, TR is right temporal, TL is left temporal, CR is right cheek, CL is left cheek, NR is right nsolabial, NL is left nasolabial [2].

The following biochemical tests were carried out: fasting blood sugar (FBS), fasting insulin, total cholesterol, triglyceride which determined by enzymatic methods, growth hormone and serum leptin enzyme immunoassay for the quantitative determination in human serum were used. DRG international Inc. USA is done by ELISA test and the results were correlated with the severity of acanthosis nigricans (Sharquie's ANSI score) using coefficient correlation.

Twenty seven healthy control individuals with age and gender matching with the patients of acanthosis nigricans of the face were studied for the same biochemical blood changes.

Data were statistically described in terms of range, mean, standard deviation (±SD), mode of frequencies (number of cases) and relative frequencies (percentages). Comparison between investigations of patients and controlled individuals was done using Chi square (x^2) test. A probability value (p value) less than 0.05 was considered significant. All statistical calculations were done using computer programs SPSS ver. 20 (Statistical Package for the Social Science; SPSS Inc. Chicago, IL, USA).

3. Results

Twenty seven patients with acanthosis nigricans of the face were included in this study, 26 (96.6%) males and 1 (3.3%) female, with a male to female ratio was 26:1. Their ages ranged from 16 - 58 years with a mean ± SD of 39 ± 4.9 years. The third and fourth decades of life were the commonest age groups affected. The duration of the disease ranged from 1 - 8 years with a mean ± SD of 3.34 ± 5.67 years. All patients had bilateral symmetrical distribution of acanthosis nigricans on the face (**Figure 1**) in addition to acanthois nigricans of neck and axillae. No patients with underling malignancies, clinical diabetes or other important medical conditions were noted.

Twenty seven healthy control were assessed, 25 males and 2 females, their ages ranged from 18 - 56 years with a mean ± SD of 40 ± 2.93 years. the body mass index was ranged from 23 - 29.3 with a mean ± SD of 27 ± 0.93 (**Table 1**).

Normal weight was seen in 4 (13.3%) patients while overweight seen in 10 (33.3%) patients, and obese in 16 (53.3%) patients. The body mass index (BMI) ranged from 24.1 - 38 with a mean ± SD of 32.33 ± 0.72. So BMI was found to be highly significant elevated in patients with acanthosis nigricans of the face in comparison with healthy control individuals with P value = 0.00545.

Fasting blood sugar (P value = 0.00141), fasting serum insulin (P value = 0.00150), Homa-insulin resistance (P value = 0.00157), growth hormone (P value = 0.061446), Serum leptin (P value = 0.01550), total cholesterol (P value = 0.0014) and triglyceride (P value = 0.0032) were statistically significantly elevated in comparison with healthy control. Also, cardiac risk ratio (CRR) (P value = 0.001) and atherogenic coefficient (AC) (P value = 0.005) and atherogenic index plasma (AIP) (P value = 0.003) were highly significantly elevated (**Table 1**).

Sharquie's ANSI score was ranged from 4 - 62 and was positively correlated with the following parameter: serum insulin (r = 0.925), total cholesterol (r = 0.968), AIP (r = 0.95), AC (r = 0.976), serum leptin (r = 0.889) growth hormone (r = 0.945) and fasting blood sugar (r = 0.943), while there was negative correlation with HDL (r = 0.913) (**Figures 2-6**). (r = *coefficient correlation*).

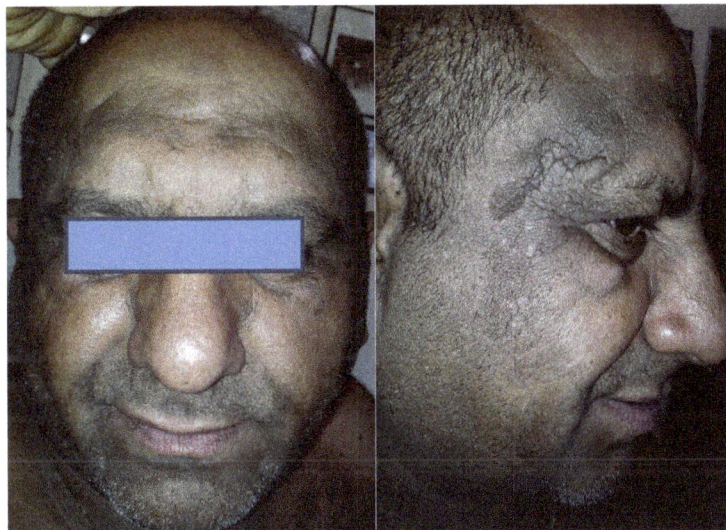

Figure 1. Bilateral symmetrical distribution of acanthosis nigricans on the face.

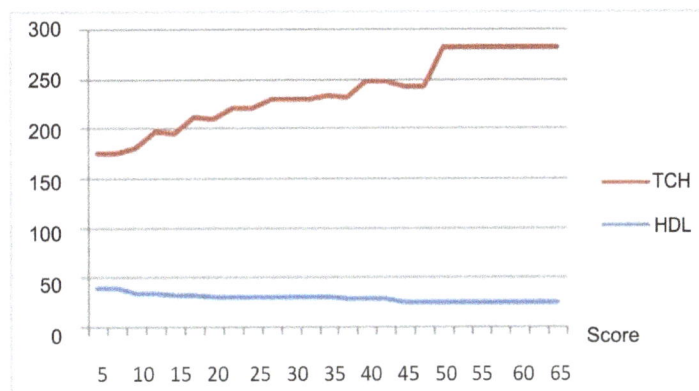

Figure 2. Showing the correlation between ANSI score & HDL & TCH levels.

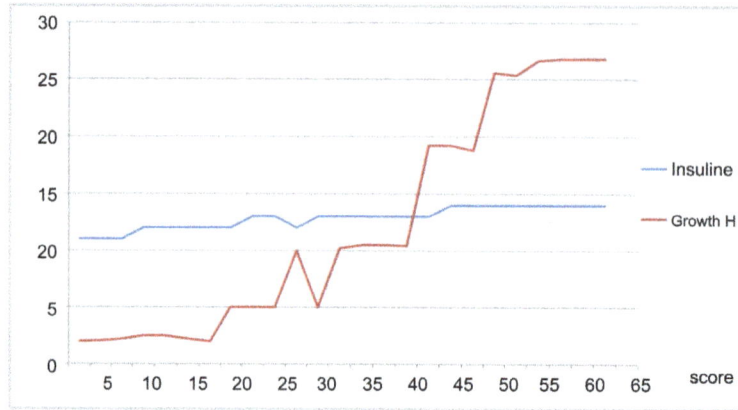

Figure 3. Showing the correlation between ANSI score & insulin & growth hormone levels.

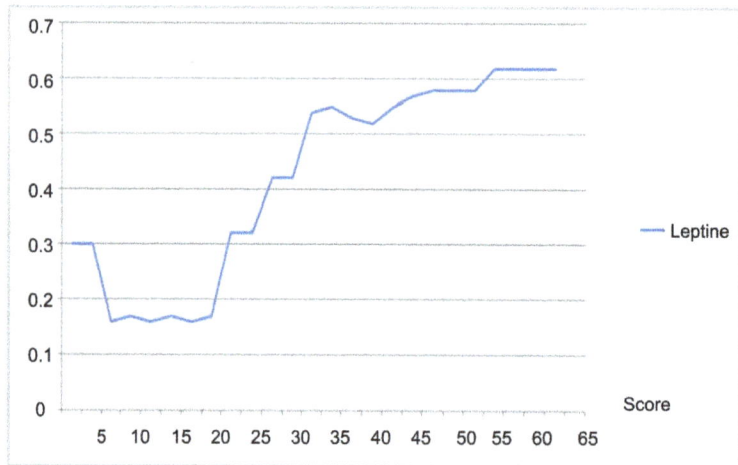

Figure 4. Showing the correlation between ANSI score & leptin level.

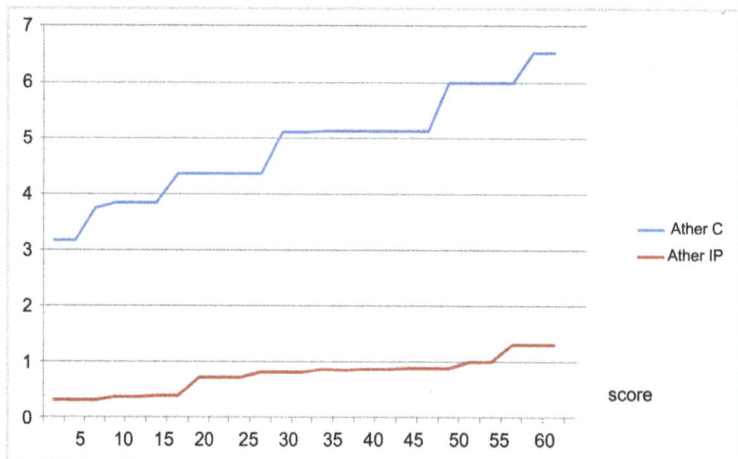

Figure 5. Showing the correlation between ANSI score & AC & AIP levels.

4. Discussion

Acanthosis nigricans is commonly associated with obesity and might be associated with many metabolic disturbances like diabetes mellitus, elevated cholesterol and HBA1c [2]. No malignancies or drugs induced acanthosis

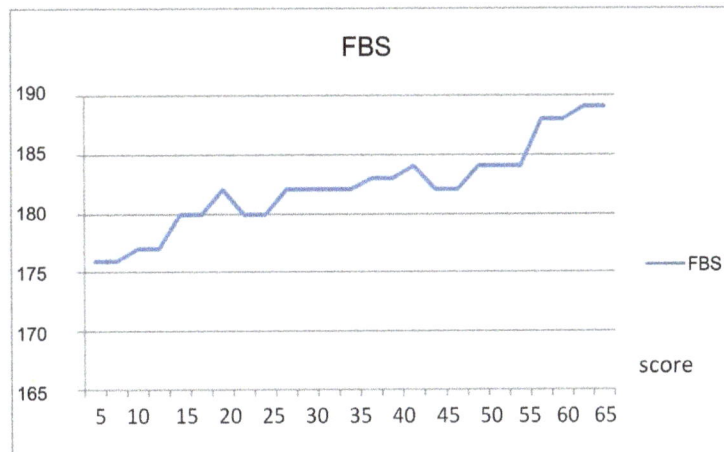

Figure 6. Showing the correlation between ANSI score & FBS levels.

Table 1. The result of fasting blood sampling from 27 patients with acanthosis nigricans of the face in comparison with 27 healthy controls.

	Control	Patients	P-value
Age	40 ± 2.93	39 ± 4.97	NS
BMI (Kg/m^2)	27 ± 0.93	32.33 ± 0.72	HS
FBG (mg/dl)	96.4 ± 3	180.3 ± 2.16	HS
Insulin (μIU/ml)	10.76 ± 0.4	12.3 ± 0.9	HS
Homa-IR	2.57 ± 0.1	5.46 ± 0.36	HS
Leptin (mg/dl)	0.38 ± 0.25	0.479 ± 0.07	S
CRP (mg/dl)	2.078 ± 0.432	$1.68 \pm o.79$	S
GH (ng/ml)	5.66 ± 0.10	13.16 ± 9.43	S
TC (mg/dl)	187.3 ± 10.78	191.75 ± 34.34	HS
TG (mg/dl)	121 ± 9.55	223 ± 44	HS
HDL-C (mg/dl)	49.8 ± 6.78	33.12 ± 3.9	HS
CRR	3.80 ± 0.31	5.70 ± 1.21	HS
AC	2.80 ± 0.31	4.82 ± 1.03	HS
AIP	0.39 ± 0.03	0.85 ± 0.24	HS

nigricans were included in the present work.

The present study showed that Sharquie's ANSI score of acanthosis nigricans of the face was well correlated with the severity of acanthosis nigricans and body mass index. This score was also statistically significantly correlated with the following biochemical changes: FBS, fasting insulin, total cholesterol, triglyceride, growth hormone and serum leptin.

The present work also showed patients with acanthosis nigricans of the face had hyperinsulinemia and insulin resistance and this explain the pathogenesis of acanthosis nigricans like thickening of the epidermis and increased melanin deposition as was similarly reported about ordinary acanthosis nigricans [10], similarly this study also demonstrated elevated growth hormone in majority of cases of acanthosis nigricans of the face and this hormone also increase the activity of fibroblast and keratinocyte and play a role in pathogenesis of acanthosis nigricans. Serum leptin also elevated in majority of patients in the present study and this might explain the increased obesity among patients with acanthosis nigricans [11].

Total cholesterol and triglyceride were significantly elevated in majority of patients with decreased high density lipoprotein that lead to increase in cardiac risk ratio, atherogenic coefficient andatherogenic index plasma. These findings are very important as you can judge the changes in these parameter just by looking at the acanthosis nigricans of the face. To the best of our knowledge these findings are for the first time to be reported.

5. Conclusion

In conclusion, acanthosis nigricans of the face is an important cause of facial melanosis among Iraqi males where its clinical pictures and associated manifestations were similar to acanthosis nigricas of the body. Also, acanthosis nigricans of the face is a marker for many metabolic and biochemical changes in blood like elevated fasting blood sugar and lipid. Sharquie's ANSI scoring of acanthosis nigricans of the face was positively correlated with all biochemical changes.

Disclosure

This study was an independent study and not funded by any drug companies.

References

[1]   Houp, K.R. and Crus, P.D. (1999) Acanthosis Nigricans. In: Fitzpatrick, T.B., Freedberg, I.M., Eison, A.Z., Wolff, K., Austen, K.F., Gold Smith, L.A. and Katz, S.I., Eds., *Fitzpatrick's Dermatology in General Medicine*, 5th Edition, McGraw-Hill Book Company, New York, **40**, 244-252.

[2]   Sharquie, K.E., Noaimi, A.A. and Al-Ogaily, S.M. (2015) Acanthosis Nigricans as a Cause of Facial Melanosis (Clinical and Histopathological Study). *IOSR Journal of Dental and Medical Science*, **14**, 84-90.

[3]   Sharquie, K.E. and Noaimi, A.A. (2014) Gazelle Eye like Facial Melanosis (Clinico-Histopathological Study). *Journal of Pigmentary Disorders*, **2**, 111.

[4]   Judge, M.R., Mclean, W.H.I. and Munro, C.S. (2010) Disorder of Keratinization. *Tony B. Stephen B. Rook Textbook of Dermatology*, 8th Edition, Wiley-Blackwell, 119-120.

[5]   Torley, D., Bellus, G.A. and Munro, C.S. (2002) Genes, Growth Factors and Acanthosis Nigricans. *British Journal of Dermatology*, **147**, 1096. http://dx.doi.org/10.1046/j.1365-2133.2002.05150.x

[6]   Skiljevic, D.S., Nikolic, M.M. and Jakovljevic, A. (2001) Generalized Acanthosis Nigricans in Early Childhood. *Pediatric Dermatology*, **18**, 213-218. http://dx.doi.org/10.1046/j.1525-1470.2001.018003213.x

[7]   Kahn, C.R., Flier, J.S. and Bar, R.S. (1999) The Syndromes of Insulin Resistance and Acanthosis Nigricans: Insulin Receptor Disorders in Man. *New England Journal of Medicine*, **294**, 739-754. http://dx.doi.org/10.1056/NEJM197604012941401

[8]   Haase, I. and Hunzelmann, N. (2002) Activation of Epidermal Growth Factor Receptor, ERK Signaling Correlates with Suppressed Differentiation in Malignant Acanthosis Nigricans. *Journal of Investigative Dermatology*, **118**, 891-893. http://dx.doi.org/10.1046/j.1523-1747.2002.17631.x

[9]   Cruz, P.D.G. and Hud, J.A.J. (1992) Excess Insulin Binding to Insulin-Like Growth Factor Receptor: Proposed Mechanism for Acanthosis Nigricans. *Journal of Investigative Dermatology*, **98**, 825-855. http://dx.doi.org/10.1111/1523-1747.ep12462293

[10]   Habif, T.P. (2004) Cutaneous Manifestations of Internal Disease: Acanthosis Nigricans. Clinical Dermatology: A Color Guide to Diagnosis and Therapy, 4th Edition, Mosby Company, Philadelphia, **10**, 900-901.

[11]   Considine, R.V. Sinha, M.K., Heiman, M.L., Kriauciunas, A., Stephens, T.W., Nyce, M.R., Ohannesian, J.P., Marco, C.C., Mckee, L.J., Bauer, T.L. and Caro, J.F. (1996) Serum Immunoreactive-Leptin Concentration in Normal-Weight and Obese Humans. *New England Journal of Medicine*, **334**, 292-295. http://dx.doi.org/10.1056/NEJM199602013340503

23

Treatment of Basal Cell Carcinoma by Topical 25% Podophyllin Solution

Khalifa E. Sharquie[1]*, Adil A. Noaimi[1], Mohammad S. Al-Zoubaidi[2]

[1]Department of Dermatology, College of Medicine, University of Baghdad Iraqi and Arabic Board of Dermatology, Baghdad, Iraq
[2]Department of Dermatology, Baghdad Teaching Hospital, Medical City, Iraq
Email: *ksharquie@ymail.com, adilnoaimi@yahoo.com, mkhrabit@yahoo.com

Academic Editor: Reich Adam, Wroclaw Medical University, Poland

Abstract

Background: Basal cell carcinoma is the most common malignancies of the skin. Numerous modalities of treatment are available. Podophyllin is an antimitotic and caustic agent that has been used in treatment of genital warts. Objective: To test the effectiveness and safety of topical 25% podophyllin in treatment of basal cell carcinoma. Patients and Methods: Thirty eight patients with basal cell carcinoma enrolled in this open labeled interventional study that had been enrolled in Department of Dermatology-Baghdad Teaching Hospital, Baghdad, from January 2010 to October 2011. History and physical examination was performed to all patients regarding all demographics detail related to the disease. Exclusion criteria: were pregnancy, recurrent tumors, aggressive deep subtypes, morpheaic type, and size more than 2 cm^2 in diameter. Biopsies for all patients were done for histopathological examination at the first visit, and after clinical cure of the lesions. Lesions were treated with 25% topical podophyllin solution once weekly for 6 weeks. Follow up after clinical cured was done every 3 months up to 18 months to recording any sign and symptom of recurrent. Results: Thirty five patients with basal cell carcinoma completed the study: 28 (80%) males and 7(20%) females with males to females ratio 4:1, their ages ranged from 30 - 87 (64.114 ± 12.68) years, and the duration of the disease ranged from 2 months to 30 years (6.88. ± 4.83) years. The size of lesions ranged from 0.8 - 1.9 (1.454 ± 0.239) cm. The total podophyllin applications number ranged from 2 - 6 (4.65 ± 1.055) sessions. The total numbers of treated lesions were 100 lesions: 64 (64%) nodular, 31(31%) pigmented, 3(3%) Basosquamous, and 2 (2%) superficial. Ninety six (96%) lesions in 32 patients showed complete cure with 2 - 6 sessions, while 4 lesions in 3 patients showed partial response with 6 sessions. Biopsy from 21 cured lesions in 21 patients showed complete clearness apart from one with residual malignant cells. All the patients did not show clinical recurrence, during the follow up period up to 18 months. Inflammatory reactions were noted in all treated lesions as redness, edema and juicy skin 36 - 72 hours after topical po-

---

*Corresponding author.

dophyllin applications. After 3 - 5 days, the reaction became more exaggerated and ulceration developed, ended with crust formation. No evidence of systemic side effects was seen and this had been confirmed clinically and by laboratory during the sessions and one month later. Minimal or no scarring was noticed. Conclusions: Topical 25% podophyllin solution is a new, effective therapeutic modality in treatment of basal cell carcinoma which gives 96% cure, and it is highly recommended as alternative therapy in all type of basal cell carcinoma, single and multiple and for all ages especially for elderly patients and those who have surgeries phobia.

Keywords

BCC, Podophyllin, Topical Therapy

1. Introduction

Basal cell carcinoma (BCC) is the most common malignancy in worldwide [1], account for approximately 75% of all skin cancers [2]. It emerges from keratinocytes stem cells, in hair follicles, sebaceous glands, or interfollicular basal cells. Generally, most BCC cases are sporadic, but it may also appear in genetic disorders such as Goblin's syndrome and xeroderma pigmentosum [3] [4]. The majority of sporadic cases are induced by sunlight, specifically ultraviolet-B rays [5]. It commonly appears on the head and neck, or the back, but uncommon on the back of the hands and forearm. There is no known "precursor" lesion for basal cell carcinoma [6]. The incidence rate of this disease has been estimated to have increased between 20% - 80% worldwide over the last three decades [1]. Mortality rate is low but basal cell carcinoma may occasionally grow aggressively causing extensive tissue destruction [2]. It is usually slowly growing and rarely metastasizing, and the metastatic potential rates are ranging from 0.0028% - 0.1%. The metastasis commonly occurs in the regional lymph nodes and lungs [7]. The major risk factor for BCC development is a patient's cumulative exposure to ultraviolet light [8].

There are many standard therapeutic modalities which have been used in treatment of basal cell carcinoma including surgical excision [9], curettage with electrodessication [10], cryotherapy [11], and radiotherapy [12]. Moh's micrographic surgery [13], photodynamic therapy (PDT) [14], laser therapy [15], intralesional interferon [16] and intralesional zinc sulphate 2% [17]. Moreover, topical remedies such as Imiquimod [18], 5-flurouracil [18] and tazarotene [19] also have been used. However, many side effects were encountered with this medication [18] [19].

Podophyllin is the dried resin extracted from the roots and rhizomes of *Podophyllum peltatum* known as American mandrake, May apple, Ducks' foot and Indian apple. It is an antimitotic and caustic agent, a lipid-soluble compound with cytotoxic properties that easily cross cell membranes leads to inhibit cell mitosis and DNA synthesis by reversibly binding to tubulin; the protein subunit of the spindle microtubules thereby prevents polymerization of tubulin into microtubules; cell division is arrested and other cellular processes are impaired. It often causes local necrosis and death of tumor cells and erosion of the tissues. Podophyllin is indicated for the treatment of condyloma acuminatum (venereal warts), seborrhoeic, actinic, and roentgen ray keratoses; and juvenile papilloma of the larynx [20]-[25]. There is a local side effects associated with topical podophyllins such as erythema, tenderness, pruritus, burning, erosions, pain, and swelling [20] [26]. There are systemic side effects if extensive podophyllin treatment is used for large area, sub-dermal injection or ingestion [27] [28].

Accordingly, the aim of the present study is to use 25% podophyllin as topical therapy for treatment of different types of basal cell carcinoma.

2. Patients and Methods

Thirty eight patients with basal cell carcinoma enrolled in this open, labeled interventional study had been enrolled in Department of Dermatology and Venereology-Baghdad Teaching Hospital, Baghdad, Iraq, from January 2010 - October 2011.

History was taken from each patient regarding to: age, gender, site, duration, smoking, and alcohol intake. Close clinical examination was done for each patient. Skin photo-type was established for all patients according to Fitzpatrick's classification and any signs of sun damage were recorded. Basal cell carcinoma lesions were assessed including their numbers, site, morphology, size, color and lymph nodes examination was performed to all patients. Exclusion criteria: were pregnancy, recurrent tumors and those with more aggressive subtypes, morpheaic type of BCC, and size more than 2 cm^2 in diameter. Shave or incision biopsies were done for clinical and histopathological examination for all patients at the first visit, and after clinical cure of the lesions.

Formal consent was taken before the start the therapy, after full explanation about the nature of the disease, course, the procedure of treatment, follow up, prognosis and the need for pre and post treatment photographs. Also, ethical approval was performed by the Scientific Council of Dermatology and Venereology-Iraqi Board for Medical Specializations. Digital photographs were taken using SONY Cyber-Shot T300 10.1 MP for each patient in good illumination.

The lesions treated with 25% topical podophyllin solution once weekly for 6weeks. And the follow up was done after clinical cure every 3 months up to 18 months to record recurrence rate of the lesions after clinical cured.

2.1. Preparation of Topical 25% Podophyllin Solution and the Way of Use

Podophyllum Resin 25% Topical Solution USP prepared by mixing 25 grams of the alcohol-soluble extract of podophyllum resin in alcohol and 10 grams of the alcohol-soluble extract of benzoin in alcohol, and diluting with alcohol to make 100 ml The solution was applied by a wood stick applicator and the lesion was covered with thin layer of solution. The amounts used in each session depend on the size of lesion but always not exceeding 0.5 ml. The solution was allowed to dry in approximately 3 minutes and patients were instructed to wash off it after 5 hours. The solution was applied once weekly for maximum of 6 weeks and the number of applications depend on rate of response of the lesions [20].

2.2. Statistical Descriptive

1) Excel program has been used for the statistical analysis.
2) Mean, standard deviation, and percentage of the treated cases calculated to show the values of the results.
3) Table and figure has been used to present the results.

3. Results

Thirty five patients with basal cell carcinoma completed the study: 28 (80%) males and 7 (20%) females with males to females ratio 4:1, their ages ranged from 30 - 87 (64.114 ± 12.68) years, and the duration of the disease ranged from 2 months to 30 years (6.88. ± 4.83) years. The size of lesions ranged from 0.8 - 1.9 cm (1.454 ± 0.239) cm. The total podophyllin applications number ranged from 2 - 6 (4.65 ± 1.055) sessions. The total numbers of treated lesions were 100 lesions: 64 (64%) nodular, 31 (31%) pigmented (**Figures 1-7**), 3 (3%) Basosquamous (**Figure 8**), and 2 (2%) superficial.

Ninety six (96%) lesions in 32 patients showed complete clinical cure with 2 - 6 (4.65 ± 1.055) sessions. while 4 lesions in 3 patients showed partial response with 6 sessions. Biopsy from 21 lesions in 21 patients showed complete clearness apart from one with residual malignant cells (4.76%). All the patients did not showed any clinical recurrence, up to 18 months.

Inflammatory reaction was noted in all treated lesions as redness, edema and juicy skin 36 - 72 hours after topical podophyllin. After 3 - 5 days, the reaction became more exaggerated and ulceration developed, ended with crust formation.

No evidence of systemic side effects was seen, and this had been confirmed clinically and by laboratory during the sessions and 1months later.

Although all lesions recovered completely after podophyllin application, but we noticed that different types of BCC might respond differently as superficial and ulcerative BCC responded more quickly within 4.5 ± 1.09 sessions (**Figure 6** and **Figure 7**), while the nodular type needed much longer time and more application in order to achieve full cure and usually with 5.15 ± 0.812 sessions (**Figures 1-5**, **Figure 8** and **Figure 9**).

Regarding the side effects, no evidence of systemic side effects was found in any of these cases, and this had been confirmed by clinical examination and laboratory results including blood picture, liver, and renal function tests. Minimal or no scarring was noticed in all lesions but postinflammatory hyperpigmentation was observed in 3 cases and one patient developed transient hypopigmentation. But generally this therapy gave nice cosmetic result.

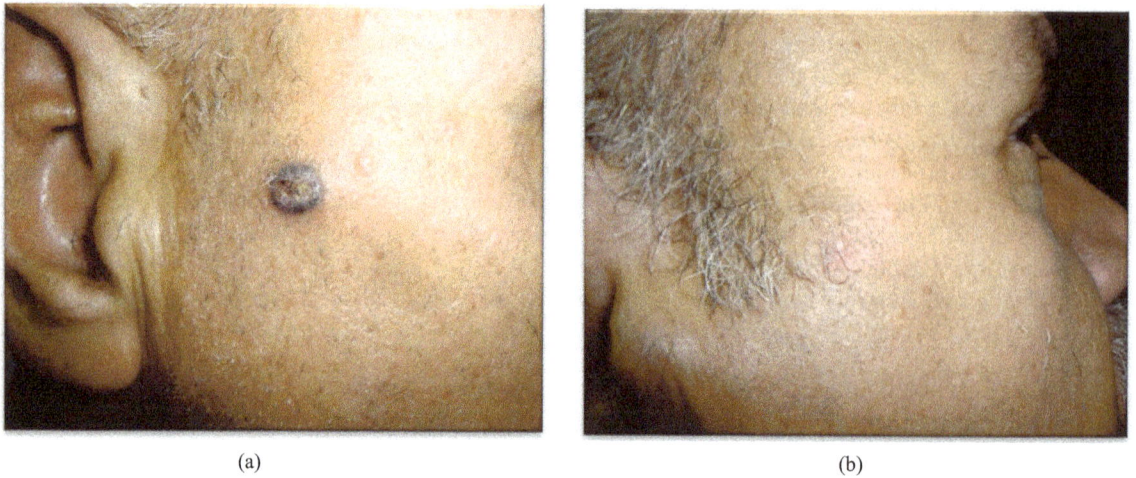

Figure 1. (a) Pigmento-nodular BCC before treatment with podophyllin, (b) the same lesion above after podophyllin application, after 4 sessions.

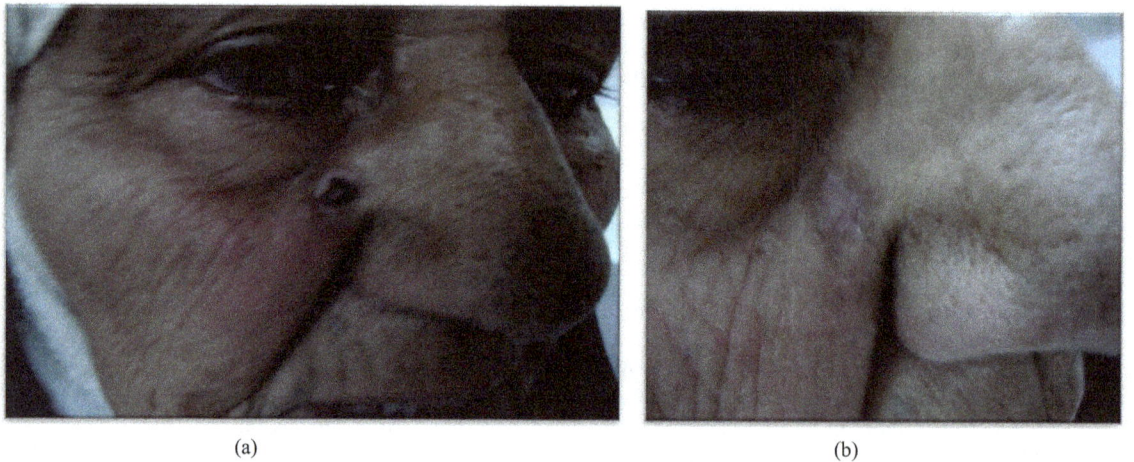

Figure 2. (a) Nodulopigmented BCC on the nasolabal fold, (b) the same patient with full clinical cure after podophyllin application, after 5 sessions.

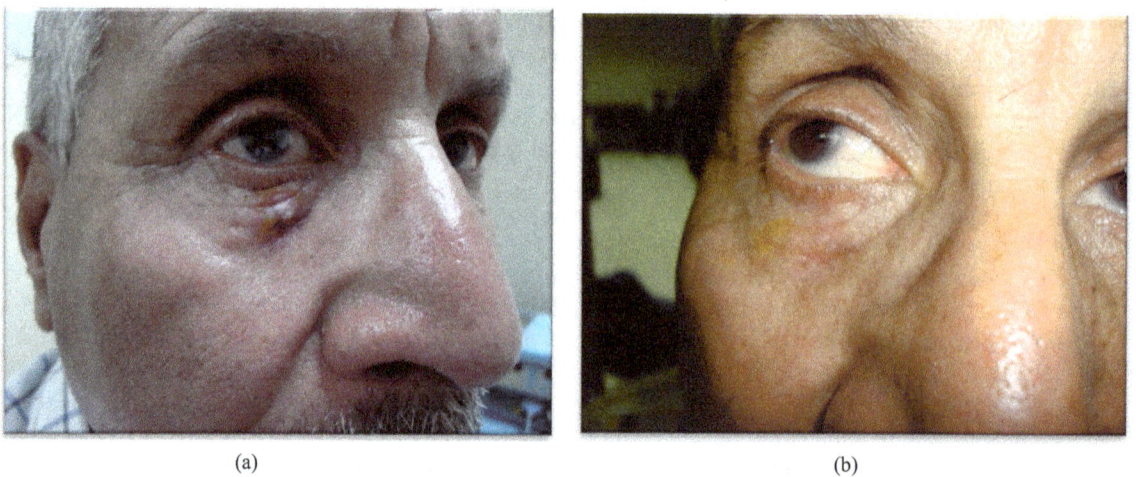

Figure 3. (a) Showing 65 years old patient with nodular BCC near eye lid before podophyllin application, (b) the same patient above after podophyllin application. After 5 sessions.

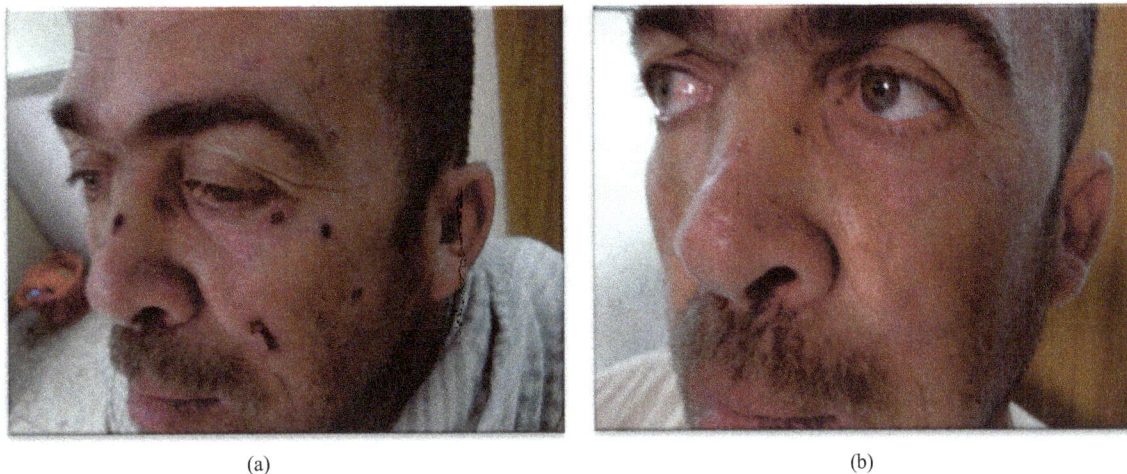

Figure 4. (a) Showing 30 years old male presenting with Gorlin's syndrome and multiple BCC before podophyllin application, (b) the same patient with Gorlin's syndrome after 6 sessions of podophyllin application.

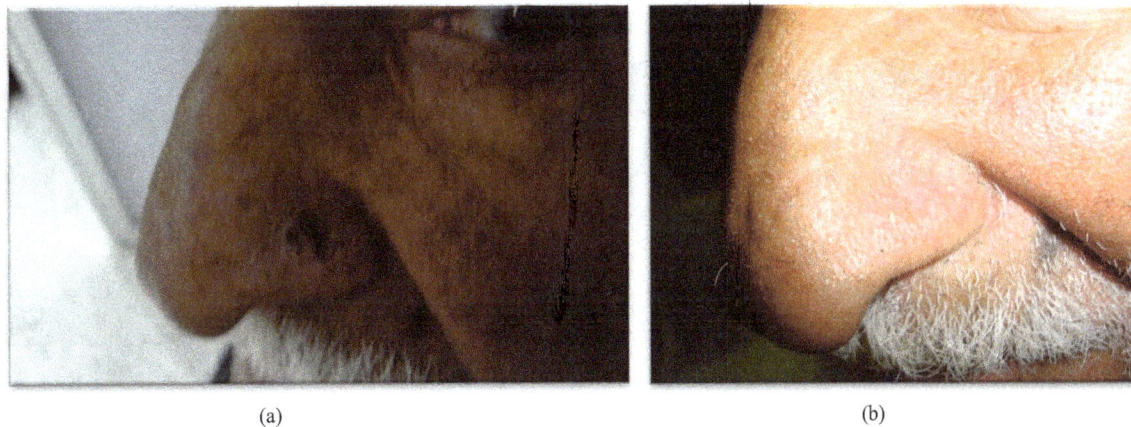

Figure 5. (a) A 75 years old male showing nodular BCC on ala nasi before podophyllin application, (b) the same patient above after 4 session of podophyllin application.

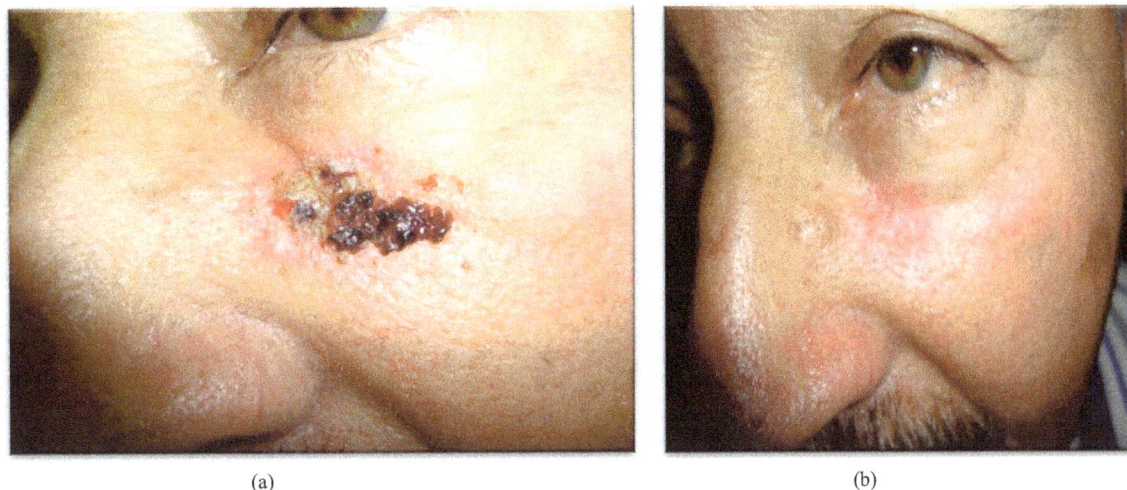

Figure 6. (a) Showing ulcerative BCC on face before treatment with topical podophyllin, (b) the same patient above after podophyllin application. After 4 sessions.

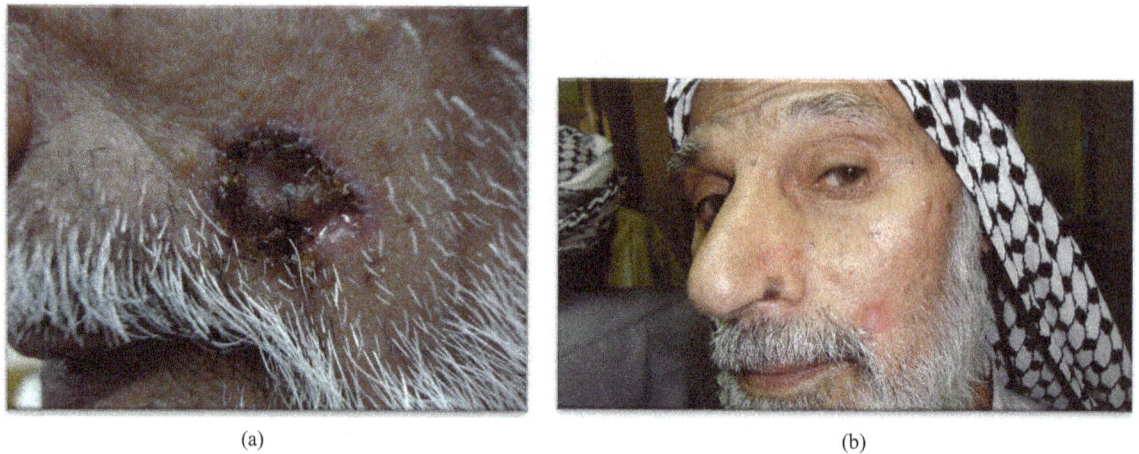

Figure 7. (a) Noduloulcerative BCC nasolabial before podophyllin application, (b) the same patient after podophyllin application. After 4 sessions.

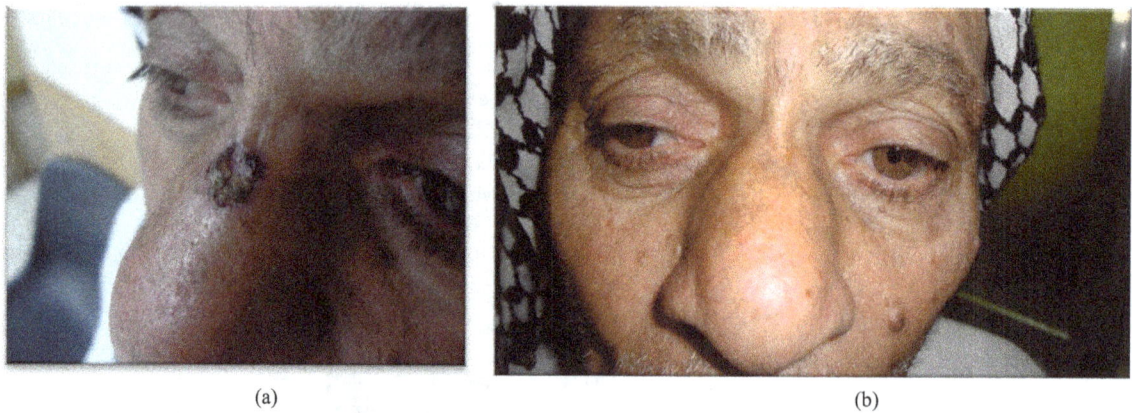

Figure 8. (a) Showing patient with Basosquamous cell carcinoma on the nose before treatment with podophyllin, (b) the same patient showing a full cure after with podophyllin application. After 6 sessions treatment.

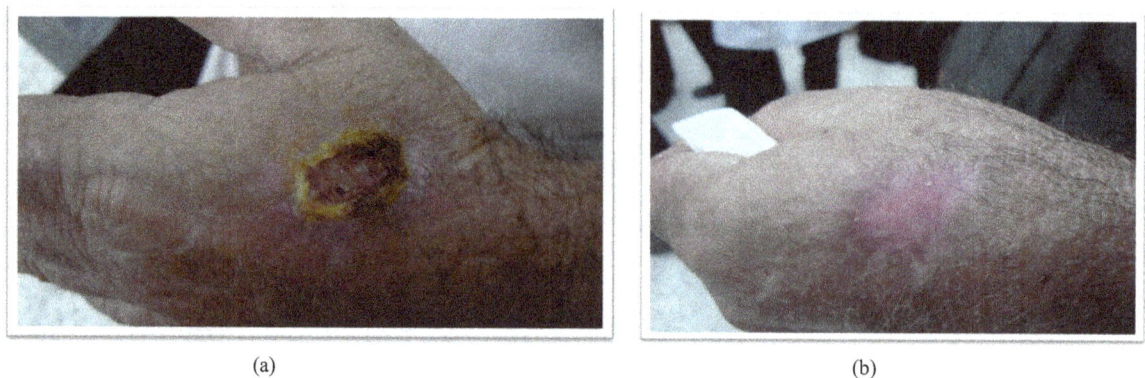

Figure 9. (a) BCC on dorsum of the left hand before podophyllin application, (b) the same patient showing a full cure after podophyllin application after 5 sessions.

4. Discussion

There are controversies whether to use surgical or non surgical therapy for basal cell carcinoma but the clinicians always search for simple, non costly, easy procedure in order to achieve cure. There are many standard therapeutic modalities used in treatment of BCC including surgical excision [9], curettage with electrodessication [10], cryotherapy [11], and radiotherapy [12]. Moh's micrographic surgery [13], photodynamic therapy (PDT) [14], laser therapy [15], intralesional interferon [16], and intralesional zinc sulphate 2% [17]. Moreover topical remedies such as Imiquimod [18], 5-flurouracil [18], tazarotene [19], also have been used. However many side effects were encountered with this medication [18] [19].

Topical Imiquimod is approved by food and drug administration (FDA) only for superficial BCCs as large as 2 cm in diameter located on the neck, trunk, or extremities. Cure rates for nonaggressive subtypes of BCC have ranged from 60% - 100% [29] [30]. Local side effects include erythema, hardened skin, edema, and vesiculation, and erosion, ulceration, scabbing, and flaking. It can have systemic effects such as headache, gastrointestinal disturbances, nausea, and vomiting. Therefore, topical 5% Imiquimod cream applied once daily 5 days per week for at least 6 weeks [31] [32].

Topical 5-FU is usually used in cases of low-risk BCCs especially superficial BCCs. 5-FU can be used for multiple BCCs on the trunk and extremities, but it is not indicated for nodular BCCs. However, this compound is not strong enough to eliminate tumors with extensive invasion or involving a patient' follicles [33] [34]. It can cure up to 95% of superficial BCCs [15]. Solution and cream formulations of 5% 5-FU application twice daily for at least 6 weeks, for superficial BCCs, However , therapy may be required for as long as 10 to 12 weeks [31].

Tazarotene has been preliminarily shown to be efficacious in the regression of small superficial and nodular BCC when applied topically in 0.1% gel formulation over a range of 6 weeks to 8 months, with one study reporting complete regression without recurrence to be 30.5% at 3-year follow-up [19].

The present work is the first well established extensive study to be reported as it is showed 96% cure and it is a superior when compared with other topical therapies like Imiquimod, 5-FU, and tazarotene as gave a high cure rates, no relapse, recovery with short time, no post treatment scarring and no systemic and minimal topical side effects.

Topical 25% podophyllin solution had been used in treatment of superficial, nodular, ulcerative, pigmented BCCs in head, neck, and all over the body, for the single and multiples BCCs in sporadic and genodermatosis one, with diameter equal or less than 2 cm^2. All the lesions of BCC that treated with topical podophyllin has been cured by 2 to 6 session with cure rates 96%. The side effects that had seen in this work are local side effects and as follow: erythema, edema, ulceration, with or without slight pain following by crust formation. No systemic toxicity has been shown.

Cure rate in the present study was 96% which is high, in comparison with other topical therapeutic modalities used in the treatment of basal cell carcinoma: as the treatment for nonaggressive subtypes of BCC with topical Imiquimod 5% cream have cure rates ranged from 60% to 100%, and this topical medication is approved by FDA only for superficial BCCs as large as 2 cm in diameter located on the neck, trunk, or extremities [29] [30]. while we using the topical podophyllin in all areas of the head, face, the neck, trunk, and the extremities. In addition Imiquimod need more application and it is costly in comparison to the podophyllin. The comparison the topical 5-FU in treatment BCC with topical podophyllin, we found that the topical 5-FU is usually used in cases of low-risk BCCs specially superficial BCCs [33], and it can be used for multiple BCCs on trunk and extremities, but it not indicated for nodular BCC [34]. It can cure up to 95% of superficial BCC, and therapy may be required for as long as 6 to 10 weeks [15], while we using the topical podophyllin for superficial and nodular BCC in high and low-risk areas and for 6 weeks once weekly. Topical podophyllin has fewer side effects than topical Imiquimod and 5-FU. Topical podophyllin is much superior to Imiquimod and 5-FU.and the side effects of podophyllin is could be considered as part of mechanism of action as unless there is a reaction, there will be not cure. Accordingly these are not side effects.

5. Conclusion

Topical 25% podophyllin solution is a new, effective therapeutic modality in treatment of basal cell carcinoma which gives 96% cure in all varieties of basal cell carcinoma. It is highly recommended for any age and any type of basal cell carcinoma but especially for elderly patients and those who have surgeries phobia.

References

[1]   Mikilineni, R. and Weinstock, M.A. (2001) Epidemiology of Skin Cancer. In: *Atlas of Clinical Oncology: Skin Cancer*, BC Decker, London, 1-15.

[2]   Akinci, M., Aslan, S., Morkoc, F. and Cetin, A. (2008) Metastatic Basal Cell Carcinoma. *Acta Chirurgica Belgica*, **108**, 269-272.

[3]   Lacour, J.P. (2002) Carcinogenesis of Basal Cell Carcinoma: Genetics and Molecular Mechanism. *British Journal of Dermatology*, **146**, 17-19. http://dx.doi.org/10.1046/j.1365-2133.146.s61.5.x

[4]   Kogerman, P., Krause, D. and Rahnama, F. (2002) Alternative First Exons of *PTCH*1 Are Differentially Regulated *in Vivo* and May Confer Different Functions to the PTCH1 Protein. *Oncogene*, **21**, 6007-6016. http://dx.doi.org/10.1038/sj.onc.1205865

[5]   Kim, M., Park, H.J. and Baek, S. (2002) Mutations of the P53 and PTCH Gene in Basal Cell Carcinoma: UV Mutation Signature and Strand Bias. *Journal of Dermatological Science*, **29**, 1-6.

[6]   Nouri, K., Christopher, J., Ballard, B.S., Asha R., Patel, B.S. and Brasie, R.A. (2008) Basal Cell Carcinoma. Skin Cancer, The McGraw-Hill Companies.

[7]   Ting, P.T., Kasper, R. and Arlette, J.P. (2005) Metastatic Basal Cell Carcinoma: Report of Two Cases and Literature Review. *Journal of Cutaneous Medicine and Surgery*, **9**, 10-15.

[8]   Hoban, P.R., Ramachandran, S. and Strange, R.C. (2002) Environment, Phenotype and Genetics: Risk Factors Associated with BCC of the Skin. *Expert Review of Anticancer Therapy*, **2**, 570-579. http://dx.doi.org/10.1586/14737140.2.5.570

[9]   Grabski, W.J. and Salasche, S.J. (1998) Positive Surgical Excision Margins of A Basal Cell Carcinoma. *Dermatologic Surgery*, **24**, 921-924. http://dx.doi.org/10.1111/j.1524-4725.1998.tb04276.x

[10] Nouri, K., Spencer, J. and Taylor, J. (1999) Does Wound Healing Contribute to the Eradication of Basal Cell Carcinoma Following Curettage and Electrodessication? *Dermatologic Surgery*, **25**, 183. http://dx.doi.org/10.1046/j.1524-4725.1999.08128.x

[11] Kaur, S., Thami, G.P. and Kanwar, A.J. (2003) Basal Cell Carcinoma-Treatment with Cryosurgery. *Indian Journal of Dermatology, Venereology and Leprology*, **69**, 188-190.

[12] Mendenhall, W.M., Amdur, R.J., Hinerman, R.W., Cognetta, A.B. and Mendenhall, N.P. (2009) Radiotherapy for Cutaneous Squamous and Basal Cell Carcinomas of the Head and Neck. *The Laryngoscope*, **119**, 1994-1999. http://dx.doi.org/10.1002/lary.20608

[13] Tierney, E.P. and Hanke, C.W. (2009) Cost Effectiveness of Mohs Micrographic Surgery: Review of the Literature. *Journal of Drugs in Dermatology*, **8**, 914-922.

[14] Foley, P. (2005) Clinical Efficacy of Methyl Aminolevulinate Photodynamic Therapy in Basal Cell Carcinoma and Solar Keratosis. *Australasian Journal of Dermatology*, **46**, S8-S10.

[15] Padgett, J.K. and Hendrix, J.D. (2001) Cutaneous Malignancies and Their Management. *Otolaryngologic Clinics of North America*, **34**, 523-553. http://dx.doi.org/10.1016/S0030-6665(05)70004-9

[16] Kim, K.H., Yavel, R.M. and Gross, V.L. (2004) Intralesional Interferon Alpha-2b in the Treatment of Basal Cell Carcinoma and Squamous Cell Carcinoma: Revisited. *Dermatologic Surgery*, **30**, 116-120.

[17] Sharquie, K.E., Al-Nuaimy, A.A. and Al-Shmary, F.A. (2005) New Intralesional Therapy for Basal Cell Carcinoma by 2% Zinc Sulphate Solution. *Saudi Medical Journal*, **26**, 359-361.

[18] Love, W.E., Bernhard, J.D. and Bordeaux, J.S. (2009) Topical Imiquimod or Fluorouracil Therapy for Basal and Squamous Cell Carcinoma: A Systematic Review. *Archives of Dermatology*, **145**, 1431-1438. http://dx.doi.org/10.1001/archdermatol.2009.291

[19] Bianchi, L., Orlandi, A., Campione, E., Angeloni, C., Costanzo, A. and Spagnoli, L.G. (2004) Topical Treatment of Basal Cell Carcinoma with Tazarotene: A Clinicopathological Study on a Large Series of Cases. *British Journal of Dermatology*, **151**, 148-156. http://dx.doi.org/10.1111/j.1365-2133.2004.06044.x

[20] United State Pharmacopeia Committees (Eds.) (2004) Podophyllin. In: United State Pharmacopeia Committees, Eds., *Drug Information for the Health Care Professional*, 24th Edition, Rev. US Convention Inc., Thomason Micromedex, 2341-2348.

[21] Podophyllum (Topical). Drugs.com. Know More Be Sure. Update 3 August 2000. http://www.drugs.com/mmx/podocon-25.html

[22] Katzung, B.G. (1992) Basic and Clinical Pharmacology. 5th Edition, Appleton and Lange, Norwalk, 884.

[23] Martin, E.C., Christy, L., Cowan, M.C., Marshal, S.W., Dawson, A.H., Seifert, S.A., Schon, W.S., Yip, L., Keyes, D.C., Hurlbut, K.M. and Erdman Arm Dart, R.C. (Eds). (2004) Medical Toxicology. 3rd Edition, Chap. 255, Walters Kluwer Company, Philadelphia, 1690-1691.

[24] Lin, M.C., Cheng, H.W., Tsai, Y.C., Liao, P.L. and Kang, J.J. (2009) Podophyllin Induced Genotoxicity *in Vitro* and *in Vivo* through ROS Production. *Drug and Chemical Toxicology*, **32**, 68-76.

http://dx.doi.org/10.1080/01480540802433757

[25]   Rahman, A.U., Ashraf, M., Choudhary, M.I., Rehman, H.U. and Kazmi, M.H. (1995) Antifungal Aryltetralin Lignans from Leaves of *Podophyllum hexandrum*. *Phytochemistry*, **40**, 427-431. http://dx.doi.org/10.1016/0031-9422(95)00195-D

[26]   Beutner, K.R. and Ferenczy, A. (1997) Therapeutic Approaches to Genital Warts. *The American Journal of Medicine*, **102**, 28-37. http://dx.doi.org/10.1016/S0002-9343(97)00181-2

[27]   Moore, M.M. and Strober, B.E. (2008) Topical and Intralesional Cytotoxic Agent. In: Wolff, K., Goldsmith, L.A., Katz, S.I., Gilchrest, B.A., Paller, A.S. and Leffell, D.J., Eds., *Fitzpatrick's Dermatology in General Medicine*, 7th Edition, Chap. 220, McGraw-Hill-Company, New York, 2124.

[28]   Habif, T.P. (2004) Sexually Transmitted Viral Infection. In: Habif, T.P., Ed., *Clinical Dermatology*, 4th Edition, Chap. 11, Mosby Inc., Toronto, 336-342.

[29]   Huber, A., Huber, J.D. and Skinner, R.B. (2004) Topical Imiquimod Treatment for Nodular Basal Cell Carcinomas: An Open-Label Series. *Dermatologic Surgery*, **30**, 429-430. http://dx.doi.org/10.1097/00042728-200403000-00023

[30]   Vidal, D., Matias-Guiu, X. and Alomar, A. (2004) Open Study of the Efficacy and Mechanism of Action of Topical Imiquimod in Basal Cell Carcinoma. *Clinical and Experimental Dermatology*, **29**, 518-525. http://dx.doi.org/10.1111/j.1365-2230.2004.01601.x

[31]   Efudex (Fluorouracil) Topical Solution and Cream (Product Pamphlet). ICN Pharmaceuticals, Inc., Costa Mesa, 2000.

[32]   Berman, B., Sullivan, T. and De Araujo, T. (2003) Expression of Fas-Receptor on Basal Cell Carcinomas after Treatment with Imiquimod 5% Cream or Vehicle. *British Journal of Dermatology*, **149**, 59-61. http://dx.doi.org/10.1046/j.0366-077X.2003.05634.x

[33]   Lawrence, C.M. (1999) Mohs Micrographic Surgery for Basal Cell Carcinoma. *Clinical and Experimental Dermatology*, **24**, 130-133. http://dx.doi.org/10.1046/j.1365-2230.1999.00433.x

[34]   Reymann, F. (1979) Treatment of Basal Cell Carcinoma of the Skin with 5-Fluorouracil Ointment. *Dermatologica*, **158**, 368-372. http://dx.doi.org/10.1159/000250782

24

Sarcoidosis-Lymphoma Syndrome: A Spectrum of One Disease

Khalifa E. Sharquie*, Raafa K. Al-Hayani, Waqas S. Abdulwahhab,
Abd-Allah S. Mohammed

The Scientific Council of Dermatology and Venereology-Iraqi and Arab Board for Medical Specializations,
Department of Dermatology and Venereology, Baghdad Teaching Hospital,
College of Medicine, University of Baghdad,
Baghdad, Iraq
Email: *ksharquie@ymail.com, raafahayani@yahoo.com

Abstract

Lymphoma might occur in association with sarcoidosis or sarcoidosis might be combined with lymphoma, in so called ("sarcoidosis-lymphoma syndrome"). This syndrome is well reported in medical literature. The question, which one starts before is difficult to answer, as in some cases sarcoidosis starts first then is followed by lymphoma but in other cases during the course of lymphoma sarcoid reaction might be seen. In the present report, we describe a case of 60 years male patient that is presented with a rash with classical sarcoid pathology that overtime changes into typical lymphoma ended with death.

Keywords

Sarcoidosis, Lymphoma, Granuloma

1. Introduction

Sarcoidosis is well known as a multisystem disease of unknown etiology characterized by the presence of non-caseating granuloma in affected organs. The disease may affect any organ but most commonly involves the lungs, skin, and eyes. Clinically, patients may be completely asymptomatic or experience a progressive clinical course [1].

The etiology of sarcoidosis remains unknown and the disease remains a diagnosis of exclusion. The current understanding regarding the pathogenesis of the disease involves the exposure of a genetically susceptible individual to some environmental antigenic stimulus. The genetic predisposition may affect not only the occurrence

---

*Corresponding author.

of disease but also the clinical expression and course. To date, the precise nature of the environmental stimulus remains unknown, although numerous leads and theories have been investigated and continue to be explored. Despite these efforts, the ability to identify a specific cause for this disease remains elusive [2].

Treatment is usually designed to help relieve the symptoms and thus does not directly alter the course of the disease [3]. This treatment usually consists of anti-inflammatory drugs like ibuprofen or aspirin [3]. In cases where the condition develops to the point that it has a progressive and/or life-threatening course, the treatment is most often steroid treatment with prednisolone [4]. Alternatively, drugs that are most commonly used to treat cancer and suppress the immune system, such as methotrexate, azathioprine and leflunomide, may be used [3] [4].

The disease can remit spontaneously or become chronic, with exacerbations and remissions. In some persons, it can progress to pulmonary fibrosis and death. About half of cases resolve without treatment or can be cured within 12 - 36 months, and most within five years. Some cases, however, may persist several decades [4]. Two-thirds of people with the condition achieve a remission within 10 years of the diagnosis. Overall mortality ranges from 1% - 6% [1]. When the heart is involved, the prognosis is generally less favorable, although, corticosteroids appear effective in improving AV conduction [5].

The association between lymphoma and sarcoidosis was first suggested by Bichel and Brincker in the 1960s [6]. Since then, additional descriptions of this possible connection have been published but without providing a better understanding of this relationship [1]. The sarcoidosis-lymphoma syndrome descried by Brincker [7] [8] was established on the basis of 2 different studies. In a Danish registry of patients with respiratory sarcoidosis, lymphoma occurred 11.5 times more frequently than expected in the general population [8].

Second, Brincker [7] reviewed 46 cases of lymphoma occurring in patients with sarcoidosis. He reported only 2 cases in which lymphoma preceded sarcoidosis with an additional 2 cases in a subsequent study [9]. Sarcoidosis patients are about 40% - 60% more likely to develop malignancy, including solid tumors such as non-melanoma skin cancers (three-fold risk), renal cancer, and nonthyroid endocrine tumors [10].

Cases have been published in which sarcoidosis precedes lymphoma and vice-versa, albeit they can infrequently appear simultaneously. Sarcoidosis may precede the development of a lymphoma (the "sarcoidosis-lymphoma syndrome") by 18 months to 28 years [11]. All types of lymphoma may develop, and there is an increased incidence of thyroid cancer and leukaemia [12].

In the present case report, we are describing a patient that has first sarcoidosis and then changes into lymphoma. The aim of present report is to describe atypical spectrum of sarcoidosis-lymphoma state. The consent form taken from patient's family is about the publication of his condition.

2. Case Report

We present the case of a 60 years old male patient who was being referred to the dermatological department in Baghdad Teaching Hospital from Tikrit Teaching Hospital suspecting Kaposi sarcoma and complaining of recurrent, multiple, mildly itchy skin lesions all over the body mainly on the extremities for 3 years duration. No other systemic complaints were mentioned. Physical examination revealed multiple, diffuse, well-defined brown nodules and plaques distributed all over the body excluding the face, palms, soles, scalp, and genitalia. The surfaces of those lesions were smooth, non-scaly, and dusky color. The nodules not tethered to the overlying skin **Figure 1**.

Provisional diagnosis of kaposi sarcoma was raised but to our surprise the histopathological picture was typical of granulomatous reactions that are seen in sarcoidosis **Figure 2**.

This finding alerts our attention to look for sarcoidosis. Tuberculin test was negative. Routine hematologic investigations were normal. Serum calcium, liver function tests (LFT), & renal function tests (RFT) were within the normal level. Nothing was seen by ophthalmological examination. On Chest-XR mild hilar LAP was detected. High resolution CT-Scan showed bilateral diffuse ground glass-masses, and bilateral multiple enlarged hilar and paratracheal LAP. The patient was classified as having stage II sarcoidosis. Accordingly the patient was given 30 mg/day prednisolone for 2 weeks with dramatic clearance of most of the skin lesions **Figure 3**.

However, 3 months later and suddenly after steroid tapering, the patient develop new, asymptomatic, rapidly growing solitary cutaneous lesion which reached several centimeters in size within only 2 weeks on the right side of his chest, with reactivation of another old lesion on the right leg, this new finding had brought the patient back again to our department.

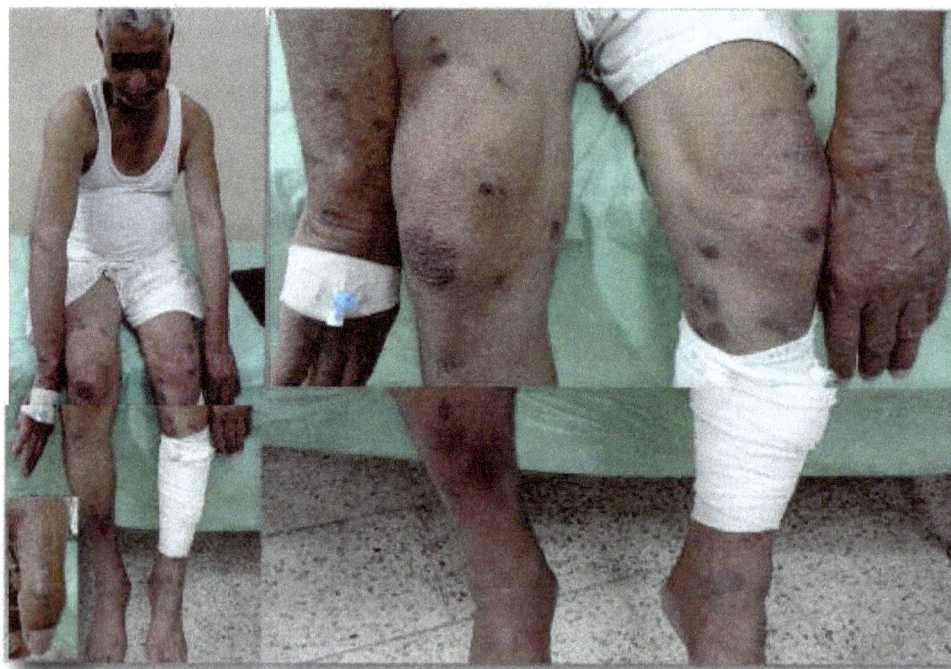

Figure 1. A 60 years old male patient with 3 years history of multiple, diffuse, well-defined brown nodules and plaques over many parts of the body, with smooth, non-scaly, and dusky color.

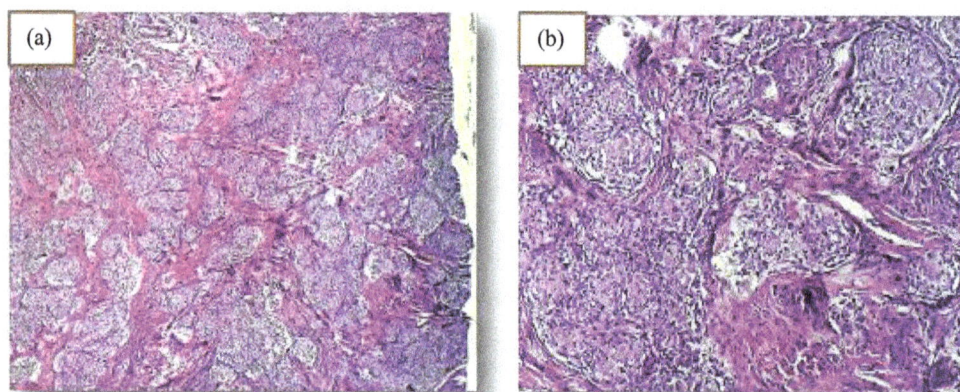

Figure 2. Hematoxylin & eosin (H & E) stained section showed typical naked granulomas involving the whole dermis; (a) original magnification ×10; (b) original magnification ×40.

Physical examination revealed solitary, about 5 cm in diameter, erythematous, smooth surface, arciform, mass located on the lower right axillary line. Another solitary, about 3 cm in diameter, hyperpigmented, with fine scaly surface, nodule was also found on the lateral aspect of the right leg. No palpable LAP **Figure 4** and **Figure 5**.

Incisional biopsy was taken from the mass on the chest for Histopathological study. Routine hematologic investigations were normal. Liver function tests (LFT), & renal function tests (RFT) were normal. Chest-XR was normal. Patient asked to repeat the course of steroid therapy (15 mg/day) plus zinc sulphate 440 mg/day until the diagnosis confirmed, and again surprisingly, the mass disappeared completely within 2 weeks of therapy. However, the histopathological study showed diffuse atypical lymphocytic infiltrate of the dermis and subcutaneous fat with frequent mitotic figures a picture of CTCL, but no granuloma was seen **Figure 6**.

Then shortly after steroid and zinc sulphate weaning, the patient develop sudden eruption of multiple, slightly itchy skin lesions involving the abdomen and thigh. Physical examination showed multiple, erythematous, subcutaneous nodules distributed symmetrically over the abdomen and both thighs, No LAP **Figure 7**.

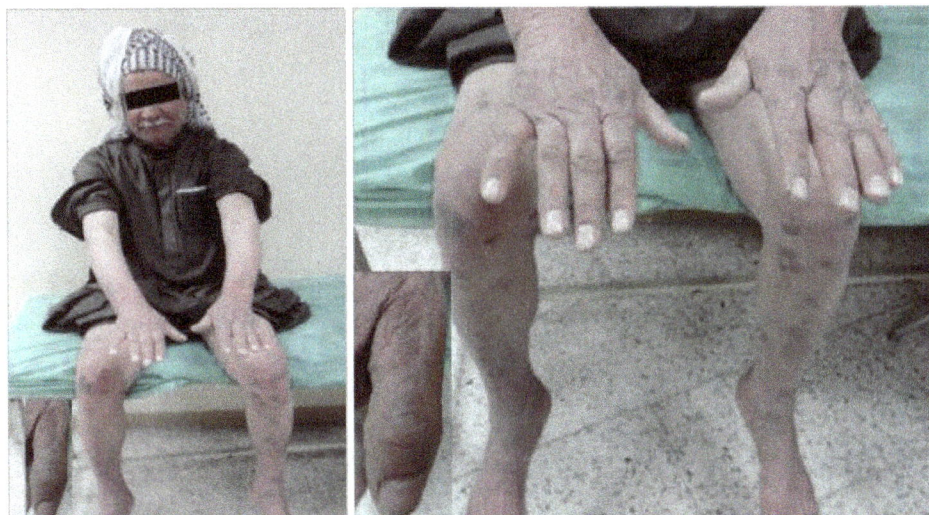

Figure 3. The same patient above after 2 weeks of treatment with 30 mg/day prednisolone with dramatic clearance of most of the skin lesions.

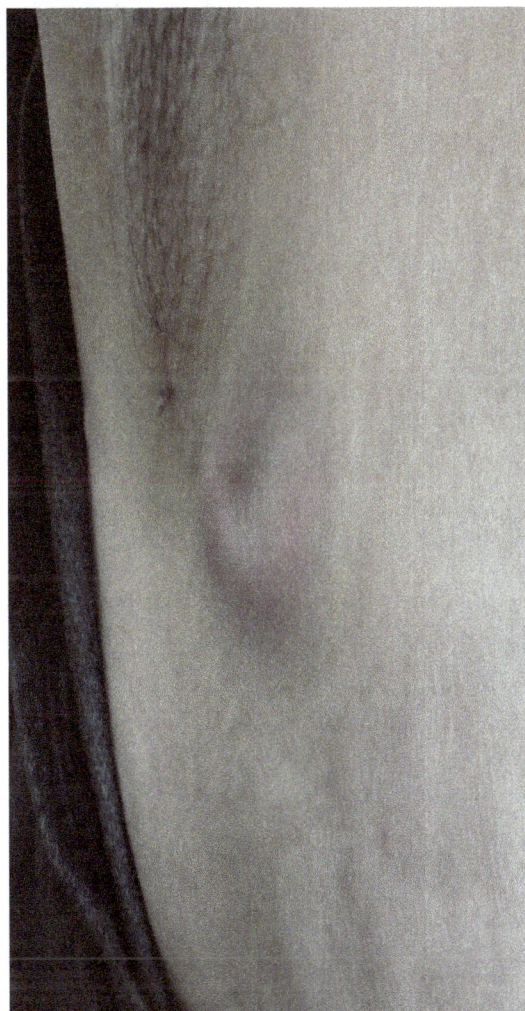

Figure 4. The patient 3 months later developed solitary, about 5 cm in diameter, erythematous, smooth surface, arciform mass located on the lower right axillary line.

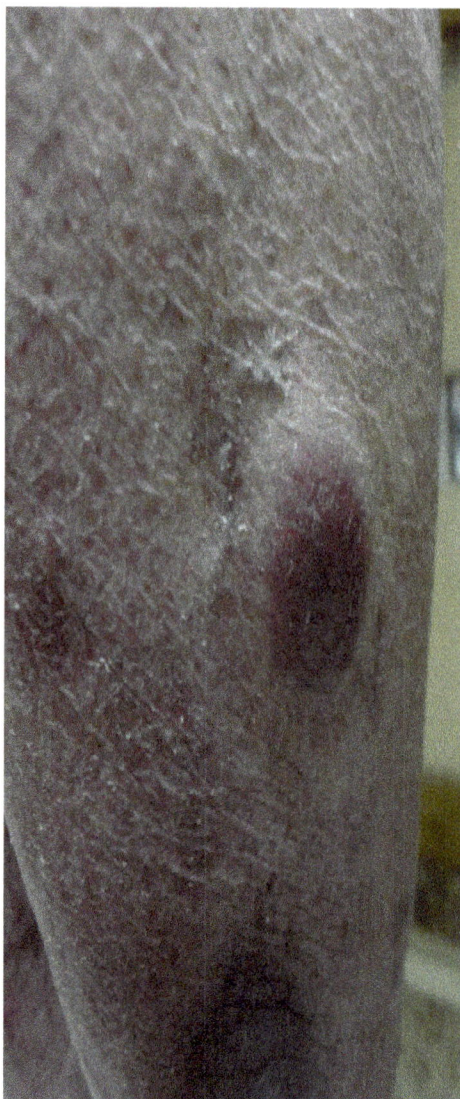

Figure 5. 3 months later developed solitary about 3cm in diameter, hyperpigmented, with fine scaly surface nodule on the lateral aspect of right leg.

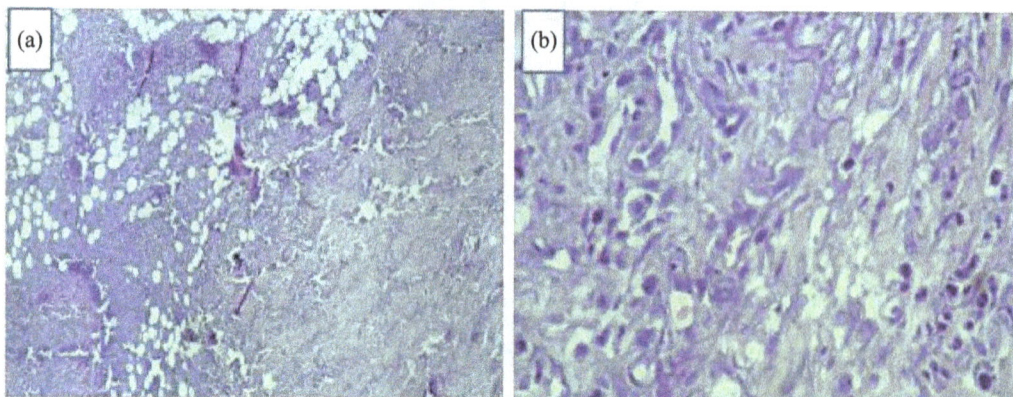

Figure 6. Hematoxylin and eosin (H & E) stained section showed diffuse atypical lymphocytic infiltration in dermis and subcutaneous fat; (a) original magnification ×10; (b) original magnification ×40.

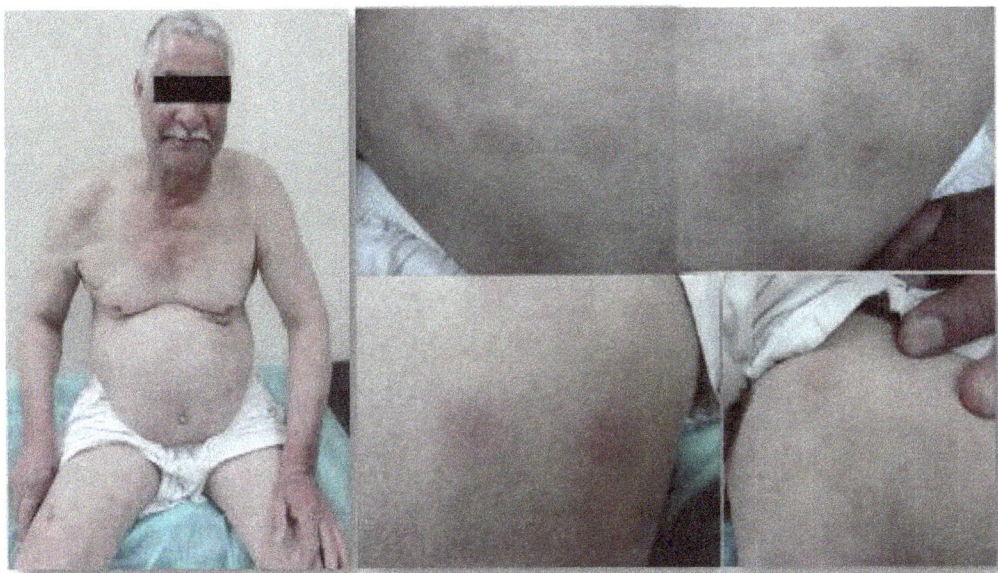

Figure 7. The same patient above after steroid and zinc sulphate weaning, the patient developed multiple, erythematous, subcutaneous nodules distributed symmetrically over the abdomen and both thighs.

Again, biopsy was done, and sent for histopathological study. Routine hematologic, and biochemical investigations were normal. Chest-XR was normal and US showed no abnormality in the abdomen. CT scan of the chest was being arranged. Patient asked to repeat the course of zinc sulphate therapy alone, to prevent masking of the original disease. After 1 month of this regimen patient noticed some improvement but clinically the subcutaneous nodules still there. Biopsy was done again and revealed a picture of diffuse atypical lymphocytic infiltration of dermis and picture goes with T-cell lymphoma.

Consultation to the hematologist was done who decide to make bone marrow aspiration and waiting the result of CT scan to start therapy for CTCL. Bone marrow aspirations reveal no lymphocytic infiltration.

However, while the patient waiting the appointment of CT scan, Patient develop another non tender, rapidly growing skin lesion on his shoulder. By repeating the physical examination we notice large, erythematous, smooth surface mass with irregular nodularity located on the right shoulder, associated with bilateral axillary and left inguinal firm, non tender lymphadenopathy. The patient looks tired, a bit toxic, and feels really ill. Abdominal examination showed for the first time multiple irregular masses but no hepatosplenomegally **Figure 8**.

Another incisional biopsy was taken from the shoulder mass and showed infiltration of deep dermis and subcutaneous fat by atypical large lymphoid cells with frequent mitosis, and CD markers were positive for CD30, CD43, and ALK-1 which is the marker of large anaplastic T-Cell lymphoma. The result of CT scan of the chest now is ready and showed bilateral axillary and Para-aortic LAP, with increased thickness of the abdominal wall **Figure 9**.

The final diagnosis now was established as the patient having large anaplastic T-Cell lymphoma, and accordingly chemotherapy was started, but unfortunately, patient condition rapidly deteriorated and patient died after 2 weeks of the initial chemotherapy cycle.

3. Discussion

Sarcoidosis in Iraq is a very rare and even the reported cases are not well documented. Accordingly we are very surprised to diagnose this patient as a case of sarcoidosis, while lymphoma is a common disease encountered in clinical practice. So from reviewing the literatures and the finding in the reported previous cases we can think that no proper cases of sarcoidosis seen and all patients react to same antigens probably virus that overtime change either into sarcoid reaction first and then develop to lymphoma, or lymphoma appear first and sarcoid reaction appear during the course of the disease [13]. Accordingly, we can hypothesize that there are no pure cases of sarcoidosis and all the reported patients with sarcoid, are either remain as a sarcoidosis for years or transfer rapidly to a stage of lymphoma.

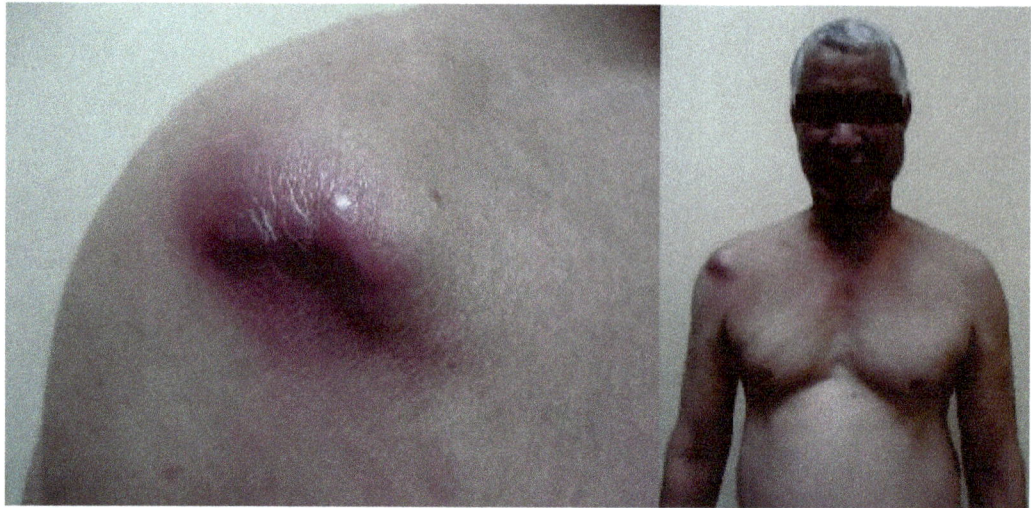

Figure 8. The same patient above developed Large, erythematous, smooth surface mass with irregular nodularity located on the right shoulder.

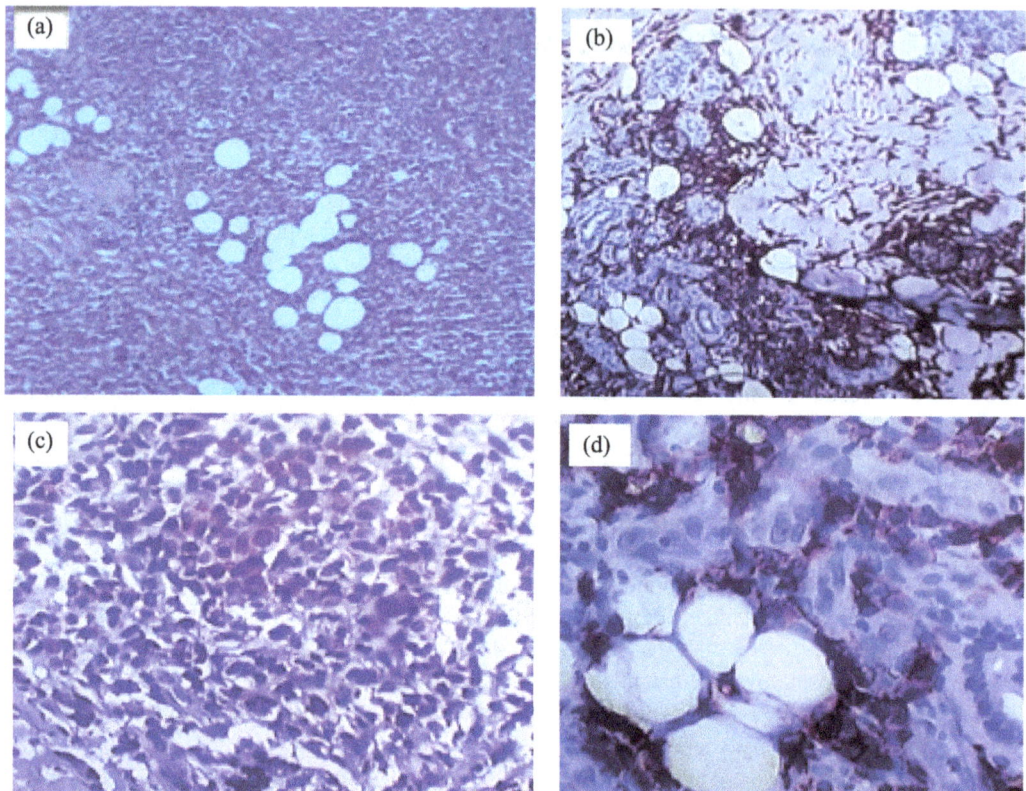

Figure 9. Hematoxylin and eosin (H & E), CD markers stained section showed infiltration of deep dermis and subcutaneous fat by atypical large lymphoid cells with frequent mitosis. (a) H & E original magnification ×10; (b) CD43 original magnification ×10; (c) CD30 original magnification ×10; (d) ALK-1 original magnification ×40.

So we can suggest that there is a state of spectrum with two poles one is the sarcoidosis and the other is lymphoma and there are mixed cases with overlapping features in the middle and all sharing same etiopathological factors in which viruses are the most incriminated agents.

In countries where sarcoidosis is a common problem every doctor should be aware about the spectrum of sarcoidosis-lymphoma state otherwise either the pole of the spectrum will be missed and wrongly managed. Further researches in this field are mandatory in order to reach out the final decision of the strange clinical and pathological conditions.

4. Conclusion

In conclusion, we agree to use the term ("sarcoidosis-lymphoma syndrome") or ("lymphoma-sarcoidosis syndrome") to all cases of so called sarcoidosis/lymphoma and watch the patient by frequent examination, histopathological testing, and doing CD markers in order to detect any further change from one pole to another one.

Disclosure

This study is an independent study and not funded by any of the drug companies.

References

[1]   Joint Statement of the American Thoracic Society (ATS), the European Respiratory Society (ERS) and the World Association of Sarcoidosis and Other Granulomatous Disorders (WASOG) (1999) Statement on Sarcoidosis. *American Journal of Respiratory and Critical Care Medicine*, **160**, 736-755.

[2]   McGrath, D.S., Goh, N., Foley, P.J. and duBois, R.M. (2001) Sarcoidosis: Genes and Microbes-Soil or Seed. *Sarcoidosis Vasculitis Diffuse Lung Disease*, **18**, 149-164.

[3]   King, C.S. and Kelly, W. (2009) Treatment of Sarcoidosis. *Disease-A-Month*, **55**, 704-718.
http://dx.doi.org/10.1016/j.disamonth.2009.06.002

[4]   Nunes, H., Bouvry, D., Solar, P. and Valeyre, D. (2007) Sarcoidosis. *Orphanet Journal Rare Disease*, **2**, 46.
http://dx.doi.org/10.1186/1750-1172-2-46

[5]   Sadek, M.M., Yung, D., Birnie, D.H., Beanlands, R.S. and Nery, P.B. (2013) Corticosteroid Therapy for Cardiac Sarcoidosis: A Systemic Review. *Canadian Journal of Cardiology*, **29**, 1034-1041.
http://dx.doi.org/10.1016/j.cjca.2013.02.004

[6]   Goswami, T., Siddique, S., Cohen, P. and Cheson, B.D. (2010) The Sarcoid-Lymphoma Syndrome. *Clinical Lymphoma, Myeloma & Leukemia*, **4**, 241-247.

[7]   Brincker, H. (1986) The Sarcoidosis-Lymphoma Syndrome. *British Journal Cancer*, **54**, 467-473.
http://dx.doi.org/10.1038/bjc.1986.199

[8]   Brinker, H. and Wilbek, E. (1974) The Incidence of Malignant Tumours in Patients with Respiratory Sarcoidosis. *British Journal Cancer*, **29**, 247-251. http://dx.doi.org/10.1038/bjc.1974.64

[9]   Brincker, H. (1995) Sarcoidosis and Malignancy. *Chest*, **108**, 1472-1474. http://dx.doi.org/10.1378/chest.108.5.1472

[10] William, D., Timothy, G. and Dirk, M. (2011) Sarcoidosis in Andrews Disease of the Skin, Clinical Dermatology. 11th Edition, Saunders *Alsevier*, **31**, 700-707.

[11] Karakantza, M., Matutes, E., MacLennan, K., *et al.* (1996) Association between Sarcoidosis and Lymphoma Revisited. *Journal Clinical Pathology*, **49**, 208-212. http://dx.doi.org/10.1136/jcp.49.3.208

[12] Cohen, P.R. and Kurzrock, R. (2007) Sarcoidosis and Malignancy. *Clinical Dermatology*, **25**, 326-323.
http://dx.doi.org/10.1016/j.clindermatol.2007.03.010

[13] Maayan, H., Ashkenazi, Y., Nagler, A. and Izbicki, G. (2011) Sarcoidosis and Lymphoma: Case Series and Literature Review. *Sarcoidosis Vascular Diffuse Lung Disease*, **28**, 146-152.

25

Topical Application of Tenshino-Softgel™ Reduces Epidermal Nerve Fiber Density in a Chronic Dry Skin Model Mouse

Atsushi Noguchi[1*], Mitsutoshi Tominaga[1*], Kyi Chan Ko[1], Hironori Matsuda[1], Yasushi Suga[2], Hideoki Ogawa[1], Kenji Takamori[1,2#]

[1]Institute for Environmental and Gender Specific Medicine, Juntendo University Graduate School of Medicine, Urayasu, Japan
[2]Department of Dermatology, Juntendo University Urayasu Hospital, Urayasu, Japan
Email: atnogu@juntendo.ac.jp, #ktakamor@juntendo.ac.jp

Abstract

Background: Dry skin induces antihistamine-resistant itch, as well as epidermal hyperinnervation, which is partly responsible for peripheral itch sensitization. In acute dry skin, topical application of emollients prevents the penetration of nerve fibers into the epidermis. However, the effects of emollients on itch and epidermal hyperinnervation in individuals with chronic dry skin are poorly understood. Objective: This study examined the effects of Tenshino-softgel™ (TSG) on itch-related behavior, epidermal hyperinnervation and skin barrier function in a chronic dry skin model mouse. Methods: Chronic dry skin was induced by application of acetone/ether (1:1) mixture and water (AEW) to the rostral parts of the back of hairless mice twice daily for six consecutive days. As treatment, TSG or, as control, Vaseline (V) was applied to the same areas twice daily. Skin barrier function was evaluated by measuring transepidermal water loss (TEWL) before each treatment. Scratching behavior was recorded and analyzed using a SCLABA®-real system, and skin samples were collected for immunohistochemical assays. Results: TEWL tended to be lower and scratching bouts fewer in AEW + TSG- than in AEW-treated mice. The numbers of protein gene product 9.5-immunoreactive fibers and substance P-immunoreactive fibers were each significantly lower in the epidermis of AEW + TSG- than of AEW-treated mice, but the expression of nerve growth factor in epidermis was similar in the three groups. Semaphorin 3A expression was significantly higher in the epidermis of AEW + TSG- than of AEW- and AEW + V-treated mice. Conclusion: Topical application of TSG may attenuate itch induced by chronic dry skin through a mechanism involving the inhibition of epidermal hyperinnervation.

---

*They contributed equally to this work.
#Corresponding author.

Keywords

Dry Skin, Emollient, Epidermal Nerve Fiber, Itch, Skin Barrier

1. Introduction

Dry skin, as observed in patients with senile xerosis and atopic dermatitis, is a very common dermatologic problem frequently presenting with pruritus, defined as an unpleasant sensation and a desire to scratch frequently [1] [2]. Dry skin is induced by decreased water-holding capacity, which is controlled by cutaneous barrier function in the stratum corneum (SC). Skin dryness, as characterized by reduction of SC hydration and transepidermal water loss (TEWL), has been found to induce pruritus [3] [4], as well as epidermal hyperinnervation, which is partly responsible for peripheral itch sensitization [5]. Increased density of nerve fiber in the epidermis is mainly caused by an imbalance between nerve elongation factors such as nerve growth factor (NGF) and nerve repulsion factor such as semaphorin 3A (Sema3A) [6]. These factors may also affect keratinocytes, immune cells and vascular endothelial cells, possibly relating to the modulation of itch [7].

Tenshino-softgel^{TM} (TSG) is a gel-like moisturizing lotion made by Ina Food Industry Co., Ltd. TSG contains water, glycerin, urea, methyl paraben, propyl paraben and agar. Agar is widely used as a food and gelling agent in Asian countries. Solutions of glycerol and/or urea in water are not sufficiently viscous, but the addition of agar was found to enhance the viscosity of TSG. Although agar may have moisturizing and/or anti-inflammatory actions [8], the effectiveness of TSG in treating pruritus due to dry skin is currently unclear. This study therefore evaluated the effects of TSG on itch-related behavior, skin barrier function, epidermal hyperinnervation, and epidermal expression level of axon guidance molecules in mice with chronic dry skin.

2. Materials & Methods

2.1. Animals

Male HR-1 hairless mice (Hoshino Laboratory Animal Inc., Ibaragi, Japan), aged 10 weeks, were maintained under clean conditions, with a 12 h light: 12 h dark cycle at 22°C - 24°C and food and tap water provided *ad libitum*. Care and handling of these mice conformed to the NIH guidelines for animal research. All animal procedures were approved by the Institutional Animal Care and Use Committee at Juntendo University Graduate School of Medicine.

2.2. Reagents

TSG was obtained from Ina Food Industry Co., Ltd. (Nagano, Japan), hydrophilic petrolatum (Vaseline, ointment base) from Maruishi Seiyaku Inc. (Osaka, Japan), optimal cutting temperature (O.C.T.) compound from Sakura Finetechnical Co., Ltd. (Tokyo, Japan), normal donkey serum (NDS) from Merck Millipore (Darmstadt, Germany), bovine serum albumin (BSA) from Sigma-Aldrich (St. Louis, MO, USA), Vectashield mounting medium with DAPI from Vector Laboratories Ltd. (Peterborough, UK), and sevoflurane from Abbott Japan (Osaka, Japan).

2.3. Antibodies

Primary antibodies used in this study included rabbit anti-protein gene product 9.5 (PGP 9.5, 1:400 dilution; Enzo Life Sciences Inc., Farmingdale, NY, USA), rat anti-substance P (SP, 1:100 dilution; Merck Millipore), rabbit anti-NGF (1:500 dilution; Merck Millipore), and rabbit anti-Sema3A (1:200 dilution; Abcam Inc., Cambridge, MA, UK). Secondary antibodies conjugated with Alexa Fluor dye (1:300 dilution) were purchased from Molecular Probes (Eugene, OR, USA).

2.4. Induction of Dry Skin and Application of Emollients

Acetone/ether (1:1) mixture (AE), followed by water (AEW) was applied cutaneously as described [9]. Briefly, cotton (2 × 2 cm) soaked with AE was placed on the rostral parts of the back of mice for 15 seconds under sevoflurane anesthesia, followed within 5 seconds by placement on the same areas of cotton soaked with distilled water for 30 seconds. Within five seconds after each AEW treatment, TSG or Vaseline (V) was applied to the same area as a therapy or control, respectively. These procedures were performed twice daily for six consecutive days. The number of mice used in this study is as follows: untreated (n = 8), AE (n = 8), AEW (n = 7), AEW + V (n = 7), AEW + TSG (n = 7).

2.5. Measurement of TEWL

Before each of the AEW treatment, TEWL of the treated area (the rostral parts of the back of mice) was measured under sevoflurane anesthesia using a Tewameter®TM210 (Courage & Khazawa, Cologne, Germany), as described [5].

2.6. Measurement of Scratching Behavior

Following the second treatment on the sixth day, the behavior of the mice was recorded using a SCLABA®-Real system (Noveltec Inc., Kobe, Japan), as described [10]. After an acclimation period of at least one hour, the behavior of animals was recorded for two hours with no experimenters present in the observation room. The number of scratching bouts was defined as that of periodical lower limb movements lasting more than 150 millisecond search [11].

2.7. Immunohistochemistry

Skin from the dorsal neck of each mouse was taken under sevoflurane anesthesia on the seventh day. Half of each skin sample was fixed in 4% paraformaldehyde in 0.1 M phosphate buffer (pH 7.4) for 4 hours. After washing with phosphate-buffered saline (PBS, pH7.4), small pieces of the skin were immersed in PBS containing 20% sucrose overnight at 4°C. The skin specimens were embedded in O.C.T. compound, frozen on dry ice, and cut into cryosections (20 μm thick for PGP9.5 and SP staining or 8 μm thick for NGF) using a CM1850 cryostat (Leica Microsystems, Wetzlar, Germany). The sections were mounted onto silane-coated glass slides. After blocking in PBS containing 5% NDS, 2% BSA and 0.2% TritonX-100 (blocking solution), the sections were incubated with primary antibodies overnight at 4°C. The next day, the sections were washed with PBS containing 0.05% Tween 20(PBS-T) and incubated with secondary antibodies for one hour at room temperature. After washing with PBS-T, the sections were mounted in Vectashield mounting medium with DAPI.

For immunofluorescence staining of Sema3A, the other half of each skin sample was embedded in O.C.T. compound without fixation, and cut into cryosections (8 μm thick) using a CM1850 cryostat, mounted onto silane-coated glass slides. The sections were fixed in ice-cold acetone for 10 minutes at −20°C, rehydrated in PBS-T, blocked in blocking solution, and then incubated with anti-Sema3A antibody overnight at 4°C. The next day, the sections were washed with PBS-T, incubated with secondary antibody for one hour at room temperature. After washing with PBS-T, the sections were mounted in Vectashield mounting medium with DAPI.

2.8. Semi-Quantification of Nerve Fibers in Epidermis

Six random fields per mouse were viewed with a confocal laser-scanning microscope (DMIRE2; Leica Microsystems), with optical sections 0.9 μm thick scanned through the z-plane of the stained specimens (thickness 20 μm). Three-dimensional images were reconstructed using Leica Confocal Software (Leica Microsystems). The numbers of nerve fibers penetrating into the epidermis and intraepidermal nerve fibers were hand-counted separately. The average number of six observed fields per mouse was calculated and used for statistical analysis.

2.9. Quantitative Measurements of the Fluorescence Intensities of NGF and Sema3A

Six random fields per mouse were observed with a confocal laser-scanning microscope, with exposure and acquisition settings such that no signal saturation occurred. The sum of the fluorescence intensity of the epidermis and the area of the epidermis in each observed field was measured using Leica Confocal Software. Fluorescence intensity per unit area was calculated and used for statistical analysis.

2.10. Statistical Analysis

Data were analyzed using Prism 5 (Graph Pad software Inc., La Jolla, CA, USA). Statistical analyses were performed by analysis of variance (ANOVA) followed by Bonferroni's multiple comparison test, with P < 0.05 regarded as statistically significant.

3. Results

3.1. Evaluation of a Chronic Dry Skin Model Mouse Induced by AEW

Repeated AEW treatment induced the symptoms of dry skin, such as scaling and deep wrinkles (**Figure 1(a)-(c)**). Beginning on the second day of the treatment, TEWL was significantly higher in AEW-treated than in untreated mice, whereas the difference between AE-treated and untreated mice was not significant (**Figure 1(d)**). AEW treatment also significantly increased scratching behavior compared with untreated and AE-treated mice (**Figure 1 (e)**).

3.2. Effects of Tenshino-Softgel™ on TEWL and Scratching Behavior in AEW-Treated Mice

TEWL tended to be lower in AEW + TSG-treated mice, becoming significantly lower in AEW + TSG-treated than in AEW-treated mice on the fourth day (**Figure 2(a)**). The number of scratching bouts was also lower in AEW + TSG-treated mice, but not significantly when compared with the other groups (**Figure 2(b)**).

3.3. Effect of Tenshino-Softgel™ on Epidermal Nerve Fibers in AEW-Treated Mice

The density of PGP9.5-immunoreactive (PGP9.5$^+$) fibers in epidermis was examined immunohistochemically in each group using confocal microscopy (**Figure 3(a)**). The PGP9.5$^+$ fiber density was significantly lower in the AEW + TSG group than in the AEW and AEW + V group (**Figure 3(b)**, **Figure 3(c)**). Assessment of the density

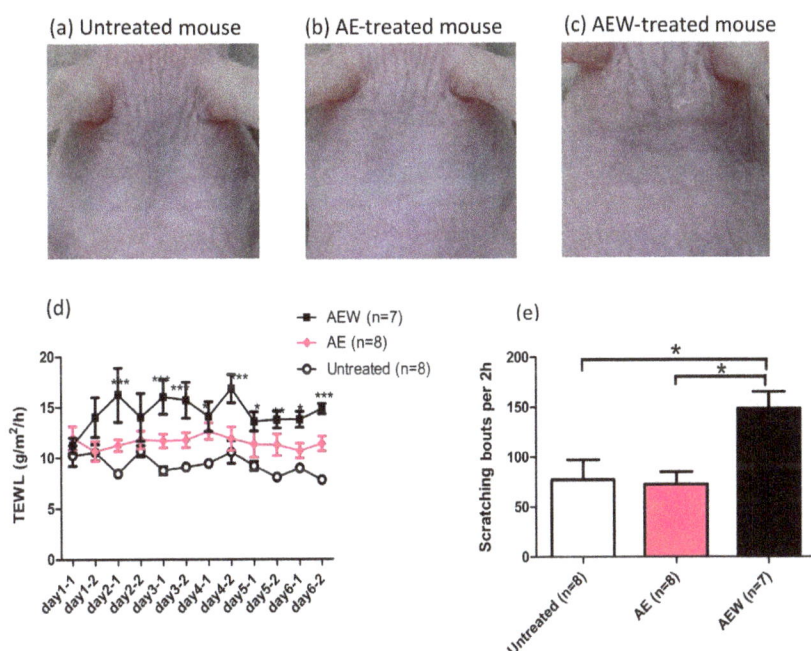

Figure 1. Evaluation of a mouse model of chronic dry skin induced by repeated applications of AEW. (a) Untreated mice showed no abnormalities. (b) Acetone/ether (1:1) mixture (AE)-treated mice showed slight scaling and wrinkling. (c) Mice treated with AE followed by water (AEW) showed scaling and deep wrinkles. (d) Transepidermal water loss (TEWL) was significantly higher in mice receiving repeated AEW treatment than in untreated mice. AE treatment slightly increased TEWL. Results are shown as means ± SEM (standard error of the mean) and compared by two-way ANOVA with Bonferroni's multiple comparison test. *P < 0.05, **P < 0.01, ***P < 0.001. (e) The number of scratching bouts for two hours was significantly higher in AEW-treated mice than in untreated and AE-treated mice. Results are shown as means ± SEM and compared by one-way ANOVA with Bonferroni's multiple comparison test. *P < 0.05.

(a)   (b)

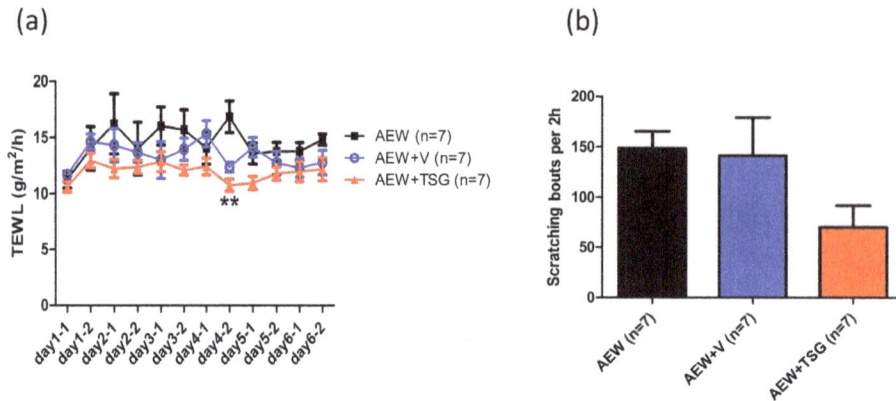

Figure 2. Effects of Tenshino-softgel^{TM} on TEWL and scratching behavior in AEW-treated mice. (a) Compared with acetone/ether (1:1) mixture and water (AEW)-treated mice, AEW + Tenshinosoftgel^{TM}-treated mice showed slight improvements in transepidermal water loss (TEWL). Results are shown as means ± SEM and compared by two-way ANOVA with Bonferroni's multiple comparison test. **$P < 0.01$. (b) Scratching behavior was attenuated in AEW + TSG-treated mice compared with AEW- and AEW + Vaseline-treated mice, but the differences were not significant. Resultsare shown as means ± SEM and compared by one-way ANOVA with Bonferroni's multiple comparison test.

of SP-immunoreactive (SP$^+$) fibers in the epidermis (**Figure 3(d)**) also showed that the SP$^+$ fiber density was significantly lower in the AEW + TSG group than in the AEW group (**Figure 3(e)**, **Figure 3(f)**).

3.4. Effects of Tenshino-Softgel™ on the Expression of NGF and Sema3A in the Epidermis of AEW-Treated Mice.

Immunohistochemical examination for the effects of TSG on epidermal NGF and Sema3A expression showed that the expression level of NGF in the epidermis was similar in mice treated with AEW, AEW + V, and AEW + TSG (**Figure 4(b)**). In contrast, the expression level of Sema3A in the epidermis was higher in AEW + TSG-treated mice than in AEW- and AEW + V-treated mice (**Figure 4(d)**).

4. Discussion

This study showed that topical application of TSG significantly reduced the densities of PGP9.5$^+$- and SP$^+$-epidermal nerve fibers in a mouse model of chronic dry skin (**Figure 3**). In addition, our data showed that topical application of TSG tended to suppress scratching behavior (**Figure 2(b)**). According to the previous study, skin barrier disruption alters epidermal innervation and increases nerve density in the skin [5]. This hyperinnervation is indicative of increases in sensory receptive areas responsive to exogenous triggers of itch, suggesting that hyperinnervation is at least partly responsible for peripheral itch sensitization [12]. Thus, TSG may be therapeutically effective for pruritus in dry skin through inhibiting the epidermal hyperinnervation associated with skin barrier dysfunction. This inhibition in the AEW + TSG group may be due to the increased expression level of Sema3A in the epidermis (**Figure 4(d)**), although the mechanisms underlying the regulation of Sema3A expression in skin remain unclear.

In this study, emollients were applied immediately after skin barrier disruption by AEW treatment. Application of emollients such as heparinoid cream to mice with acute dry skin resulted in greater improvements in epidermal nerve fiber density and epidermal NGF levels, but had no effect on epidermal Sema3A levels [13]. In addition, the increased number of epidermal nerve fibers was lowered more by immediate than delayed application of emollients to dry skin, suggesting that prompt application of emollients is more effective in normalizing epidermal hyperinnervation and epidermal expression of axon guidance molecules [13].

This study showed that repeated AEW treatment elicited spontaneous scratching (**Figure 1(e)**), concomitant with an increase in TEWL (**Figure 1(d)**). Repeated application of AEW to the cheek skin of mice was found to generate itch without pain [14]. Moreover, AEW treatment induced spontaneous scratching in mast cell-deficient mice, indicating that mast cells may not be involved in AEW-induced scratching behavior [9]. Although

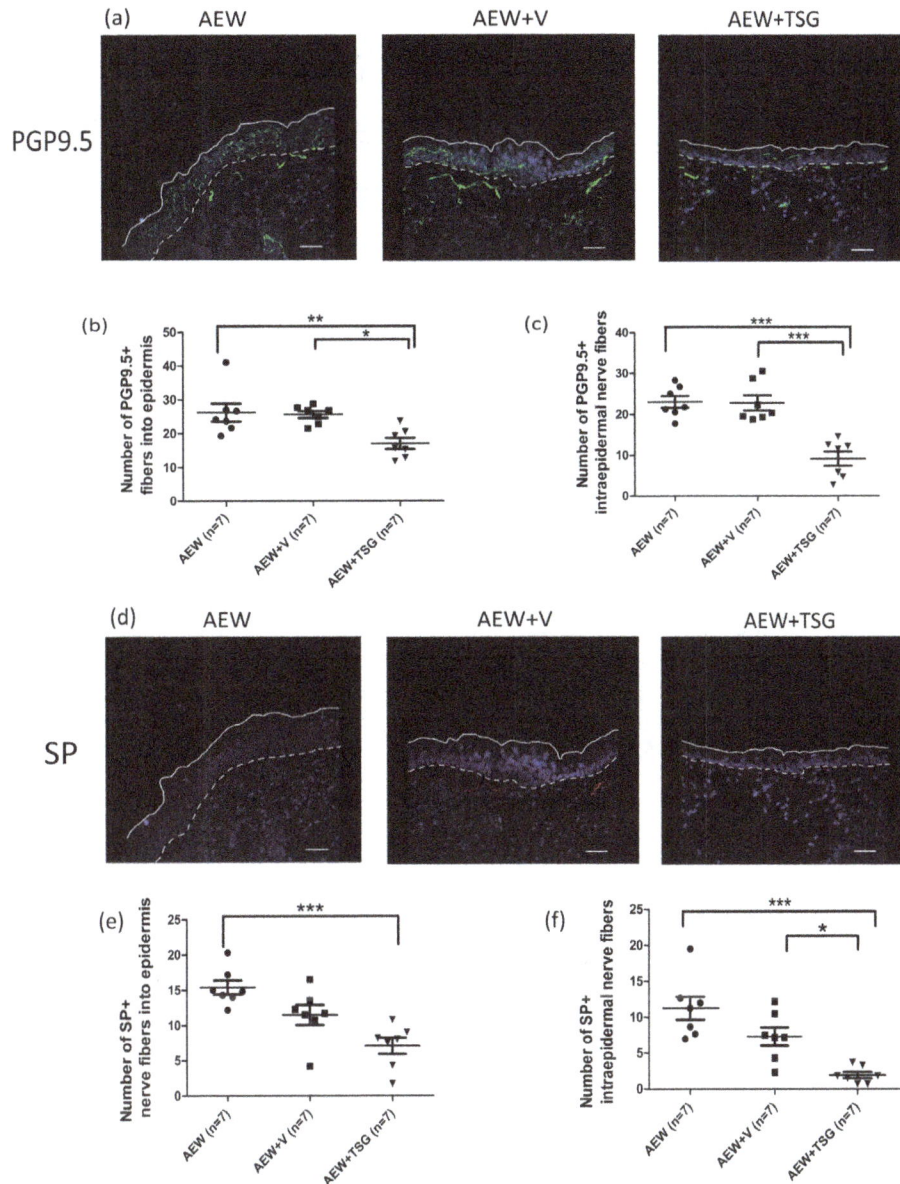

Figure 3. Effect of Tenshino-softgel^{TM} on epidermal nerve fibers in AEW-treated mice. (a) Immunolabeling with anti-protein gene product 9.5 (PGP9.5) antibody (green) of epidermal nerve fibers on lesional skin after application of acetone/ether (1:1) mixture and water (AEW), AEW + Vaseline (V), and AEW + Tenshino-softgel^{TM} (TSG). Images of nerve fibers are superimposed on differential interference microscopic images. White and broken lines indicate the skin surface and the border between the epidermis and dermis (basement membrane), respectively. Scale bars, 100 μm. (b, c) Numbers of PGP9.5-immunoreactive (PGP9.5$^+$) fibers (b) penetrating into and (c) within the epidermis were lower in AEW + TSG-treated mice than in AEW- and AEW + V-treated mice. (d) Immunolabeling with anti-substance P (SP) antibody (red) of epidermal nerve fibers on lesional skin after application of AEW, AEW + V, and AEW + TSG. Images of nerve fibers are superimposed on differential interference microscopic images. White and broken lines indicate the skin surface and the border between the epidermis and dermis (basement membrane), respectively.Scale bars, 100 μm. (e) Numbers of SP-immun-oreatctive (SP$^+$) fibers penetrating into the epidermis were lower in AEW + TSG-treated mice than in AEW-treated mice. (f) Numbers of SP$^+$fibers within the epidermis were lower in AEW + TSG-treated mice than in AEW-and AEW + V-treated mice. Results are shown as means ± SEM (n = 7 per group) and compared by one-way ANOVA with Bonferroni's multiple comparison tests. *P < 0.05, **P < 0.01, ***P < 0.001.

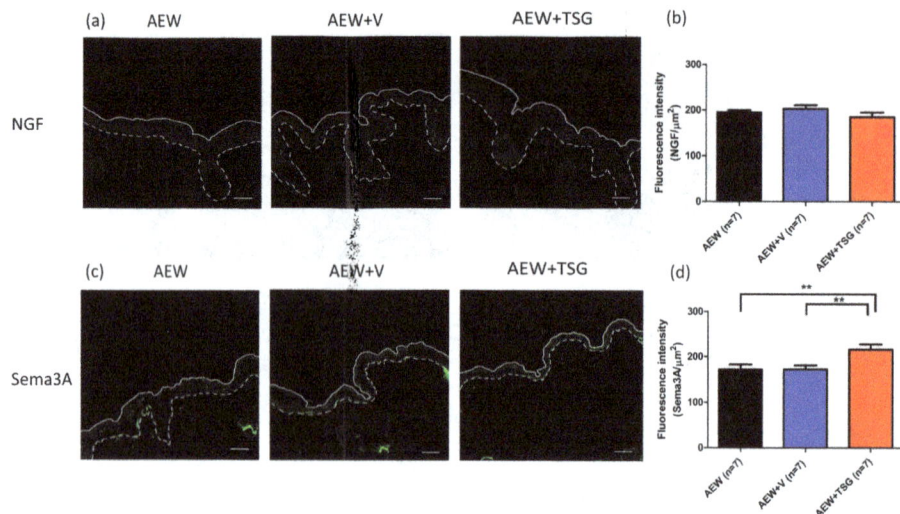

Figure 4. Effects of Tenshino-softgel[TM] on the expression of NGF and Sema3A in epidermis. (a) Immunolabeling with anti-nerve growth factor (NGF) antibody (green) ofmouse skin after application of acetone/ether (1:1) mixture and water (AEW), alone or plus Vaseline (V) or Tenshino-softgel[TM] (TSG). (b) Epidermal NGF expression levels were similar in the three groups. (c) Immunolabeling with anti-Sema3A antibody (green) of mouse skin after application of AEW, alone or plus Vaseline or TSG. (d) Epidermal Sema3A expression levels were significantly higher in the AEW + TSG group than in the AEW- and AEW + V-treated groups. White and broken lines in each panel indicate the skin surface and the border between the epidermis and dermis (basement membrane), respectively. Scale bars, 100 μm. Results are shown as means ± SEM (n = 7 per group) and compared by one-way ANOVA with Bonferroni's multiple comparison tests. **$P < 0.01$.

the mechanisms are unclear, scratching behavior in mast cell-deficient mice may be caused, at least in part, by increases in epidermal nerve fibers or pruritogens secreted by other dermal cells and/or keratinocytes [15]. Alternatively, spontaneous scratching may be induced by water treatment following AE, but not by organic solvents alone. Water can remove natural moisturizing factors important for skin hydration, impairing SC hydration and flexibility [16]. Water may also induce transient swelling of the SC followed by a drying out of the surface layers. Physical swelling and shrinking of SC may act as mechanical stimuli of C-fibers in upper epidermis and evoke itch. This idea may be supported by the finding that mechanical stimuli induced the sprouting of cutaneous sensory nerve fibers [17].

5. Conclusion

In conclusion, these findings suggest that topical application of TSG restrains the progression of barrier disruption and improves the imbalance of axon guidance molecule by increasing the expression of Sema3A, possibly resulting in a decrease in epidermal nerve fiber density. TSG may therefore be useful as antipruritic therapy in patients with dry skin-based skin diseases.

Acknowledgements

We thank Ina Food Industry Co., Ltd. for providing TSG and valuable scientific support. This work was partly supported by a grant Strategic Research Foundation Grant-aided Project for Private Universities from MEXT (Grant number S1311011).

Conflict of Interest

The authors state no conflict of interest.

References

[1]   Di Nardo, A., Wertz, P., Giannetti, A. and Seidenari, S. (1998) Ceramide and Cholesterol Composition of the Skin of

Patients with Atopic Dermatitis. *Acta Dermato Venereologica*, **78**, 27-30.
http://dx.doi.org/10.1080/00015559850135788

[2]   Thaipisuttikul, Y. (1998) Pruritic Skin Diseases in the Elderly. *The Journal of Dermatology*, **25**, 153-157.
http://dx.doi.org/10.1111/j.1346-8138.1998.tb02371.x

[3]   Long, C.C. and Marks, R. (1992) Stratum Corneum Changes in Patients with Senile Pruritus. *Journal of the American Academy of Dermatology*, **27**, 560-564. http://dx.doi.org/10.1016/0190-9622(92)70222-2

[4]   Morton, C.A., Lafferty, M., Hau, C., Henderson, I., Jones, M. and Lowe, J.G. (1996) Pruritus and Skin Hydration during Dialysis. *Nephrology Dialysis Transplantation*, **11**, 2031-2036.
http://dx.doi.org/10.1093/oxfordjournals.ndt.a027092

[5]   Tominaga, M., Ozawa, S., Tengara, S., Ogawa, H. and Takamori, K. (2007) Intraepidermal Nerve Fibers Increase in Dry Skin of Acetone-Treated Mice. *Journal of Dermatological Science*, **48**, 103-111.
http://dx.doi.org/10.1016/j.jdermsci.2007.06.003

[6]   Tominaga, M., Tengara, S., Kamo, A., Ogawa, H. and Takamori, K. (2009) Psoralen-Ultraviolet A Therapy Alters Epidermal Sema3A and NGF Levels and Modulates Epidermal Innervation in Atopic Dermatitis. *Journal of Dermatological Science*, **55**, 40-46. http://dx.doi.org/10.1016/j.jdermsci.2009.03.007

[7]   Tominaga, M. and Takamori, K. (2014) Itch and Nerve Fibers with Special Reference to Atopic Dermatitis: Therapeutic Implications. *The Journal of Dermatology*, **41**, 205-212. http://dx.doi.org/10.1111/1346-8138.12317

[8]   Enoki, T., Okuda, S., Kudo, Y., Takashima, F., Sagawa, H. and Kato, I. (2010) Oligosaccharides from Agar Inhibit Pro-inflammatory Mediator Release by Inducing Heme Oxygenase 1. *Bioscience, Biotechnology, and Biochemistry*, **74**, 766-770. http://dx.doi.org/10.1271/bbb.90803

[9]   Miyamoto, T., Nojima, H., Shinkado, T., Nakahashi, T. and Kuraishi, Y. (2002) Itch-Associated Response Induced by Experimental Dry Skin in Mice. *The Japanese Journal of Pharmacology*, **88**, 285-292.
http://dx.doi.org/10.1254/jjp.88.285

[10]   Tanaka, A., Amagai, Y., Oida, K. and Matsuda, H. (2012) Recent Findings in Mouse Models for Human Atopic Dermatitis. *Experimental Animals*, **61**, 77-84. http://dx.doi.org/10.1538/expanim.61.77

[11]   Nie, Y., Ishii, I., Yamamoto, K., Orito, K. and Matsuda, H. (2009) Real-Time Scratching Behavior Quantification System for Laboratory Mice Using High-Speed Vision. *Journal of Real-Time Image Processing*, **4**, 181-190.
http://dx.doi.org/10.1007/s11554-009-0111-7

[12]   Tominaga, M. and Takamori, K. (2013) An Update on Peripheral Mechanisms and Treatments of Itch. *Biological and Pharmaceutical Bulletin*, **36**, 1241-1247. http://dx.doi.org/10.1248/bpb.b13-00319

[13]   Kamo, A., Tominaga, M., Negi, O., Tengara, S., Ogawa, H. and Takamori, K. (2011) Topical Application of Emollients Prevents Dry Skin-Inducible Intraepidermal Nerve Growth in Acetone-Treated Mice. *Journal of Dermatological Science*, **62**, 64-66. http://dx.doi.org/10.1016/j.jdermsci.2011.01.008

[14]   Valtcheva, M.V., Saminen, V.K., Golden, J.P., Gereau 4th, R.W. and Davidson, S. (2015) Enhanced Nonpeptidergic Intraepidermal Fiber Density and An Expanded Subset of Chloroquine-responsive Trigeminal Neurons in a Mouse Model of Dry Skin Itch. *The Journal of Pain*, **16**, 346-356. http://dx.doi.org/10.1016/j.jpain.2015.01.005

[15]   Akiyama, T., Carstens, M.I. and Carstens, E. (2010) Enhanced Scratching Evoked by PAR-2 Agonist and 5-HT but Not Histamine in a Mouse Model of Chronic Dry Skin Itch. *Pain*, **151**, 378-383.
http://dx.doi.org/10.1016/j.pain.2010.07.024

[16]   Yosipovitch, G. (2004) Dry Skin and Impairment of Barrier Function Associated with Itch—New Insights. *International Journal of Cosmetic Science*, **26**, 1-7. http://dx.doi.org/10.1111/j.0142-5463.2004.00199.x

[17]   Yamaoka, J., Di, Z.H., Sun, W. and Kawana, S. (2007) Erratum to "Changes in Cutaneous Sensory Nerve Fibers Induced by Skin-scratching in Mice". *Journal of Dermatological Science*, **47**, 172-182.
http://dx.doi.org/10.1016/j.jdermsci.2006.12.012

26

Higher Cell Viability and Enhanced Sample Quality Following Laser-Assisted Liposuction versus Mechanical Liposuction

Alexander Levenberg[1]*, Mickey Scheinowitz[2], Orna Sharabani-Yosef[2]

[1]Department of Plastic Surgery, Tel Aviv Sourasky Medical Center, Tel Aviv, Israel
[2]Department of Biomedical Engineering, Faculty of Engineering, Tel Aviv University, Tel Aviv, Israel
Email: *leveplas@netvision.net.il

Abstract

Background: Despite the popularity of autologous fat transfer applications, high resorption rates, and consequential volume loss, have been reported. Viable adipocyte content has been defined as a key determinant of fat transfer longevity. Moreover, traces of blood, free oil fat and fibrotic tissue accelerate adipocyte degradation. Objective: To compare the effectiveness of a 1470 nm, radial emitting laser-assisted liposection device to a mechanical liposection device in maintaining adipocyte viability in fat tissue harvests. Methods: Bilateral subcutaneous adipose tissue samples were harvested from ten female patients. Fat was harvested from one side using the LipoLife laser-assisted liposuction device and from the other side with a Byron mechanical aspirator. Samples were visually analyzed and blood:fat ratios and cell viability were determined. Results: Laser-harvested samples separated into two distinct phases, with a negligible blood phase at the bottom (1.1%) and a significant adipose phase at the top (98.9%), containing small, uniform-sized cells, of which 95.7% ± 2.7% proved viable. Mechanically harvested samples separated into blood (18%), adipose (60%) and lipid (22%) phases. The adipose phase contained significant amounts of connective tissue, large adipose tissue fragments, large oil droplets and a mean 79.7% ± 18.3% viable adipocytes. Conclusions: Laser liposuctioning was superior to mechanical liposuctioning, providing both higher cell viability and enhanced sample quality. The 1470 nm diode laser bears the potential of improving long-term clinical outcomes of fat transfer procedures. Improved purity of the harvested sample and heightened preadipocyte content are projected to provide for extended graft longevity.

Keywords

Laser Liposuction, Cell Viability, Fat Transfer, Preadipocyte

---

*Corresponding author.

1. Introduction

The dramatic evolution of contemporary plastic surgery has brought liposuction to become the fifth-most popular aesthetic procedure performed in Britain in 2014, with a 7% rise in prevalence from the preceding year [1]. The procedure is performed to recontour defects of a spectrum of severities and, when harnessed toward autologous fat transfer applications, supports tissue reconstruction, radiation-induced necrosis of the chest wall, breast augmentation, volume enhancement in the facial area and wrinkle repair [2]. Autologous fat transfer circumvents complications associated with allogenic fillers and implants, is more readily available, more cost-effective, incurs minimal donor-site morbidity and provides a more durable outcome [3]. The constantly improving fat injection techniques have transformed autologous fat transfer into a minimally invasive, outpatient procedure.

However, highly variable resorption rates have been reported, averaging 45% graft weight retention within one year of transplantation [4] [5], where volume loss as high as 70% has also been reported [6] [7], lending to overcorrection and reinjection sessions, and subsequent fat necrosis and calcification. Peer *et al.* established that the viable adipocyte content is the key determinant of fat transfer longevity [8]. Thus, minimization of the liquefied fat and serosanguinous fluid in the fat sample, increases the relative ratio of viable adipocytes, preventing early resorption as well as inflammatory reactions [9] [10]. Furthermore, while injection of fat specimens with high fibrous tissue content provides an immediate volumizing effect, postsurgical fibrosis positively correlates with adipocyte absorption and a short-lived clinical effect [11] [12]. Moreover, traces of blood, free oil fat and fibrotic tissue in transferred fat are said to accelerate adipocyte degradation [11], via increased inflammatory responses to the graft [13]. Thus, the ideal fat graft, containing a high adipocyte count and low contaminant content, has been the focus of harvesting optimization efforts for decades. Isolation solutions designed to maximize cell yield and viability, will inevitably ensure more durable clinical results and reduce the need for correction procedures.

As laser-assisted liposuction has often been charged with detrimental effects on cell viability, continuous efforts are being invested in design of a device that can maximize viable adipocyte yields. This study presents experience with a novel laser liposuction device featuring a 1470 nm diode laser and a radial emitting fiber. Specimen content and preadipocyte cell viability when harvested via laser-assisted lipolysis versus mechanical liposuctioning were compared. Laser-assisted liposuction proved more effective in preserving preadipocyte viability, while ensuring as fewer blood and connective tissue contaminations in the collected adipose tissue.

2. Materials and Methods

Donors: Human subcutaneous adipose tissue samples were obtained from the abdomen, thighs and inner thighs of 10 female subjects who had provided informed consent. All procedures were performed under general anesthesia and the average volume aspirated was 1.5 liters. Maximum aspired material was 3.5 liters. Minimum was 600 cc.

Surgical procedure: Patients were prepped with betadine. Saline, supplemented with lidocaine 20% (30 cc per liter saline) and adrenaline (0.5 ml per liter saline) was introduced to the treated area via mechanical infusion (Byron Medical Inc.). Standard puncture holes were made at the treated areas with a #11 surgical blade, to allow fat laser aspiration. The ratio of injected liquid (Tumescent) to aspirated material was 2:1. For fat aspiration, Mercedes 3 mm and 4 mm cannulas specially designed with a swivel handle (LipoLife, Alma Lasers) were used. The 1470 nm, 600 micron, radial emitting laser fiber (Alma Lasers, Ltd.) was advanced through the cannula and positioned in the center of the distal opening of the cannula.

Mechanical aspiration was then performed on the opposite side and by the same physician using 3 mm - 4 mm Mercedes liposuction cannulas (Byron Medical Inc.). Temperature in the treated area was measured throughout the procedure and was maintained below 40°C.

Adipose tissue harvesting: Fat samples were collected with a laser-assisted liposuction device (LipoLife, Alma) from one side of the patient and with a mechanical liposuction device (Byron) from the other side of the patient. Samples were not manipulated or washed in any way and were allowed to stand at room temperature to allow for phase separation. Samples were analyzed within 12 hours of collection.

Calculation of fat:blood phase ratios: The following formulation was applied to calculate the ratios between the phases into which specimens separated following liposuction:

The volume of a cone is given by the formula:

$$V = 1/3\pi(R_1^2 + R_2^2 + R_1 R_2)$$

Where:

$R_1 \cdot R_2$ is the upper and lower radius, respectively

H is the cone height

A volume percentage is given by:

$$V_1(\%) = 100* V_1/(V_1 + V_2)$$

$$V_2(\%) = 100* V_2/(V_1 + V_2)$$

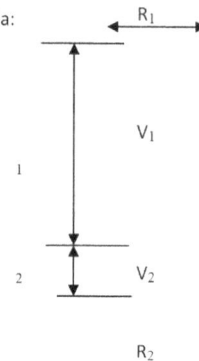

Cell yield, viability and morphology: Viable cell yield after isolation was determined using the trypan blue staining test. To assess the number of stem cells, the adherent cells were removed by proteolysis with trypsin C (Biological Industries, Israel). Cells were then stained with 0.4% trypan blue solution (10 µl cells: 10 µl dye) and counted in a hemocytometer, viewed under a phase contrast microscope (Nikon). Duplicates samples from each specimen were evaluated. In addition, cell diameter, and connective tissue content were visually estimated.

Preadipocyte isolation: Preadipocytes were isolated after tissue harvesting. Fibrous structures and visible vessels were removed, and then washed up to seven times in phosphate-buffered saline (PBS) (Biological industries, Israel). After centrifugation (300 g, 10 min) the tissue pellet was enzymatically digested with 2 mg/mL collagenase Type I (Sigma-Aldrich) dissolved in an equal volume of PBS solution (37°C, 60 min). Collagenase was inactivated with 10% fetal bovine serum (FBS) (Biological Industries, Israel), followed by redistribution of the mixture into 50 ml conicals and centrifugation (1000 g, 10 min) to separate the oil and remaining fat lobules from the stromal vascular fraction (SVF). The red blood cells in the SVF pellet were then lysed in 160 mM NH4Cl (room temperature (RT), 10 min). The sample was then washed twice in PBS and centrifuged (300 g, 5 min, RT). The adherent cell population was then isolated by culturing the cells overnight in flasks (DMEM F-12, 10% fetal calf serum, 2 mM L-Glutamine, 0.1% penicillin/streptomycin (Biological Industries, Israel)). The non-adherent cells and debris were washed away with PBS and the adipose stem cells were grown and expanded as monolayers. Cell viability was determined using trypan blue.

Statistical analysis: Comparative analyses between mechanical liposuction samples and laser liposuctioned samples were performed. Mean values and standard deviations are presented. Significance was determined using a one-sided Student's T-test.

3. Results

3.1. Phase Separation of Collected Samples

Samples harvested using laser lipolysis separated into two distinct phases, with a blood phase at the bottom of the canister, that contained only a small amount of blood, and a smooth, uniform, yellowish-pink adipose tissue phase at the top (**Figure 1(a)**). This latter phase consisted primarily of adipose cells, a minimal amount of connective tissue and very small lipid droplets (10 - 30 µm diameter; **Figure 2**). Samples harvested by mechanical liposuction, separated into three distinct phases, which included, a blood phase at the bottom of the canister, adipose tissue phase in the middle and an oil phase at top (**Figure 1(b)**). The adipose tissue phase contained a significant amount of connective tissue, large adipose tissue fragments and large droplets (diameter 20 µm - 100 µm, **Figure 2**).

3.2. Blood:Fat Ratios

The blood, lipid droplets and adipose tissue phases of samples collected via mechanical liposuction comprised approximately 18%, 22% and 60% of the total sample, respectively. In contrast, laser liposuction samples separated into a 1.1% blood phase and 98.9% adipose tissue phase (**Figure 1**). These calculations were further supported by the significantly higher red blood cell content observed in samples collected by mechanical liposuc-

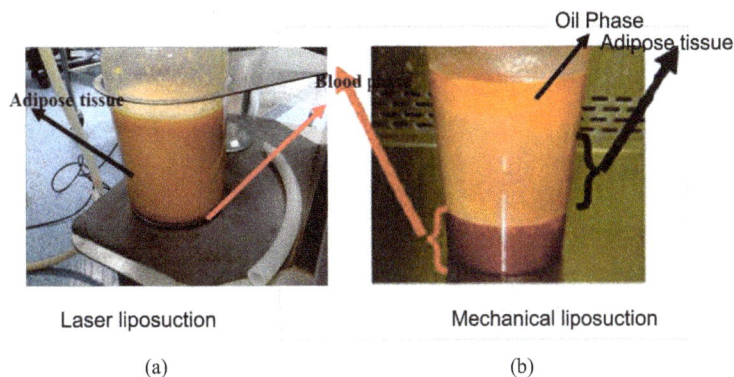

Figure 1. Human fat tissue aspirates Specimens were collected by (a) Laser lipolysis or (b) mechanical liposuction and separated into two and three phases, respectively.

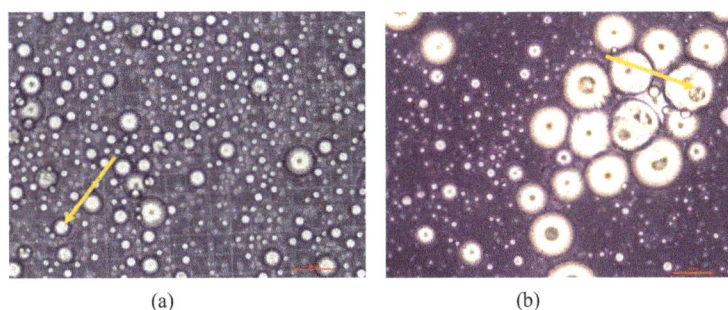

Figure 2. Microscopic analysis of the adipose phase of fat tissue aspirates Fat specimens were collected by (a) laser lipolysis or (b) mechanical liposuction and observed under a phase contrast microscope. The diameter of lipid droplets in the laser lipolysis-collected samples was much smaller than in mechanical liposuction samples (yellow arrows) (Magnification ×100).

tion (**Figure 3(b)**).

3.3. Cell Viability

Cell viability in the tissue harvested by mechanical liposuction (n = 9) was 79.7% ± 18.3%, while the laser liposuction samples (n = 10) consistently contained more viable cells, averaging 95.7% ± 2.7% per sample (**Figure 4**, **Table 1**, one-sided T-test p = 0.005).

3.4. Stem Cell Isolation from Adipose Tissue

There were no significant differences in the number of viable stem cells isolated from adipose tissue harvested by way of laser liposuction vs. mechanical liposuction, although typical morphological features were better maintained among cells obtained by way of laser liposuction (**Figure 5**).

3.5. Trauma Induced by Laser versus Mechanical Liposuction

Laser liposuction decreased likelihood of burns and internal scarring, while the rounded cannula tip minimized tissue trauma (**Figure 6**) when compared to mechanical liposuction. Following mechanical liposuction, hemorrhages were still observed one week after treatment and more subcutaneous scarring was apparent.

4. Discussion

While no consensus has been reached regarding the best means of obtaining fat samples, it is largely agreed that long-term clinical effectiveness of adipose tissue grafts is heavily contingent upon the overall ratio of viable

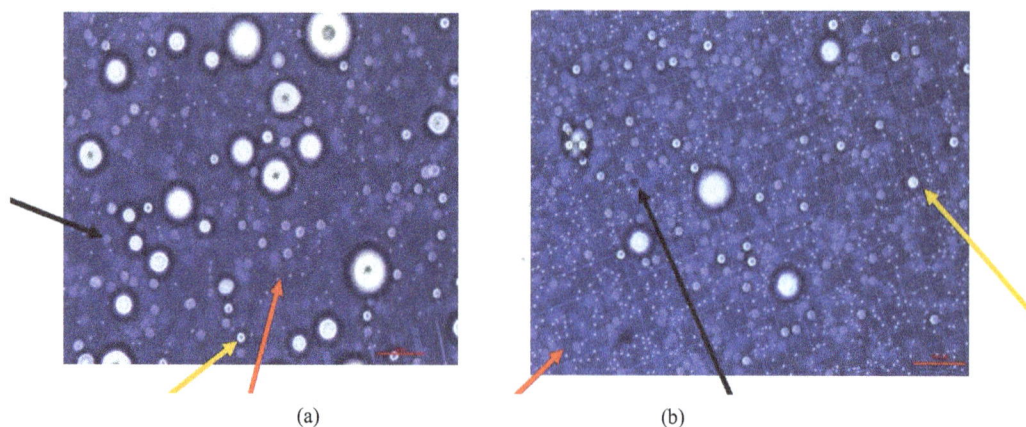

Figure 3. Adipose phase, trypan blue-stained specimens Fat specimens were collected by (a) laser lipolysis or (b) mechanical liposuction and stained with trypan blue before being observed and counted under a phase-contrast microscope. Viable cells (yellow arrows) have a clear cytoplasm whereas nonviable cells have a blue-stained cytoplasm (black arrows). Red blood cells are indicated by red arrows and were more prevalent in the mechanical liposuctioned specimens.

Table 1. Cell viability in the adipose phase of harvested adipose tissue samples.

Sample #	Laser	Mechanical
1	98%	96%
2	96%	92%
3	96%	91%
4	95%	50%
5	96%	66%
6	99%	88%
7	95%	55%
8	96%	90%
9	96%	89%
10	90%	
Average	95.7%	79.7%
SD	2.36	18.33

adipocytes [8]. Over the years, the various liposuction techniques have been refined, in efforts to minimize mechanical and ischemic trauma, incidence of fat and pulmonary emboli, and reduced hemoglobin levels, and to enhance both short- and long-term specimen viability [14]. Laser-assisted liposuction induces both thermal and micromechanical lipolysis of the adipose tissue, improving skin contraction and reducing the need for traumatic aspiration forces and pressures and consequential patient pain [15], blood loss [16], hematomas and overall risk [17]. The added thermal component, overcomes the key limitation of mechanical liposuction, by melting connective tissue, coagulating vasculature, and stimulating neocollagen deposition, promoting skin contraction at the treatment site [17] [18].

The presented LipoLife device was designed with a 1470 nm diode laser, illuminating tissues at a wavelength effectively absorbed by cellular water, rendering it ideal for soft tissues by reducing the risk of tissue burn. In addition, its radial emitting fiber reduces the emission intensity in the surgical region, with decreased likelihood of burns and internal scarring, while the rounded cannula tip minimizes tissue trauma (**Figure 5**). In contrast, flat-tipped fibers deliver very high power densities, while the radial fiber delivers approximately 1/10 the power density.

This study demonstrated that laser liposuction of fat tissue with the LipoLife device, provides an ultimate and

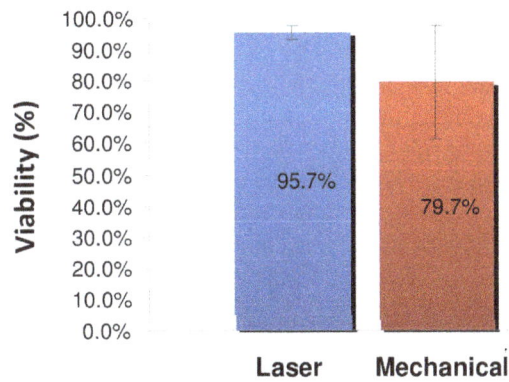

Figure 4. Cell viability in adipose phase samples Fat specimens were collected by laser lipolysis (n = 10) or mechanical liposuction (n = 9) and stained with trypan blue before being counted in a hemocytometer. The results represent the average of the samples ± standard deviation.

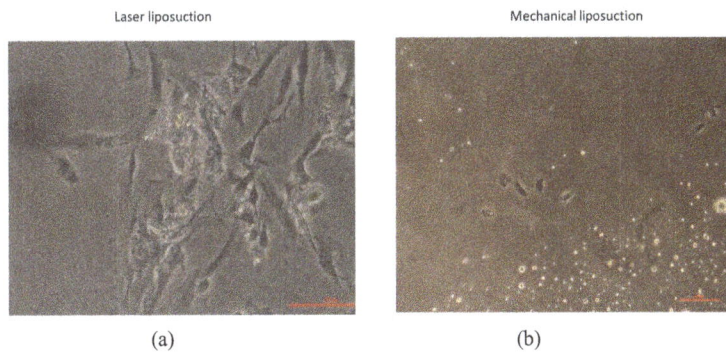

Figure 5. Morphology of stem cells isolated from adipose tissue collected by laser lipolysis versus mechanical liposuction Adipose tissue (20 ml) was grown in a flask, as described in the methods section and photographed after three days in culture.

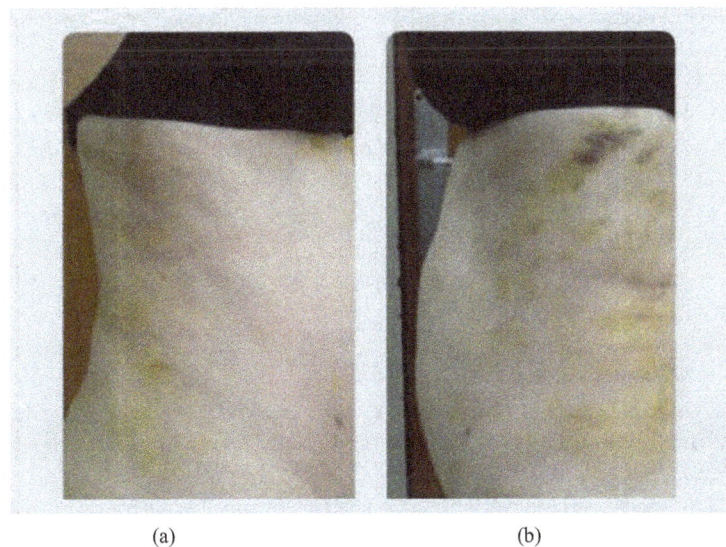

Figure 6. Trauma induced by laser versus mechanical liposuction Photographs taken one week after treatment with (a) laser liposuction and (b) mechanical liposuction.

consistent source of preadipocytes, surpassing the quality and viability obtained by mechanical liposuction. The consistently higher cell yield, integrity and viability suggest that this extraction method avoids cell damage to the aspired adipose tissue. In addition, the low fibrous and blood, further promotes the clinical value of this harvesting method, by both minimizing patient risk and maximizing the potential of the preadipocyte specimen. Furthermore, the LipoLife laser liposuction harvesting yielded a more homogenous sample with less variable and more predictable results, as demonstrated by the uniform lipid droplet size and the lower standard deviations between samples, respectively. Overall, the improved purity of the harvested sample and heightened preadipocyte content, are projected to provide for extended graft longevity, reducing the incidence of overcorrection, and the need for repeat grafting and recontouring sessions. In addition, the high-quality samples bear significant potential in regenerative laboratories and in various clinical applications founded on the progenitor cell content in adipose tissue [19]. These early findings warrant further study of the functional advantage of the isolated specimens.

References

[1]   http://www.plasticsurgerypractice.com/2015/01/baaps-data-plastic-surgery-falls-across-pond/

[2]   Atiyeh, B., Costagliola, M., Illouz, Y.G., *et al.* (2015) Functional and Therapeutic Indications of Liposuction: Personal Experience and Review of the Literature. *Annals of Plastic Surgery.*

[3]   Banyard, D.A., Salibian, A.A., Widgerow, A.D. and Evans, G.R. (2015) Implications for Human Adipose-Derived Stem Cells in Plastic Surgery. *Journal of Cellular and Molecular Medicine*, **19**, 21-30. http://dx.doi.org/10.1111/jcmm.12425

[4]   Peer, L.A. (1950) Loss of Weight and Volume in Human Fat Grafts. *Plastic and Reconstructive Surgery*, **5**, 217. http://dx.doi.org/10.1097/00006534-195003000-00002

[5]   Etzkorn, J.R., Divine, J.M., Lopez, J.J., *et al.* (2011) Autologous Fat Transfer: Techniques, Indications and Future Investigation. *Cosmetic Dermatology*, **24**, 470-476.

[6]   Kaufman, M.R., Miller, T.A., Huang, C., *et al.* (2007) Autologous Fat Transfer for Facial Recontouring: Is There Science behind the Art? *Plastic and Reconstructive Surgery*, **119**, 2287-2296. http://dx.doi.org/10.1097/01.prs.0000260712.44089.e7

[7]   Fournier, P.F. (2000) Fat Grafting: My Technique. *Dermatologic Surgery*, **26**, 1117-1128. http://dx.doi.org/10.1046/j.1524-4725.2000.00272.x

[8]   Peer, L.A. (1956) The Neglected Free Fat Graft, Its Behavior and Clinical Use. *American Journal of Surgery*, **92**, 40-44. http://dx.doi.org/10.1016/S0002-9610(56)80009-3

[9]   Fagrell, D., Enestrom, S., Berggren, A., *et al.* (1996) Fat Cylinder Transplantation: An Experimental Comparative Study of Three Different Kinds of Fat Transplants. *Plastic and Reconstructive Surgery*, **98**, 90-96, 97-98. http://dx.doi.org/10.1097/00006534-199607000-00014

[10]   Coleman, S.R. (1995) Long-Term Survival of Fat Transplants: Controlled Demonstrations. *Aesthetic Plastic Surgery*, **19**, 421-425. http://dx.doi.org/10.1007/BF00453875

[11]   Sommer, B. and Sattler, G. (2000) Current Concepts of Fat Graft Survival: Histology of Aspirated Adipose Tissue and Review of the Literature. *Dermatologic Surgery*, **26**, 1159-1166. http://dx.doi.org/10.1046/j.1524-4725.2000.00278.x

[12]   Har-Shai, Y., Lindenbaum, E., Ben-Itzhak, O., *et al.* (1996) Large Liponecrotic Pseudocyst Formation Following Cheek Augmentation by Fat Injection. *Aesthetic Plastic Surgery*, **20**, 417-419. http://dx.doi.org/10.1007/BF02390317

[13]   Carpaneda, C.A. (1996) Study of Aspirated Adipose Tissue. *Aesthetic Plastic Surgery*, **20**, 399-402. http://dx.doi.org/10.1007/BF02390314

[14]   Heymans, O., Castus, P., Grandjean, F.X., *et al.* (2006) Liposuction: Review of the Techniques, Innovations and Applications. *Acta Chirurgica Belgica*, **106**, 647-653.

[15]   Prado, A., Andrades, P., Danilla, S., *et al.* (2006) A Prospective, Randomized, Double-Blind, Controlled Clinical Trial Comparing Laser-Assisted Lipoplasty with Suction-Assisted Lipoplasty. *Plastic and Reconstructive Surgery*, **118**, 1032-1045. http://dx.doi.org/10.1097/01.prs.0000232428.37926.48

[16]   Abdelaal, M.M. and Aboelatta, Y.A. (2014) Comparison of Blood Loss in Laser Lipolysis vs Traditional Liposuction. *Aesthetic Surgery Journal*, **34**, 907-912. http://dx.doi.org/10.1177/1090820X14536904

[17]   Badin, A.Z., Moraes, L.M., Gondek, L., *et al.* (2002) Laser Lipolysis: Flaccidity under Control. *Aesthetic Plastic Surgery*, **26**, 335-339. http://dx.doi.org/10.1007/s00266-002-1510-3

[18]   Goldman, A. (2006) Submental Nd:Yag Laser-Assisted Liposuction. *Lasers in Surgery and Medicine*, **38**, 181-184.

http://dx.doi.org/10.1002/lsm.20270

[19] Yoshimura, K., Shigeura, T., Matsumoto, D., *et al.* (2006) Characterization of Freshly Isolated and Cultured Cells Derived from the Fatty and Fluid Portions of Liposuction Aspirates. *Journal of Cellular Physiology*, **208**, 64-76.
http://dx.doi.org/10.1002/jcp.20636

27

Evolution of Post-Surgical Scars Treated with Pure Rosehip Seed Oil

Pedro Valerón-Almazán[1], Anselmo J. Gómez-Duaso[1], Néstor Santana-Molina[1], Miguel A. García-Bello[2], Gregorio Carretero[1]

[1]Dermatology Service, Hospital Universitario de Gran Canaria Dr. Negrin, Las Palmas, Spain
[2]Research Unit, Hospital Universitario de Gran Canaria Dr. Negrin, Las Palmas, Spain
Email: maria.matabuena@invitrotecnia.com

Abstract

The rosehip seed oil (RHO), obtained from different plant species of the genus Rosa, is one of the compounds used empirically for cosmetic improvement of skin scarring. Despite its widespread use in clinical practice, there are few studies evaluating the activity of this compound on the clinical course of cutaneous scars. The aim of this study was to determine the effect of Repavar® rosehip oil on improvement of post-surgical skin scars. One comparative, single-center, prospective clinical trial was carried out in 108 patients undergoing cutaneous surgery procedures in the Dermatology Service of University Hospital of Gran Canaria Dr. Negrín (Spain). Subjective parameters (erythema, discoloration, atrophy and hypertrophy) were evaluated at 6 and 12 weeks on 76 adults who treated scars with pure RHO twice a day (test group), 32 patients with not treatment (control group), and completed the study. Lesser degree of erythema was observed at 6 and 12 weeks in treated-patients compared with the control group and decreased discoloration and atrophy at 12 weeks, with statistically significant differences in all cases (p < 0.05). This study demonstrates that the RHO Repavar® is useful for cosmetic improvement on erythema, discoloration and atrophyof post-surgical skin scars, getting a better overall evolution and appearance thereof.

Keywords

Healing, Skin Scar, Rosa Mosqueta, Rosehip Seed Oil, Skin Surgery

1. Introduction

Healing is a natural and dynamic process in which body has to regenerate tissues after injury. This process develops along three phases, comprising inflammation, granulation tissue formation and maturation/remodeling [1]-[3]. In the inflammatory phase, platelet degranulation, cell-recruitment migration, and extracellular matrix formation are initiated, all mediated by multiple cytokines and growth factors [4]. The proliferative phase starts several days after the initial injury, and it is characterized by angiogenesis, collagen deposition, formation of granulation tissue and epithelialization and contraction of the scar [5]. In the remodeling phase, tissue enzymes remove excess of extracellular matrix and collagen, and remained fibrils are realigned along the tension lines. This remodeling process occurs during 6 - 12 months but may persist for years after initial injury [3].

Clinically, cutaneous scars are defined as macroscopic alterations of the architectural structure of the skin, as a final result of the healing process. The affected area may be displayed as an elevated or depressed area, which has also variations in consistency, color, vascularization and/or innervation. Although many therapies have been tried to improve the clinical appearance of skin scars, no treatment has clearly shown its efficacy and still considers prevention as the most important attitude to avoid the appearance of hypertrophic scars or keloids [6].

"Rosa mosqueta" or "Rosehip", is a generic name which covers about 70 different species of plants of the genus *Rosa*, as *Rosa rubiginosa*, *Rosa moschata* and *Rosa canina* [7]. The rosehip seed oil (RHO) is extracted from the seed of the fruit of the wild plant. Some studies have examined before the chemical composition of this compound, where the high content of polyunsaturated fatty acid highlights: linoleic acid (54%), linolenic acid (17%) and oleic acid (16%) between others [8]. Lesser amounts of other saturated fatty acids and small amounts of other dermatological active interest like transretinoic acid or natural tretinoin (between 0.01% and 0.1%) have also been identified [9].

In the medical field, the RHO has been used for decades to treat wounds and/or scars. The beneficial effect of this oil has been attributed to its high content of essential fatty and unsaturated acids abovementioned, which play a key role in the permeability of cell membranes and injuries repair mechanisms [10]. Despite its theoretical utility in these processes, there are few studies that evaluate the activity of this compound on the clinical course of healing [11] [12].

The aim of this study was to analyze the clinical course of post-surgical cutaneous scars treated with pure RHO in terms of erythema, discoloration, atrophy and hypertrophy.

2. Methods

2.1. Patients

108 patients were underwent open surgical procedures for skin tumor removal of pigmented lesions between April and June (over three months), in the Dermatology Service, University Hospital of Gran Canaria Dr. Negrín, were enrolled in a comparative, single-center and prospective study.

Inclusion criteria in the study were elderly patients with sufficient level of understanding, with not-known-RHO-allergies, without any history of keloids or other healing defects.

The Clinical Research Ethics Committee of the Hospital approved the study, and all patients gave informed consent form to participate in it.

2.2. Treatment

Patients in the test group had to apply the RHO (Repavar®) twice a day on the scar, from the removal of sutures, for six weeks. Patients considered as controls did not perform any treatment.

Patients were assigned to each group randomly and the same experienced dermatologist performed the evaluation in all groups of patients, so that all observations follow the same validated criteria.

2.3. Analysis Parameters

The variables were analyzed at 6 and 12 weeks after removal of sutures, and data were recorded taking into account this classification (**Table 1**):

Table 1. Evaluation criteria of parameters erythema, discoloration, atrophy and hypertrophy.

	Erythema		Dyschromia		Atrophy		Hypertrophy
0	No erythema	0	No color change	0	No atrophy	0	No hypertrophy
1	Mild (pink)	1	Slight hyper/hypochromia	1	Slight depression	1	Slight hypertrophy
2	Intense (red)	2	Major hyper/hypochromia	2	Major depression	2	Major hypertrophy (keloid)

For the descriptive analysis, categorical variables were expressed as absolute frequencies and percentages.

2.4. Statistical Analysis

For statistical analysis, the Chi-square test was used, considering a level of statistical significance $\alpha < 0.05$.

3. Results and Discussion

A total of 160 patients were included in the trial, of whom 120 patients were treated with RHO and 40 underwent no treatment (control).

103 patients from the 120 treated patients group attended the review of 6 weeks and 76 attended the review of the 12 weeks. 32 patients from the 40 patients control group went to the reviews at 6 and 12 weeks. 108 patients completed the study.

No adverse effects were observed in any patient, neither in the treated group and the control group.

Table 2 and **Figures 1-4** summarize the results.

Table 2. Evolution of patients at 6 and 12 weeks.

		Treated-group	Control group	Total
Erythema				
6 weeks	No	61 (52.9%)	14 (43.8%)	75
	Mild	38 (36.9%)	11 (34.4%)	49
	Intense	4 (3.9%)	7 (21.9%)	11
12 weeks	No	56 (73.7%)	16 (50.0%)	72
	Mild	15 (19.7%)	9 (28.1%)	24
	Intense	5 (6.6%)	7 (21.9%)	12
Dischromia				
6 weeks	No	29 (28.2%)	10 (31.3%)	39
	Mild	67 (65.2%)	18 (56.3%)	85
	Intense	7 (6.8%)	4 (12.5%)	11
12 weeks	No	48 (63.2%)	7 (21.9%)	55
	Mild	24 (31.6%)	22 (68.8%)	46
	Intense	4 (5.3%)	3 (9.4%)	7
Atrophy				
6 weeks	No	83 (80.6%)	23 (71.9%)	106
	Mild	18 (17.5%)	7 (21.9%)	25
	Notorious	2 (1.9%)	2 (6.3%)	4
12 weeks	No	65 (85.5%)	20 (62.5%)	85
	Mild	9 (11.8%)	9 (28.1%)	18
	Notorious	2 (2.6%)	3 (9.4%)	5
Hypertrophy				
6 weeks	No	83 (80.6%)	26 (81.2%)	109
	Mild	14 (13.6%)	4 (12.5%)	18
	Intense	6 (5.8%)	2 (6.2%)	8
12 weeks	No	67 (89.3%)	25 (78.1%)	72
	Mild	7 (9.4%)	6 (18.8%)	24
	Intense	1 (1.3%)	1 (3.1%)	12

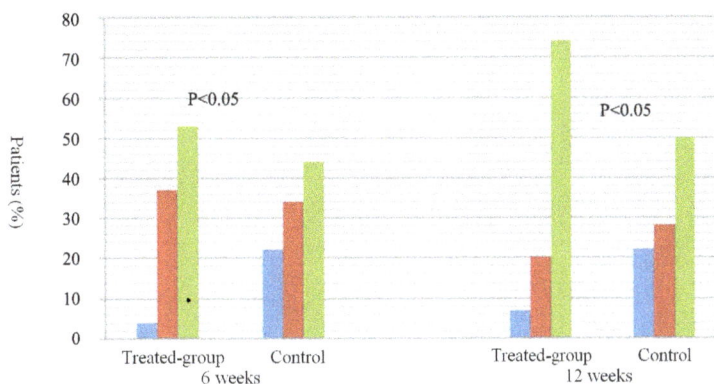

Figure 1. Subjective evaluation of erythema at 6 and 12 weeks. Blue bar, intense; red bar, mild; green bar, no erythema.

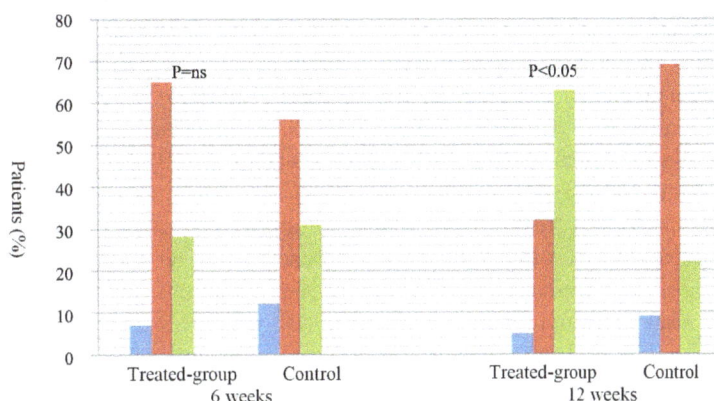

Figure 2. Subjective evaluation of discoloration at 6 and 12 weeks. Blue bar, intense; red bar, mild; green bar, no discoloration.

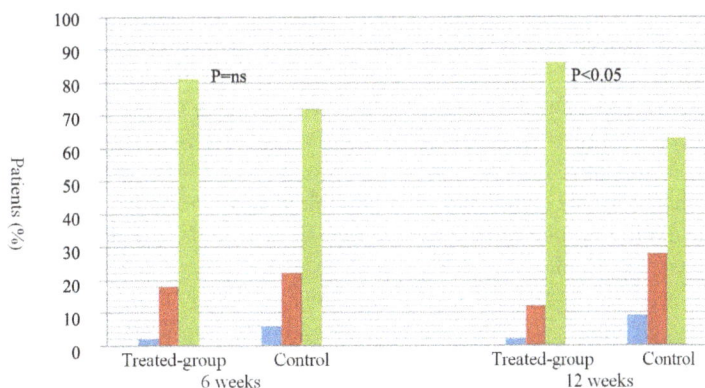

Figure 3. Subjective evaluation of atrophy at 6 and 12 weeks. Blue bar, notorious; red bar, mild; green bar, no atrophy.

In the subjective assessment of erythema carried out by the specialist (**Figure 1**), significant differences between the patients and the control group at both 6 and 12 weeks (73% of treated patients did not presented erythema at 12 weeks vs. 50% of control patients) were founded.

Concerning the colorimetric changes taken together, a higher proportion of patients treated with RHO did not shown subjective discoloration at 6 and 12 weeks, although these differences were only significant at 12 weeks (63% of treated patients without discoloration vs. 21% control) (**Figure 2**).

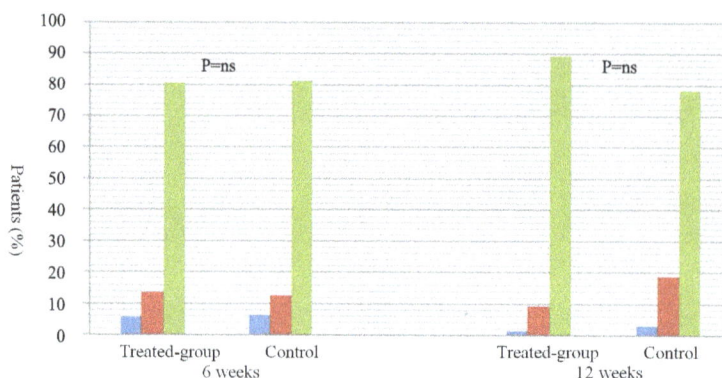

Figure 4. Subjective evaluation of hypertrophy at 6 and 12 weeks. Blue bar, notorious; red bar, mild; green bar, no hypertrophy.

The atrophy measurement (**Figure 3**) showed differences in patients treated with RHO at 6 and 12 weeks, with significant differences at the second examination (85% vs. 62% of patients without atrophy found at 12 weeks).

Finally, hypertrophy analysis showed better evolution of scars on treated-group compared to control group at 6 and 12 weeks, but no statistically significant differences (**Figure 4**).

Figure 5 and **Figure 6** show two examples of cutaneous scars treated with RHO, at the beginning of treatment (**Figure 5(A)** and **Figure 6(A)**) and after 12 weeks (**Figure 5(B)** and **Figure 6(B)**).

In daily dermatological practice, it is common that patients in whom a common surgical procedure is practiced not receive any topical treatment for cosmetic improvement after removal of sutures, beyond sunscreen always recommended. In this study, RHO showed a beneficial effect on clinical appearance of scars, in general, compared with those who were remained to their natural evolution. Our observations are concurrent with previous studies that evaluated the properties of RHO in healing injuries [11] [12].

Within the parameters analyzed, the most obvious improvement occurred in terms of erythema, with statistically significant differences in medical analysis at both 6 and 12 weeks in the RHO-treated-patients group (**Figure 1**). In the evolution of post-operative dyschromia, only significant differences at 12 weeks were found. It is possible that the scars color improvement may be associated with reduced inflammation [13] [14] and inhibition of chemotaxis [15] [16] that has been shown in *in vitro* and *in vivo* clinical trials using Rosehip seed oil.

A previous study used histological criteria to evaluate therapeutic properties of RHO [13], but we discard this possibility because the procedure was so invasive.

Several studies have found high levels of unsaturated fatty acids in RHO, mainly linoleic acid, linolenic acid and oleic acid [8] [9]. Essential fatty acids are basic components of the phospholipids in cell membranes, which are involved in numerous phosphorylation and cellular organization processes [10]. Some compounds like carotenoids and polyphenols have also been isolated from the RHO [17] [18], which are responsible for the antioxidant activity attributed to this compound. It is possible that the presence of these substances in the RHO contribute to a better evolution of the healing process, especially if it is applied early, as happened in our patients.

In the assessment of atrophy, a higher percentage of patients with outatrophy at 12 weeks, was found with significant differences, in the RHO-treated-group(85% vs. 62%). These differences may be related to the presence of derivatives of vitamin A (retinoic acid or naturally tretinoin) that have been previously identified in RHO [9]. Tretinoin topical treatment is widely used in dermatology, mainly in the context of acne vulgaris [19] and photo-induced skin damage [20], although previous references also exist about the benefit of its use in healing injury [21] [22].

With respect to the appearance of hypertrophy, no large differences were observed in treated patients, with similar percentages versus the control group. This observation is concurrent with the usual clinical experience, because, so far, no therapy has proven effective in a consistent way for the prevention or treatment of hypertrophic scars or keloids [23]. For now, early identification remains the mainstay for treatment.

4. Conclusions

As final conclusion, this study presented a group of patients in which the early application of RHO Repavar® in

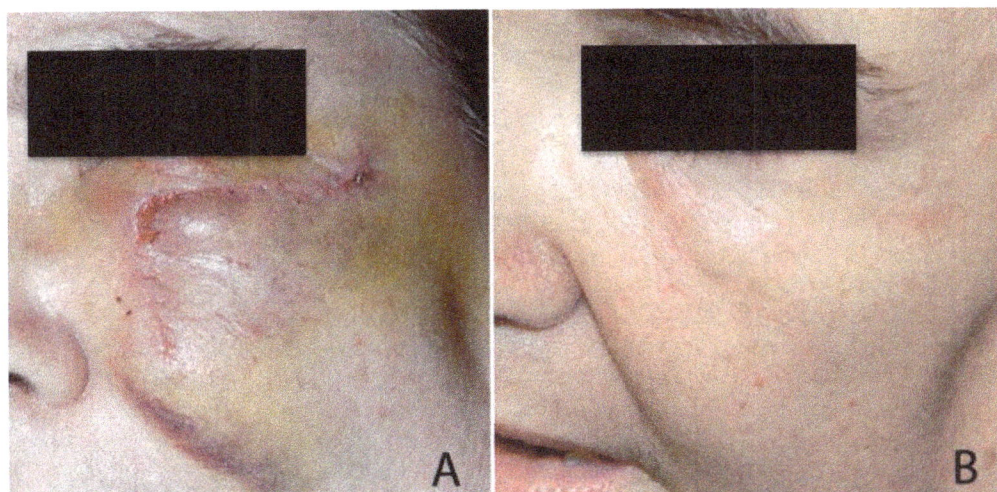

Figure 5. (A) Skin Scar on left side of the face after removal of sutures; (B) Clinical image after 12 weeks of treatment with RHO twice daily.

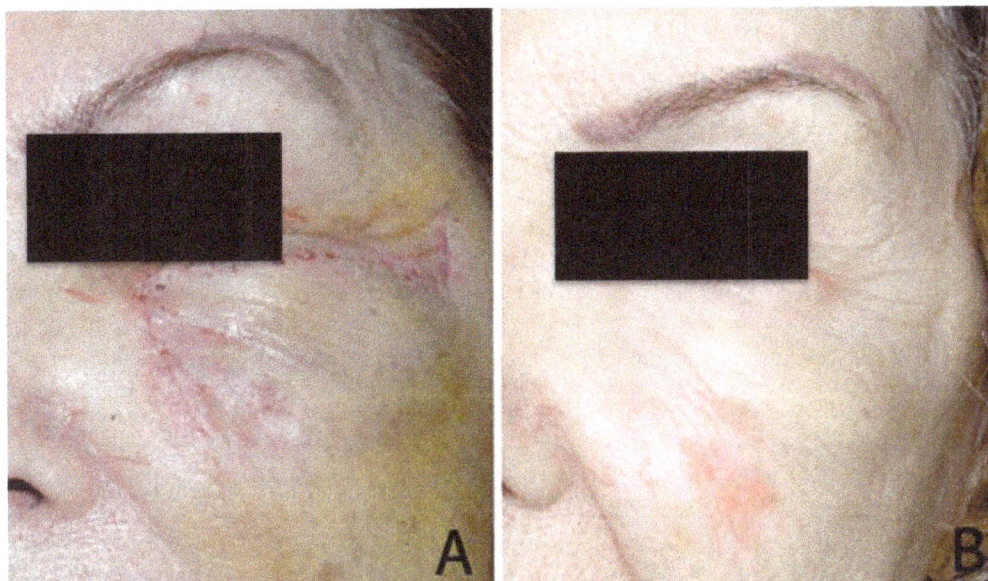

Figure 6. (A) Skin Scar on left side of the face after removal of sutures; (B) Clinical image after 12 weeks of treatment with AHM twice daily.

post-surgical scars generally resulted in a cosmetic improvement thereof. This improvement was observed subjectively, especially at the level of erythema, with significant differences at 6 and 12 weeks, and discoloration and atrophy, with significant differences at 12 weeks.

This study provides preliminary results that can support the development of other trials providing a larger number of patients and longer follow-up.

Acknowledgements

This study was sponsored by Ferrer Internacional, SA.

References

[1] Stadelmann, W.K., Digenis, A.G. and Tobin, G.R. (1998) Physiology and Healing Dynamics of Chronic Cutaneous Wounds. *American Journal of Surgery*, **176**, 26-38. http://dx.doi.org/10.1016/S0002-9610(98)00183-4

[2]   Iba, Y., Shibata, A., Kato, M. and Masukawa, T. (2004) Possible Involvement of Mast Cells in Collagen Remodeling in the Late Phase of Cutaneous Wound Healing in Mice. *International Immunopharmacology*, **4**, 1873-1880. http://dx.doi.org/10.1016/j.intimp.2004.08.009

[3]   Arndt, K.A. (2006) Scar Revision. Elsevier, Philadelphia.

[4]   McGrath, M.H. (1990) Peptide Growth Factors and Wound Healing. *Clinics in Plastic Surgery*, **17**, 421-432.

[5]   Cohen, I.K., Diegelman, R.F. and Lindblad, W.J. (1992) Wound-Healing: Biochemical and Clinical Aspects. *Annals of Surgery*, **96**, 114. http://dx.doi.org/10.1097/00006534-199211000-00034

[6]   Mustoe, T.A., Cooter, R.D., Gold, M.H., Hobbs, F.D., Ramelet, A.A. and Shakespeare, P.G. (2002) International Clinical Recommendations on Scar Management. *Plastic and Reconstructive Surgery*, **110**, 560-571. http://dx.doi.org/10.1097/00006534-200208000-00031

[7]   Dogan, A. and Kazankaya, A. (2006) Properties of Hose Hip Species Grown in Lake Van Basin (Eastern Anatolia Region). *Asian Journal of Plant Sciences*, **5**, 120-122. http://dx.doi.org/10.3923/ajps.2006.120.122

[8]   Ozcan, M. (2002) Nutrient Composition of Rose (*Rosa canina* L.) Seed and Oils. *Journal of Medicinal Food*, **5**, 137-140. http://dx.doi.org/10.1089/10966200260398161

[9]   Valladares, J., Palma, M., Sandoval, C. and Carvajal, F. (1986) Cream Hip Oil (*Rosa aff. rubiginosa* I.). Part I: Formulation, Preparation and Primary Application in Tissue Regeneration. *Annals Real Acad Farm.*, **52**, 597-612.

[10]   Santos, J.S., Vieira, A.B. and Kamada, I. (2009) The Rosehip Not Open Wounds Treatment: A Review. *Revista Brasileira de Enfermagem*, **62**, 457-462. http://dx.doi.org/10.1590/S0034-71672009000300020

[11]   Moreno, J.C., Good, J., Navas, J. and Camacho, F. (1990) Treatment of Cutaneous Ulcers with Musk Rose Oil. *Cutan Med Ibero Lat Am.*, **18**, 63-66.

[12]   Camacho, F., Moreno, J.C., Conejo-Mir, J. and Bueno, J. (1994) Treatment of Post-Surgical Scars and Pure Oil Rosehip Seed Defects. *Cutan Med Ibero Lat Am.*, **22**, 23-30.

[13]   Marchini, F.B., Martins, D.M., Teves, D.C. and Simöes, M.J. (1988) Rosehip Oil Effect on the Healing of Open Wounds. *Revista Paulista de Medicina*, **106**, 356.

[14]   Hakansson, A., Stene, C., Milhaescu, A., Molin, G., Ahrné, S. and Thorlacius, H. (2006) Rose Hip and *Lactobacillus plantarum* DSM 9843 Reduces Ischemia/Reperfusion Injury in the Mouse Colon. *Digestive Diseases and Sciences*, **51**, 2094-2101. http://dx.doi.org/10.1007/s10620-006-9170-9

[15]   Daels-Rakotoarison, D.A., Gressier, B., Trotin, F., Brunet, C., Luyckx, M. and Dine, T. (2002) Effects of *Rosa canina* Fruit Extract on Neutrophil Respiratory Burst. *Phytotherapy Research*, **16**, 157-161. http://dx.doi.org/10.1002/ptr.985

[16]   Larsen, E., Kharazmi, A., Christensen, L.P. and Christensen, S.B. (2003) An Antiinflammatory Galactolipid from Rose Hip (*Rosa canina*) That Inhibits Chemotaxis of Peripheral Blood Neutrophils *in Vitro* Huma. *Journal of Natural Products*, **66**, 994-995. http://dx.doi.org/10.1021/np0300636

[17]   Robert, P., Carlsson, R.M., Romero, N. and Masson, L. (2003) Stability of Spray-Dried Encapsulated Carotenoid Pigments from Rosehip (*Rosa rubiginosa*) Oleoresin. *Journal of the American Oil Chemists' Society*, **80**, 1115-1120. http://dx.doi.org/10.1007/s11746-003-0828-4

[18]   Salminen, J.P., Karonen, M., Lempa, K., Liimatainen, J., Sinkkonen, J. and Lukkarinen, M. (2005) Characterisation of Proanthocyanidin Aglycones and Glycosides from Rose Hips by High-Performance Liquid Chromatography-Mass Spectrometry, and Their Rapid Quantification Together with Vitamin C. *Journal of Chromatography A*, **1077**, 170-180. http://dx.doi.org/10.1016/j.chroma.2005.04.073

[19]   Torok, H.M. and Pillai, R. (2011) Safety and Efficacy of Micronized Tretinoin Gel (0.05%) in Treating Adolescent Acne. *Journal of Drugs in Dermatology*, **10**, 647-652.

[20]   Ting, W. (2010) Tretinoin for the Treatment of Photodamaged Skin. *Cutis*, **86**, 47-52.

[21]   Harris, D.W., Buckley, C.C., Ostlere, L.S. and Rustin, M.H. (1991) Topical Retinoic Acid in the Treatment of Acne Scarring Fine. *British Journal of Dermatology*, **125**, 81-82. http://dx.doi.org/10.1111/j.1365-2133.1991.tb06048.x

[22]   de Limpens A.M., J. (1980) The Local Treatment of Hypertrophic Scars and Keloids with Topical Retinoic Acid. *British Journal of Dermatology*, **103**, 319-323. http://dx.doi.org/10.1111/j.1365-2133.1980.tb07251.x

[23]   Berman, B., Villa, A.M. and Ramirez, C.C. (2004) Novel Opportunities in the Treatment and Prevention of Scarring. *Journal of Cutaneous Medicine and Surgery*, **8**, 32-36. http://dx.doi.org/10.1007/s10227-004-0806-0

28

A Guide to Cheek Augmentation: Single-Point Deep Injection of Hyaluronic Acid Filler at Midface in Close Proximity to Medial Suborbicularis Oculi Fat (SOOF) Area

Chung-Pin Liang[1], Haw-Yueh Thong[2]*

[1]Department of Dermatology, Chung-Shan University Hospital, Taiwan
[2]Department of Dermatology, Shin-Kong Wu Ho-Su Memorial Hospital, Taiwan
Email: *drkellytang@gmail.com

Abstract

Loss of volume in midface can result in an aged, wasted appearance. Osseous and fat atrophy with aging may further contribute to the loss of soft tissue support and midface ptosis. In the aging of periorbital area and midface, fat atrophy occurs mostly in the suborbicularis oculi fat (SOOF) area. The authors proposed that injection of hyaluronic acid (HA) filler to support the SOOF area could counteract the aging sign due to fat atrophy, restore volume loss and achieve a more youthful appearance. The authors described the treatment of 10 female patients who received CHAP®-particle hyaluronic acid (CHAP®-HA) injections for cheek augmentation, using single-point deep injection technique at midface in close proximity to SOOF area. Such approach provides satisfactory cheek augmentation results without significant complications. The authors discussed a rationale for their choice of dermal filler and provided an injection technique for restoring volume in the midface region with CHAP®-HA. Such technique is relatively quick to perform, have little down time, and result in a high rate of patient satisfaction.

Keywords

Midface Lift, Cheek Augmentation, Fat Compartment, Suborbicularis Oculi Fat (SOOF), Single-Point Deep Injection, Hyaluronic Acid (HA) Filler, CHAP®-Hyaluronic Acid (Crosslinked Hyaluronic Acid Platform, CHAP®-HA), Hyadermis®

---

*Corresponding author.

1. Introduction

Apart from amelioration of isolated wrinkles and folds, volume restoration and contour enhancement have become the objectives of advanced injectors [1]-[3]. The value of midfacial volume restoration and enhancement has been well documented in the literature. However, when treating this area, the injector can experience adverse events, such as the significant and long-lasting complication of malar edema, nodules and lumps, visible materials, bruising, erythema, pain, infection, skin necrosis, over- and under-correction, and infraorbital nerve injuries resulting in numbness and dysesthesia have been reported [1]-[4].

Midface Volume Restoration

Hyaluronan is a naturally occurring linear polysaccharide which can be found in skin, connective, epithelial, and neural tissues. The amount of naturally occurring hyaluronan in the skin decreases with age, contributing to the development of the aging features and wrinkle formation. The new understanding of the subcutaneous tissue of the face has led to improvements in rejuvenation techniques that focus on the skin and superficial tissue, using fillers and autologous fat [5]. A major advancement that has contributed to the current state of filler injection is the knowledge that the face does not age as one homogenous object but as many dynamic compartments, which need to be evaluated, augmented, and modified as such [6]. Recent advancements in understanding the fat compartments of the face would provide additional insights to dermal filler rejuvenation techniques. By using dermal filler to support distorted fat compartments one would be able to restore a youthful appearance.

The malar fat pad is a discrete, triangular shaped area of thickened subcutaneous fat, based at the nasolabial fold with its apex at the malar eminence in the youthful face [3]. It is attached to the overlying skin and is supported by multiple fibrous septae that extend from the superficial musculoaponeurotic system (SMAS) and into the dermis. Loss of skin elasticity and weakening of these septae, as well as volume loss within the deep medial cheek fat [4], leads to a downward and forward descent of the skin and malar fat pad until it bulges against the fixed nasolabial fold. These sequelae of aging result in deepening of the nasolabial folds, progressive hollowing of the cheeks, and loss of prominence of the malar eminences. The lower eyelid lengthens, increasing the visibility of orbicularis oculi muscle, coupled with the formation of teartrough and a crescent or "V"-shaped deformity along the maxilla and zygoma, in addition to the recession of the nasal alar cheek junction. Individual fat pockets become discernable as separate entities rather than the smooth transitions from convexities to concavities seen in youth [4]. Rohrich *et al.* [7] demonstrated that when saline was injected into the deep medial fat compartment, as opposed to superficially in the area of the nasolabial fold, numerous changes occurred, including an increase in anterior projection of the midface, flattening of the nasojugal and nasolabial creases, and an overall improved appearance of the malar region. These changes could all be brought about by manipulating one fat compartment. Therefore, we postulate that the sole correction of midcheek would be an effective way for rejuvenation [4]. Based on Rohrich's proposed concept, we hypothesized that injecting dermal filler into fat compartment would provide a more youthful appearance in an aging face. The aim of this work is to evaluate the efficacy and safety of single-point deep injection of Hyaluronic acid (HA) fillers in midface in close proximity to medial SOOF for cheek augmentation.

2. Methods

2.1. Material

The Hyadermis® product line (SciVision Biotech Inc., Taiwan ROC), including Hyadermis® Blink, Hyadermis® Kiss, Hyadermis® Smile, Hyadermis® Chic, has been marketed in European Union since 2005 and Taiwan since 2010. Hyadermis® consisted of 20 mg/ml bacterium-derived non-animal stabilized HA. These HA hydrogels are developed using CHAP® (Crosslinked Hyaluronic Acid Platform, CHAP®) technology and have a high gel-to-fluid ratio which accounts for its longevity in performance. Hyadermis® Blink is mainly used to improve fine lines and as skin boosters ; Hyadermis ® Kiss is used for correcting teartrough and lip augmentation, whereas Hyadermis® Smile and Hyadermis® Chic are favorable for contouring facial structure, volumizing medium depth facial wrinkles and lifting tissues. Hyadermis® is one of the most popular dermal filler in Taiwan. In our study, 2 syringes of 1 ml Hyadermis® Smile were used (1ml for each side) for cheek augmentation.

2.2. Subjects

Ten healthy non-pregnant female individuals with mild to moderate midface ptosis, who have never received dermal filler injection received single-point deep injection of Hyadermis® smile at midface in close proximity to medial SOOF area. Treatment area with tattoos, scars, dermatitis, or open wounds and patients with a history of major diseases, diabetes mellitus, HIV infection, connective tissue disease, and malignant disease were excluded. Those with recent (within 3 months) or aesthetic laser/chemical peeling treatment and concurrent use of medication that could disrupt coagulation (e.g., aspirin, NSAIDs, warfarin) were also excluded. All patients provided written informed consent.

2.3. Preparation and Treatment

Before treatment, a thorough evaluation of the patient's medical history was conducted. Injection point on each side of cheek was chosen based on the following guidelines: gross anatomy which would be in close proximity to medial SOOF area (**Figure 1(a)** & **Figure 1(b)**) and four clinical testing, namely pushing test, smiling test, laxity evaluation and snap test (**Figure 2**), to identify the point with most volume depletion, where dermal filler could be injected with supposedly satisfactory results. Photographic imaging was performed before and after treatment.

2.4. Treatment Protocol

The treatment area was first cleansed with a mild cleanser prior to treatment. All patients were photographed prior to injection. Local anesthetics were applied for 10 minutes. Prior to injection, ultrasound imaging was performed (Philips ultrasound iU22, with L 12-5 MHz probe) to briefly evaluate the presence of blood vessels on the intended injection point. After the confirmation of an absence of major blood vessels, single point injection was performed on both cheek using either sharp needle or micro-cannula, depending on the preference of the subjects (**Figure 3**). After injection, ultrasound imaging was performed to confirm the depth of injection (**Figure 4**).

3. Assessments and Analysis

All of the patients underwent single-point deep HA filler injection at the midface region. Photographic documentation of the treated area was recorded prior to and after injection. Ultrasound imaging was also performed prior to and after injection. Efficacy was determined by photographic evaluation, while safety was determined by clinical findings and patients' report of any discomfort. Adverse events, including evaluation of patient's response and local skin reaction in the treatment area, were recorded throughout the study. A questionnaire on the pain experience and subjective satisfaction was also performed.

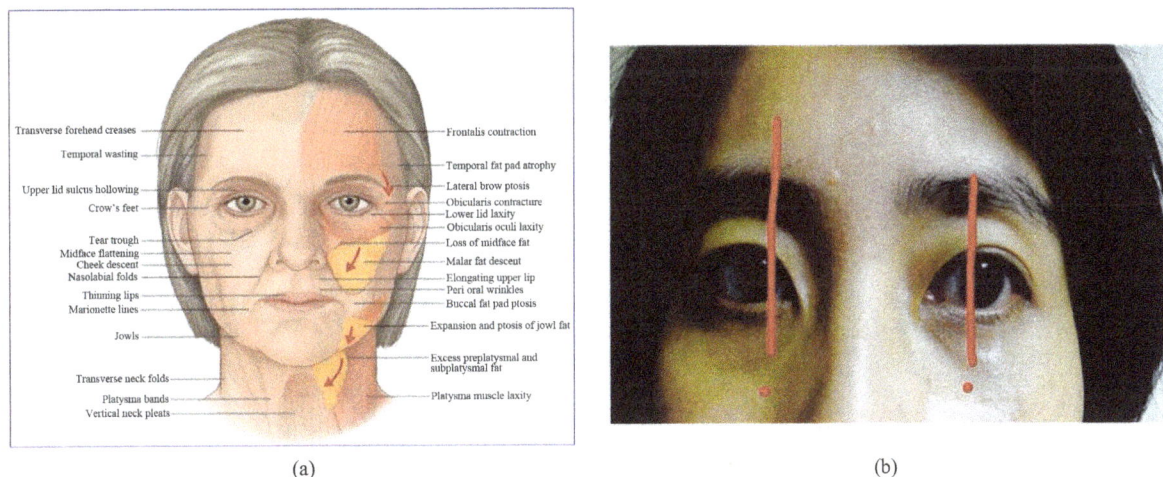

(a)   (b)

Figure 1. (a) Midface aging due to loss of midface fat and malar fat descent. *SOOF (http://www.slideshare.net/subhakantamohapatra71/facelift-surgery-36146703); (b) Injection points grossly in close proximity to medial SOOF area.

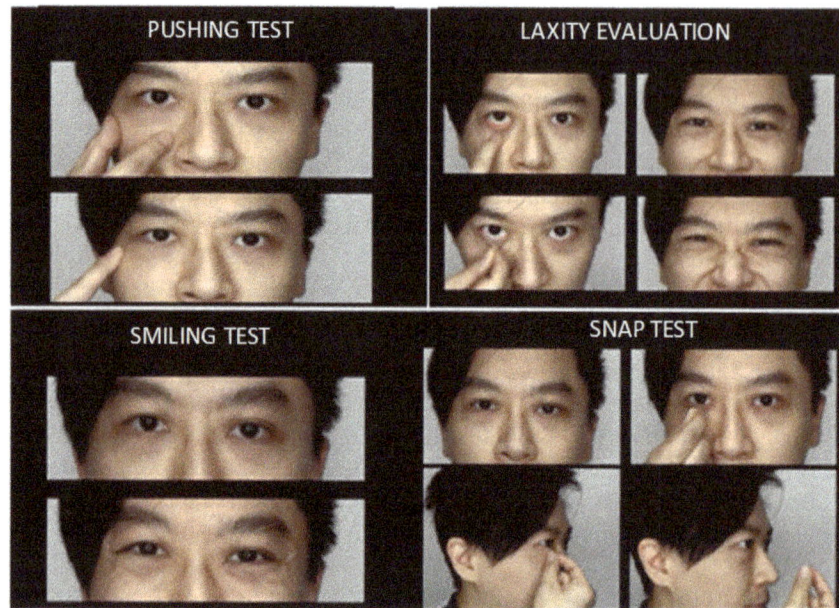

Figure 2. Pushing Test, Smiling Test, Laxity Evaluation and Snap Test are the 4 tests which could be used to identify the point with most volume depletion, where dermal fillers could be injected.

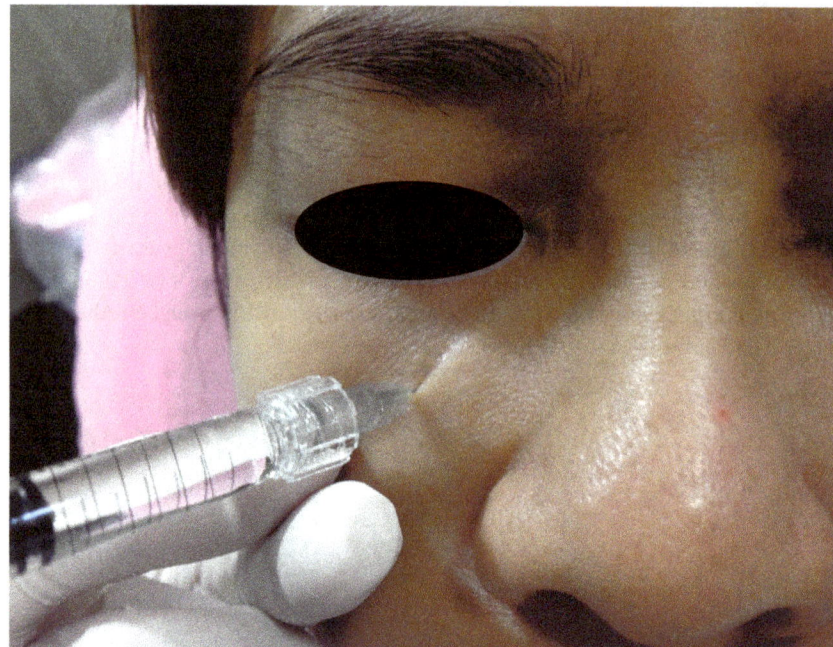

Figure 3. Single point deep injection of HA filler on treatment area using sharp needle on case 5.

4. Results

10 female subjects completed the treatments. All subjects were Taiwanese, with a mean age of 39.5 ± 6.8 years (**Table 1**). All subjects had mild to moderate midface ptosis, with or without eyebag or teartrough. All subjects received 1 ml each of Hyadermis® Smile with lidocaine, single-point injection using sharp needle or micro-cannula at their preferences, at the midface region grossly in close proximity to medial SOOF area. 6 subjects chose to be injected with sharp needle, whereas 4 subjects decided to be injected with micro-cannula.

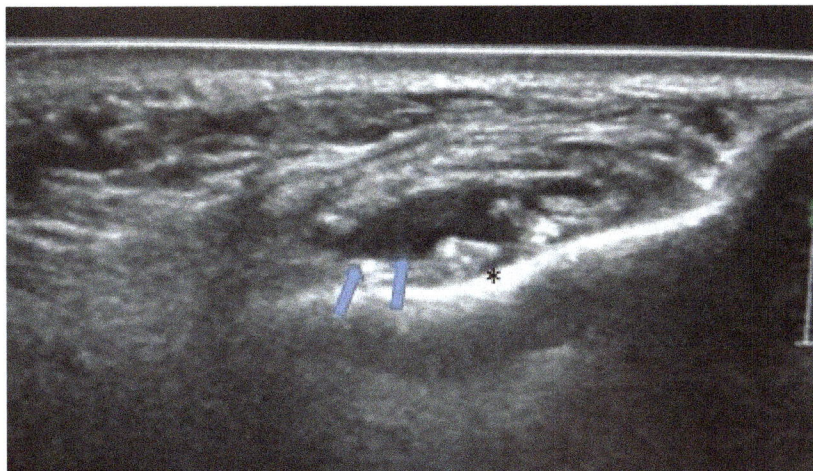

Figure 4. Ultrasound imaging of HA filler after injection to confirm depth of filler placement. Arrow = HA filler, * = periosteum.

Table 1. The basic demographics of the subjects and patient satisfaction.

Case number	Age	Injection method	Pain level on treatment	Patient satisfaction		Side effect
				Immediately after treatment	4-month with phone interview	
Case 1	40	27G Sharp Needle	No pain	Very satisfied	Very satisfied	Mild tenderness
Case 2	41	27G Sharp Needle	Acceptable	Very satisfied	Very satisfied	Mild tenderness
Case 3	50	27G Micro-Cannula	Acceptable	Very satisfied	Very satisfied	Nil
Case 4	28	27G Micro-Cannula	Acceptable	Very satisfied	Very satisfied	Nil
Case 5	39	27G Sharp Needle	Mild pain	Satisfied	Satisfied	Nil
Case 6	46	27G Sharp Needle	No pain	Very satisfied	Very satisfied	Mild tenderness
Case 7	44	27G Sharp Needle	No pain	Very satisfied	Very satisfied	Intermittent tingling sensation lasted for 3 days
Case 8	38	27G Micro-Cannula	No pain	Very satisfied	Very satisfied	Mild edema
Case 9	29	27G Sharp Needle	Acceptable	Satisfied	Satisfied	Nil
Case 10	40	27G Micro-Cannula	Acceptable	Very satisfied	Very satisfied	Nil
Average age	39.5					
Standard deviation	6.835365551					

All patients noted satisfactory cheek augmentation immediately after injection, as represented in **Table 1** and **Figure 5**. Treated subjects also noted an improvement in tear trough and eyebag (**Figure 6**). All subjects were satisfied with the treatment outcome immediately after treatment and at 4-month follow up with phone interview (**Table 1**). There was no clinically noticeable difference in the cheek augmentation effect and the degree of edema between sharp needle and micro-cannula injections.

Side effects were transient, with the most common side effect being pain and tenderness, and edema on the treatment area which typically resolved within 48 hours post treatment. Minimal bruising was noted with both sharp needle or micro-cannula injections. Pain was generally tolerable. One subject noted intermittent tingling sensation on the left cheek, which resolved within 3 days. This particular subject was injected with sharp needle. No long term complication was noted. All subjects reported to have satisfactory results with no side effects on the 4-month follow up phone interview (**Table 1**).

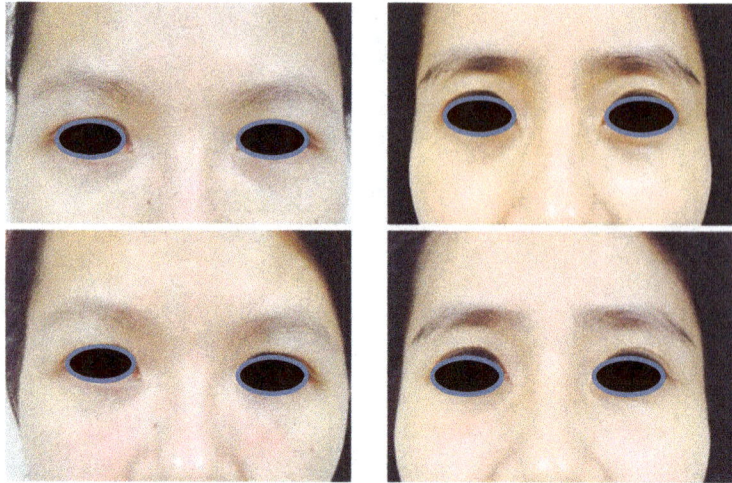

Figure 5. Before (upper) and immediately after (lower) single point deep injection of HA filler (1ml on each side) for cheek augmentation using 27 G sharp needle. Satisfactory results were noted with minimal bruising. Left: Case 2, Right: Case 7.

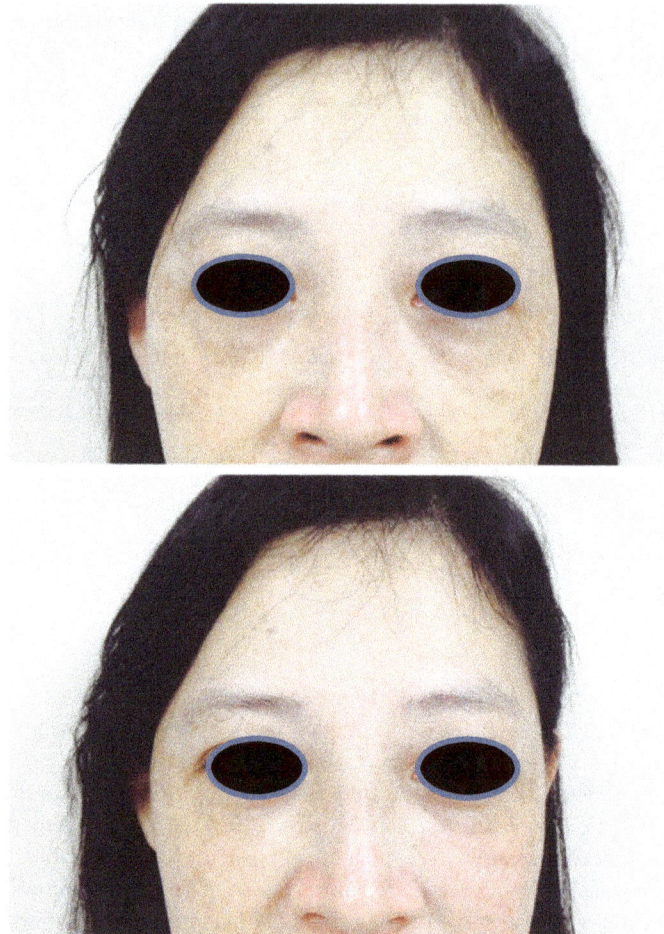

Figure 6. Case 3, before (upper) and immediately after (lower) single point deep injection of HA filler (1 ml on each side) for cheek augmentation using 27 G micro-cannula. Teartrough and eyebag could also be improved with such technique.

5. Discussion

Soft tissue augmentation with temporary dermal fillers is a continuously growing field, supported by the ongoing development and advances in technology and biocompatibility of the products marketed. We hereby presented a new technique of midface lift using a novel CHAP®-HA. Our results showed that such material is safe, and could provide satisfactory midface lifting results.

As proposed by Sandoval *et al.*, the new conceptual understanding of the facial fat will lead to new and improved methods of autologous fat injection [5]. These fat compartments may serve as the "GPS" for the injection of facial fillers. Our study has demonstrated the effect of the placement of fillers in close proximity to single fat compartment and the visual changes created by their augmentation. The safety and efficacy of such single-point deep injections has also been studied. Regrettably, with current real time imaging technology, we were unable to be certain that the filler was injected directly and solely into the SOOF area, but a placement of filler at its close proximity, with adequate injection depth as suggested by ultrasound imaging, was sufficient enough to achieve clinically satisfactory cheek augmentation. There is minimal skin texture change, irregularity, discoloration, ecchymosis, bruising and edema, allowing the subjects to resume their normal activities immediately after treatment. In the present study, adverse cutaneous events are few and range from transient tenderness to intermittent tingling sensation of the cheek possibly due to edema and irritation around the infraorbital nerve. Such complications were mild and self-limiting.

In terms of injection technique, injection with sharp needle is more precise, and less intimidating to the patients, but may have higher chance of vessel and nerve injury; whereas injection with micro-cannula is generally safer but is more technique-dependent to achieve precision. There is no difference between sharp needle and micro-cannula injection in the total amount of HA filler needed to achieve comparable cosmetic results.

6. Conclusion

Single-point deep injection of HA filler at midface in close proximity to medial Suborbicularis Oculi Fat (SOOF) area for cheek augmentation is a technique which is relatively quick and easy to perform, has little down time, and may result in a high rate of patient satisfaction. Adverse events of filler injections include intra-vascular injection, infection, nodules or granuloma formation, hypersensitivity to products and could be avoided by injecting with micro-cannula, proper injection techniques, aseptic techniques, proper plane of injection, and the selection of safe products. Ultrasound evaluation before injection could be a helpful tool to avoid inadvertent intra-vascular injection and could also be used to confirm the depth of injection. Proper patient selection and communication can lessen over-expectation and are paramount to optimize treatment outcome and patient satisfaction. This pilot study was aimed to elaborate on a simple technique for midface rejuvenation, and was limited by its few case number and hence the inability for statistic analysis. Further prospective studies may be needed to compare the efficacy, safety, and longevity of this technique to other commonly used techniques for the injection of HA fillers in this area of the face.

Disclosures

The authors have no conflict of interest to disclose. There are no funding sources for this work.

References

[1]   Werschler, W.P. (2007) Treating the Aging Face: A Multidisciplinary Approach with Calcium Hydroxylapatite and Other Fillers, Part 2. *Cosmetic Dermatology*, **20**, 791-796.

[2]   Busso, M. and Karlsberg, P.L. (2006) Cheek Augmentation and Rejuvenation Using Injectable Calcium Hydroxylapatite (Radiesse R). *Cosmetic Dermatology*, **19**, 583-588.

[3]   Pessa, J.E. and Garza, J.R. (1997) The Malar Septum: The Anatomic Basis of Malar Mounds and Malar Edema. *Aesthetic Surgery Journal*, **17**, 11-17. http://dx.doi.org/10.1016/S1090-820X(97)70001-3

[4]   Funt, D.K. (2011) Avoiding Malar Edema during Midface/Cheek Augmentation with Dermal Fillers. *Journal of Clinical and Aesthetic Dermatology*, **4**, 32-36.

[5]   Sandoval, S.E., Cox, J.A., Koshy, J.C., Hatef, D.A. and Hollier Jr., L.H. (2009) Facial Fat Compartments: A Guide to Filler Placement. *Seminars in Plastic Surgery*, **23**, 283-287. http://dx.doi.org/10.1055/s-0029-1242181

[6]   Donofrio, L.M. (2000) Fat Distribution: A Morphologic Study of the Aging Face. *Dermatologic Surgery*, **26**, 1107-1112. http://dx.doi.org/10.1046/j.1524-4725.2000.00270.x

[7]   Rohrich, R.J., Pessa, J.E. and Ristow, B. (2008) The Youthful Cheek and the Deep Medial Fat Compartment. *Plastic and Reconstructive Surgery*, **121**, 2107-2112. http://dx.doi.org/10.1097/PRS.0b013e31817123c6

29

Retrospective Study of the Use of a Fractional Radio Frequency Ablative Device in the Treatment of Acne Vulgaris and Related Acne Scars

Judith Hellman

Mt. Sinai Hospital, New York, USA
Email: jhderm@gmail.com

Abstract

Background: Acne vulgaris (AV) is a common disease that often results in disfiguring facial scarring that carries into adulthood. Here we report our experience with fractional radiofrequency (FRF) device in treatment of patients with acne and acne related scarring. Materials & Methods: We retrospectively reviewed the charts of all patients with acne scarring who completed a four treatment regimen in our clinic. Results: We identified eight patients who completed four treatments with median age of 20.5 years (range 17 - 41). All patients demonstrated significant improvement of acne lesions and acne scarring. Skin biopsies demonstrated reduction of scar depth and increased new collagen production, and repopulation of the scar tissue by elastic fibers and adnexal structures after the fourth treatment. Conclusion: FRF emerges as a safe and effective treatment modality for AV and acne related scars. Further randomized controlled studies are required to fully evaluate the magnitude of this positive effect and more basic science studies are needed in order to better characterize its mechanism of action on acne lesions.

Keywords

Acne Vulgaris, Radiofrequency, Scarring

1. Introduction

Acne vulgaris (AV) is a disease afflicting mostly adolescents and young adults, often resulting in disfiguring facial scarring that carries into adulthood. While estimates on the prevalence of acne related scarring vary substantially [1], the psycho-social morbidity is significant [2] and therefore it is crucial to effectively treat AV in order to avoid scarring. The pathogenesis of acne relates to increased sebum production in the setting of aberrant follicular keratinization and *propionibacterium acnes* proliferation and significant perifollicular inflammation [3]. This process leads to local tissue damage resulting in activation of a wound healing cascade and imbalance in collagen deposition and matrix degradation may result in permanent scarring [4].

Current treatment regimens for acne scarring include chemical peels, dermabrasion, large and small surgical excisions, subcision, as well as various lasers, each with variable reports of success and advantages as well as limitations [5]. Radiofrequency (RF) devices represent novel technology that emerged just over a decade ago and is now used routinely for treatment of rhytides, cellulite, skin laxity and AV [6]. More recently fractional RF has been used to treat these cosmetic indications. However, the effect of fractional RF on acne related scarring has not been well characterized.

Here we present our experience with fractional RF (FRF) device in treatment of eight patients with acne and acne related scarring.

2. Materials & Methods

Patients: all patients were informed about the risks, benefits and alternative treatments and all provided an informed consent based on the 1975 Declaration of Helsinki. Patients were generally young adults with history of acne scarring with or without active acne lesions. Patients with conditions considered to be contra-indicated per the manufacturer's instructions were not considered good candidates for therapy.

Treatments: we retrospectively reviewed the charts of all patients with acne scarring who completed a four treatment regimen. Each patient underwent four treatments, four weeks apart. Treatments involved only areas of the face. Pictures were taken immediately prior to the first treatment and after the fourth treatment. On average pictures were retaken 36 days after the fourth treatment (range 7 - 96 days). All patients received initial doses of 20 - 40 mJ/pin, and the doses were increased each visit, based on patient tolerance. All treated areas received one or two passes based on the treatment site and patient tolerance. Double and triple stacking of pulses was done as needed.

Prior to treatment the skin was cleansed with absolute ethanol. Treatments were performed on the affected areas, using either a regular or a coated 24 pin tip, depending on skin type. Two passes, with double or triple stacked pulses were performed with a third partial pass in the heavily scarred areas in a number of patients. Immediately following therapy, Aquaphor™ (Beiersdorf Inc. Wilton, CT) ointment was applied to the skin. Patients were instructed to continue using Aquaphor™ at home 2 - 3 times a day for a total of three days after the procedure. Concurrent treatments included topical agents (Dapsone or Clindamycin) twice a day. Patient demographics and treatment characteristics are summarized in **Table 1**.

Device: all patients were treated with an array of 24 RF conducting needles, alternating current with two long side electrodes (**Figure 1**). Each needle is 2500 µm long and 200 × 300 µm wide at the base. The coated needles are insulated along 2000 µm, leaving the distal 500 µm uncoated. The hand piece was loaded to the Fractora™ platform (also applicable to InMode™ or BodyTite™ platforms), Invasix Ltd./InMode MD Ltd., Israel).

Table 1. Study participants and treatment characteristics.

Subject	Age (yrs.)	Sex	Skin type[*]	Treatment #	Coated/uncoated
1	18	M	I	4	uncoated
2	41	F	V	4	coated
3	17	F	IV	4	coated
4	24	F	IV	4	coated
5	26	F	III	4	uncoated
6	18	F	IV	5	coated
7	19	M	III	4	uncoated
8	22	F	II	4	uncoated

[*]Fitzpatrick skin type [10].

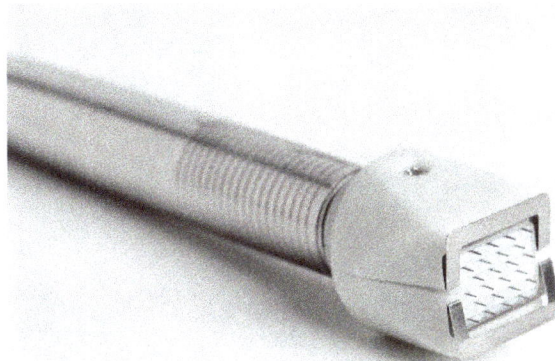

Figure 1. Fractora handpiece with 24 pin tip.

Outcome measurements: before and after pictures were qualitatively evaluated and compared for scar improvement and acne improvement. Representative skin biopsies from two patients were taken before and after treatment and examined with standard hematoxylin and eosin (H&E) stain as well as Verhoeff's Van Gieson (VVG) and Shikata stains for elastic fibers.

3. Results

We identified eight patients who completed four treatments (**Table 1**), six females and two males with a median age of 20.5 years (range 17 - 41). All patients demonstrated significant improvement of active acne lesions and acne scarring (**Figure 2**).

Histological sections of skin biopsies taken before treatment demonstrate long dermal scars 1.5 mm deep (**Figure 3(a)**) that are characterized by thick disorganized collagen fibers (**Figure 3(b)**) and lack of adnexal structures, such as hair follicles and sebaceous glands (**Figure 3(a)**), as well as lack of elastic fibers (**Figure 3(c)**).

Treatment outcome after four Fractora treatments is expressed in the reduction of scar depth to about half (**Figure 4(a)**) and appearance of new collagen fibers that pushed the scar upwards (**Figure 4(b)**). Repopulation of the scar area with adnexal structures that were devoid of the original scar tissue was also observed (**Figure 4(a)**). In addition, elastic fibers that were devoid of the original scar tissue repopulated in the treated area (**Figure 4(c)**).

4. Discussion

We report our experience with a fractional radiofrequency (FRF) device for the treatment of active acne lesions and acne scarring. Treatment with FRF led to significant improvement in the depth of the scars as demonstrated by significant improvement in clinical scoring and confirmed by pathological assay. Skin biopsies after FRF treatment demonstrated that scar thickness diminished in depth from 1.5 to 0.8 mm, having regressed higher into the superficial dermis, pushed up by the new collagen fibers. In addition, there was repopulation of adnexal structures and new elastic fibers in the superficial dermis previously occupied by scar tissue (**Figure 3**, **Figure 4**). FRF delivered electrical energy to create zones of thermal damage to the dermis in the area treated while sparing adjacent areas which serve as a reservoir for wound healing [6]. The coated pin tips used in this study feature additional epidermal protection in darker skin patients. Combination of these properties reduce the damage to the skin and result in the desired outcome with minimal downtime. In addition, the needling effect of the pins may provide additional benefit for acne scar treatment [7].

RF is hypothesized to improve AV by sebum-suppression and its effect on AV has been demonstrated elsewhere [8]. In our cohort, significant resolution of AV lesions was observed. These results suggest that FRF may be used as a modality that allows for simultaneous treatment of both active acne lesions and previous scarring.

While the treatment itself involved some discomfort, via the pins inserted through the epidermis, the overall

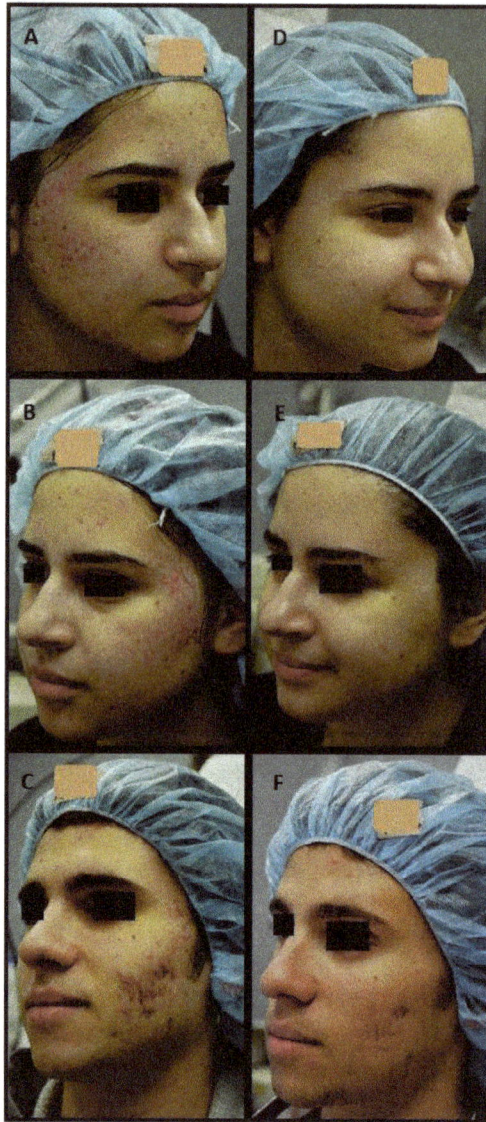

Figure 2. Active acne and acne scars before (A, B, C) and after (D, E, F) four Fractora treatments.

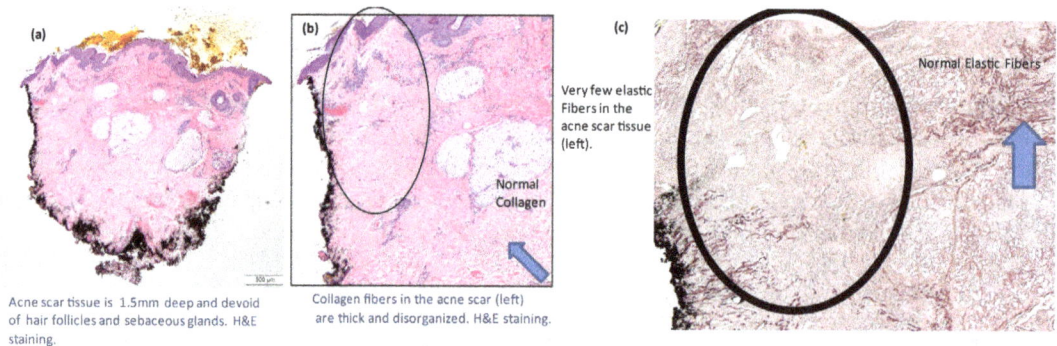

Figure 3. Histological sections of skin biopsies from a representative patient before Fractora treatments. (a) Demonstrates acne scar tissue 1.5 mm deep in the dermis, devoid of hair follicles and sebaceous glands. H&E staining. (b) Demonstrates thick and disorganized collagen fibers in the acne scar tissue (circle), as opposed to normal collagen pointed by arrow. H&E staining. (c) Demonstrates acne scar tissue mostly devoid of elastic fibers (circle), as opposed to normal elastic fibers pointed by arrow. VVG and Shikata staining.

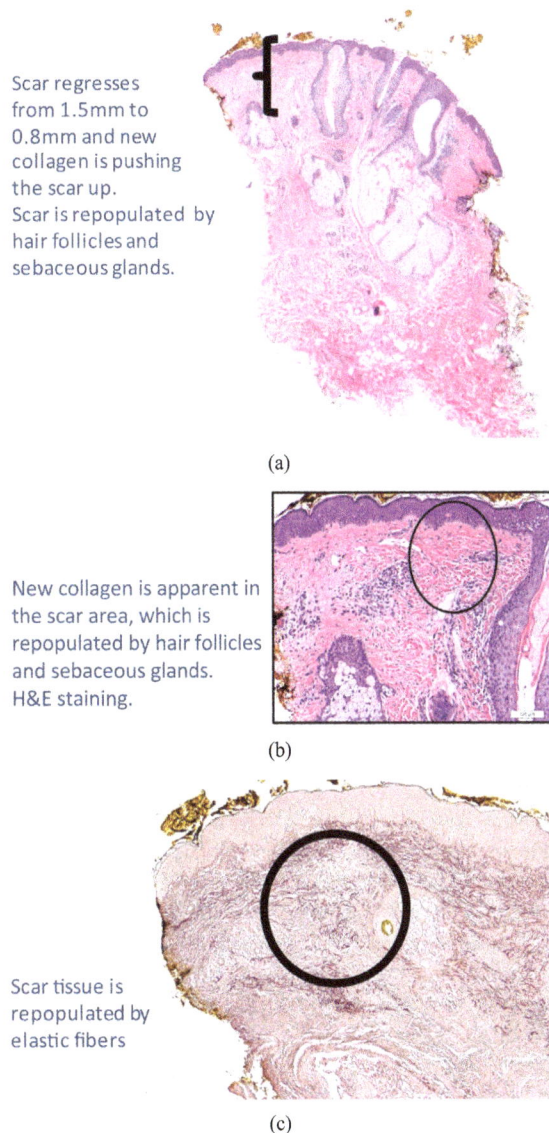

Scar regresses from 1.5mm to 0.8mm and new collagen is pushing the scar up. Scar is repopulated by hair follicles and sebaceous glands.

(a)

New collagen is apparent in the scar area, which is repopulated by hair follicles and sebaceous glands. H&E staining.

(b)

Scar tissue is repopulated by elastic fibers

(c)

Figure 4. Histological sections of skin biopsies from a representative patient after four Fractora treatments. (a) Demonstrates reduction of scar depth to 0.8 mm and repopulation of adnexal structures in the scar tissue. H&E staining. (b) Demonstrates new collagen fibers that are pushing the scar upwards (circle) H&E staining. (c) Demonstrates repopulation of the papillary dermal scar area with elastic fibers (circle). VVG and Shikata staining.

patient experience was positive without any significant adverse events reported. Some patients noted red needle marks and/or sunburn like erythema for up to 48 hours.

For the purpose of this study we arbitrarily decided on a four treatment regimen and while some patients achieved satisfactory response in four treatments, we have excluded patients with satisfactory response with fewer treatments. Other patients elected to add more treatments and we therefore conclude the total number of treatments required can be variable and depends on the goals of treatment and the patient's individual response rate.

FRF treatment has significant advantages as it is minimally invasive, has very low downtime (most patients required 3 - 4 days of recovery) and safe. We did not encounter any cases of pigment alteration and in fact can now report anecdotal use of coated tips in treatment of Fitzpatrick skin type 6 patients without adverse events (data not shown). This may be of significant value as adult acne and atrophic scarring may be more prevalent in darker skin types [9]. In addition, we have anecdotally noted some skin tightening in our patients which is a positive unintended outcome that is well received among our older patients.

Of note, our study has a few limitations since it is a single practitioner experience and it is a retrospective case series. The treatment involved significant discomfort, but the company has redesigned the pulse configuration to reduce the pain considerably. The treatment is not covered by most insurance providers.

5. Conclusion

In conclusion, FRF emerges as a safe and effective treatment modality for AV and acne related scars. Further randomized controlled studies are required to fully evaluate the magnitude of this positive effect and more basic science studies are needed in order to better characterize its mechanism of action on acne lesions.

References

[1]   Rivera, A.E. (2008) Acne Scarring: A Review and Current Treatment Modalities. *Journal of the American Academy of Dermatology*, **59**, 659-676. http://dx.doi.org/10.1016/j.jaad.2008.05.029

[2]   Thomas, D.R. (2004) Psychosocial Effects of Acne. *Journal of Cutaneous Medicine and Surgery*, **8**, 3-5. http://dx.doi.org/10.1007/s10227-004-0752-x

[3]   Del Rosso, J.Q. and Kircik, L.H. (2013) The Sequence of Inflammation, Relevant Biomarkers, and the Pathogenesis of Acne Vulgaris: What Does Recent Research Show and What Does It Mean to the Clinician? *Journal of Drugs in Dermatology: JDD*, **12**, s109-s115.

[4]   Fabbrocini, G., Annunziata, M.C., D'Arco, V., *et al.* (2010) Acne Scars: Pathogenesis, Classification and Treatment. *Dermatology Research and Practice*, **2010**, Article ID: 893080. http://dx.doi.org/10.1155/2010/893080

[5]   Goodman, G.J. (2011) Treatment of Acne Scarring. *International Journal of Dermatology*, **50**, 1179-1194. http://dx.doi.org/10.1111/j.1365-4632.2011.05029.x

[6]   Lolis, M.S. and Goldberg, D.J. (2012) Radiofrequency in Cosmetic Dermatology: A Review. *Dermatologic Surgery*, **38**, 1765-1776. http://dx.doi.org/10.1111/j.1524-4725.2012.02547.x

[7]   Alam, M., Han, S., Pongprutthipan, M., *et al.* (2014) Efficacy of a Needling Device for the Treatment of Acne Scars: A Randomized Clinical Trial. *JAMA Dermatology*, **150**, 844-849. http://dx.doi.org/10.1001/jamadermatol.2013.8687

[8]   Ruiz-Esparza, J. and Gomez, J.B. (2003) Nonablative Radiofrequency for Active Acne Vulgaris: The Use of Deep Dermal Heat in the Treatment of Moderate to Severe Active Acne Vulgaris (Thermotherapy): A Report of 22 Patients. *Dermatologic Surgery*, **29**, 333-339; discussion 9.

[9]   Perkins, A.C., Cheng, C.E., Hillebrand, G.G., Miyamoto, K. and Kimball, A.B. (2011) Comparison of the Epidemiology of Acne Vulgaris among Caucasian, Asian, Continental Indian and African American Women. *Journal of the European Academy of Dermatology and Venereology: JEADV*, **25**, 1054-1060. http://dx.doi.org/10.1111/j.1468-3083.2010.03919.x

[10]   Fitzpatrick, T.B. (1988) The Validity and Practicality of Sun-Reactive Skin Types I through VI. *Archives of Dermatology*, **124**, 869-871. http://dx.doi.org/10.1001/archderm.1988.01670060015008

Elephantiasic Pretibial Myxoedema in a Patient with Graves' Disease

Ruzhi Zhang[1]*, Yuhua Yang[1], Wenyuan Zhu[2]

[1]Department of Dermatology, The Third Affiliated Hospital of Suzhou University, Changzhou, China
[2]Department of Dermatology, The First Affiliated Hospital of Nanjing Medical University, Nanjing, China
Email: *zhangruzhi628@163.com

Abstract

Pretibial myxoedema (PM) is a late and rare manifestation of autoimmune thyroiditis, particularly in patients with Graves' disease. It occurs in 0.5% to 4.3% of patients [1], and is usually associated with high levels of thyroid hormones. The classification of PM includes four forms: non-pitting edema; plaque; nodular; or elephantiasis [1]. Mild PM often regresses spontaneously, but the severe, elephantiasic variant is typically progressive and refractory to treatment. Elephantiasic pretibial myxoedema (EPM) is characterized by massive edema, skin fibrosis and verrucous nodule formation, and it clinically resembles lymphedema. Herein, we describe a man with Graves' disease presenting with EPM for nearly 2 years. Although advanced cases have been described in the literature, to our knowledge, none have reached this level of severity.

Keywords

Pretibial Myxoedema (PM), Graves' Disease

1. Introduction

A 57-year-old Chinese man came to our clinic for advice on the cause and management of a severe skin condition of his legs. His lesions had occurred and progressed relentlessly over the past year. There was no obvious pain, but there was occasional pruritus. Once local skin was injured, it needed more than a month to heal. Physical examination revealed nonpitting edema, flesh-colored to erythematous, firm, confluent, polypoid nodules and fissured plaques extending from the shins to the heels of the feet, the dorsa of the left foot and the large toe (**Figure 1**). Initially, the disorder was thought to be the result of chronic lymphedema. However, his proptosis with eyelid retraction bilaterally reminded us to consider another diagnosis. Questioning the patient revealed that

---

*Corresponding author.

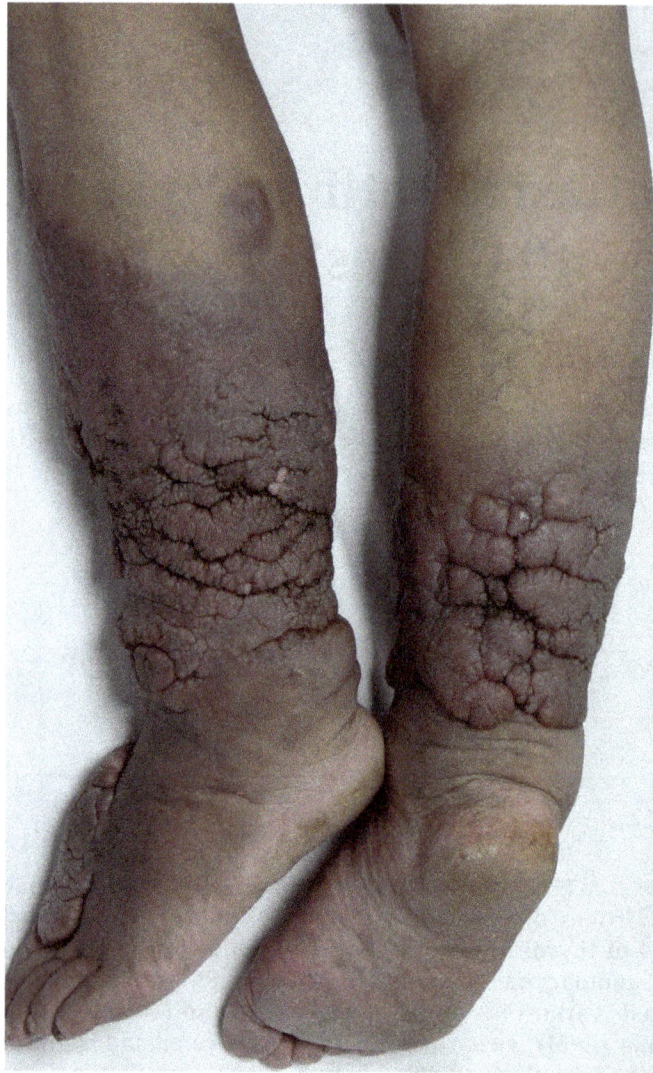

Figure 1. Nonpitting edema, flesh-colored to erythematous, firm, confluent, polypoid nodules and fissured plaques extending from the shins to the heels of the feet, the dorsum of the left foot and large toe.

he had been diagnosed with hyperthyroidism 15 years ago and treated with oral therapy for 6 months (he did not remember the details). A laboratory evaluation revealed: thyrotropin (TSH), <0.01 IU/mL (0.30 - 5.56); free thyroxine (T4), 31.01 pmol/L (11.46 - 23.17); free triiodothyronine (T3), 11.95 pmol/L (2.80 - 7.10); thyroglobulin (TG), 150 mg/ml (0.00 - 85.00); anti-thyroid peroxidase antibody (A-TPO), and 39.60 IU/ml (≤34). The patient looked healthy without evidence of other malignancy or systemic disease. He refused our request for a biopsy. Based on the clinical and laboratory results, EPM in Graves' disease was diagnosed. The patient was referred to the Department of Endocrinology to treat his hyperthyroidism, and then he was lost to follow-up.

2. Discussion

The most common presentation of dermopathy in Graves' disease is PM. The time delay from treatment of hyperthyroidism to presentation with localized myxoedema varies from 1 month to 16 years (mean 5.13 years). Clinical features are nonpitting scaly thickening and induration of the skin. In a previous report, among 150 patients with PM, 58% had nonpitting edema, 20% had the nodular variant, 21% had the plaque type, and less than 1% had either the polypoid or the elephantiasic morphologies [2]. Although several theories have been suggested, the exact pathogenesis of PM remains to be clarified [3]. It was speculated that pretibial fibroblasts may react with T cell lymphocytes via their thyrotropin receptors and then they may overproduce glycosaminogly-cans. The content of hyaluronic acid and chondroitin sulfates in the dermis is increased, causing compression of the dermal lymphatics and nonpitting edema. The predilection for localization to the pretibial area may result from trauma with the release of inflammatory cytokines and inflammatory cells or local hypoxia resulting from arterial or venous insufficiency.

The diagnosis of EPM is easily made by clinical findings and histological investigation. Our patient refused a skin biopsy. Thus differential diagnoses, including secondary edema resulting from chronic lymphatic obstruction or venous insufficiency, diabetic dermopathy, lichen amyloidosis and hypertrophic lichen planus were considered. The history of hyperthyroidism and abnormal levels of T3, T4, TG and A-TPO supported the diagnosis. Other systemic examinations excluded diabetes and vascular diseases. Therefore, the final diagnosis was made.

EPM is typically progressive and refractory to treatment. Some therapeutics are effective but are not curative. A potent topical glucocorticoid applied under occlusion is the primary treatment although intralesional steroids are sometimes used. However, local and systemic steroids very rarely give improvement. Other therapeutics have been reported. A 44-year-old woman with Graves' disease and EPM was treated in a trial of multiple recognized therapies, but had a rapid response to rituximab and plasmapheresis [4]. Another patient with PM improved significantly after treatment with I^{131} for his Graves' disease [5]. Some authors have reported using complete decongestive physiotherapy [6] or low-dose intravenous immunoglobulins [7] to treat EPM, and have obtained satisfactory results.

Acknowledgements

The authors are very grateful to Professor V. J. Hearing, Laboratory of Cell Biology, National Cancer Institute, Bethesda, MD, USA, for English-language element of this paper.

References

[1]   Chen, C.T. and Lin, J.C. (2013) Elephantiasic Pretibial Myxoedema. *Indian Journal of Medical Research*, **137**, 568.

[2]   Fatourechi, V., Pajouhi, M. and Fransway, A.F. (1994) Dermopathy of Graves Disease (Pretibial Myxedema): Review of 150 Cases. *Medicine (Baltimore)*, **73**, 1-7. http://dx.doi.org/10.1097/00005792-199401000-00001

[3]   Rapoport, B., Alsabeh, R., Aftergood, D. and McLachlan, S.M. (2000) Elephantiasic Pretibial Myxedema: Insight into and a Hypothesis Regarding the Pathogenesis of the Extrathyroidal Manifestations of Graves' Disease. *Thyroid*, **10**, 685-692. http://dx.doi.org/10.1089/10507250050137761

[4]   Heyes, C., Nolan, R., Leahy, M. and Gebauer, K. (2012) Treatment-Resistant Elephantiasic Thyroid Dermopathy Responding to Rituximab and Plasmapheresis. *Australasian Journal of Dermatology*, **53**, e1-e4. http://dx.doi.org/10.1111/j.1440-0960.2010.00693.x

[5]   Yu, H., Jiang, X., Pan, M. and Huang, R. (2014) Elephantiasic Pretibial Myxoedema in a Patient with Graves' Disease That Resolved after ^{131}I Treatment. *Clinical Nuclear Medicine*, **39**, 758-759. http://dx.doi.org/10.1097/RLU.0000000000000459

[6]   Susser, W.S., Heermans, A.G., Chapman, M.S. and Baughman, R.D. (2002) Elephantiasic Pretibial Myxedema: A Novel Treatment for an Uncommon Disorder. *Journal of the American Academy of Dermatology*, **46**, 723-726. http://dx.doi.org/10.1067/mjd.2002.119655

[7]   Dhaille, F., Dadban, A., Meziane, L., Fessier, C., Colta, L., Lok, C., *et al.* (2012) Elephantiasic Pretibial Myxoedema with Upper-Limb Involvement, Treated with Low-Dose Intravenous Immunoglobulins. *Clinical and Experimental Dermatology*, **37**, 307-308. http://dx.doi.org/10.1111/j.1365-2230.2011.04175.x

Permissions

All chapters in this book were first published in JCDSA, by Scientific Research Publishing; hereby published with permission under the Creative Commons Attribution License or equivalent. Every chapter published in this book has been scrutinized by our experts. Their significance has been extensively debated. The topics covered herein carry significant findings which will fuel the growth of the discipline. They may even be implemented as practical applications or may be referred to as a beginning point for another development.

The contributors of this book come from diverse backgrounds, making this book a truly international effort. This book will bring forth new frontiers with its revolutionizing research information and detailed analysis of the nascent developments around the world.

We would like to thank all the contributing authors for lending their expertise to make the book truly unique. They have played a crucial role in the development of this book. Without their invaluable contributions this book wouldn't have been possible. They have made vital efforts to compile up to date information on the varied aspects of this subject to make this book a valuable addition to the collection of many professionals and students.

This book was conceptualized with the vision of imparting up-to-date information and advanced data in this field. To ensure the same, a matchless editorial board was set up. Every individual on the board went through rigorous rounds of assessment to prove their worth. After which they invested a large part of their time researching and compiling the most relevant data for our readers.

The editorial board has been involved in producing this book since its inception. They have spent rigorous hours researching and exploring the diverse topics which have resulted in the successful publishing of this book. They have passed on their knowledge of decades through this book. To expedite this challenging task, the publisher supported the team at every step. A small team of assistant editors was also appointed to further simplify the editing procedure and attain best results for the readers.

Apart from the editorial board, the designing team has also invested a significant amount of their time in understanding the subject and creating the most relevant covers. They scrutinized every image to scout for the most suitable representation of the subject and create an appropriate cover for the book.

The publishing team has been an ardent support to the editorial, designing and production team. Their endless efforts to recruit the best for this project, has resulted in the accomplishment of this book. They are a veteran in the field of academics and their pool of knowledge is as vast as their experience in printing. Their expertise and guidance has proved useful at every step. Their uncompromising quality standards have made this book an exceptional effort. Their encouragement from time to time has been an inspiration for everyone.

The publisher and the editorial board hope that this book will prove to be a valuable piece of knowledge for researchers, students, practitioners and scholars across the globe.

List of Contributors

F. Atadokpédé, H. Adégbidi, J. Téclessou, C. Aholoukpé, B. Degboé, F. do Ango-Padonou and H. Yedomon
Faculté des Sciences de la Santé, Cotonou, Bénin

C. Koudoukpo
Faculté de Médecine, Université de Parakou, Parakou, Bénin

Ha Youn Lee, Amal Kumar Ghimeray and Moon Sik Chang
R & D Center, Naturalsolution Co., Ltd., Incheon, Republic of Korea

Jun Hwan Yim
Free International City Development Center (Jeju Branch), Jeju-Do, Republic of Korea

Takanori Matsubara, Saina Taniguchi, Shota Morimoto, Asami Yano and Aritsugu Hara
Isao Wataoka, Hiroshi Urakawa and Hidekazu Yasunaga
Department of Biobased Materials Science, Kyoto Institute of Technology, Kyoto, Japan

Meital Portugal-Cohen, Miriam Oron and Ze'evi Ma'or
Ahava-Dead Sea Laboratories, Lod, Israel
Dead Sea and Arava Science Center, The Laboratory for Skin Biochemistry and Biotechnology, Ein Gedi, Israel

Maria F. Dominguez
Lonza-Personal Care, South Plainfield, USA

Robert Holtz
BioInnovation Laboratories Inc., Lakewood, USA

Khalifa E. Sharquie and Adil A. Noaimi
Department of Dermatology, College of Medicine, University of Baghdad, Baghdad, Iraq
Arab Board for Dermatology and Venereology, Baghdad Teaching Hospital, Medical City, Baghdad, Iraq

Maha A. Al-Shukri
Department of Dermatology, Baghdad Teaching Hospital, Medical City, Baghdad, Iraq
Khalifa E. Sharquie and Sabeeh A. Al-Mashhadani
Department of Dermatology, College of Medicine, University of Baghdad, Iraqi and Arabic Board of Dermatology, Baghdad, Iraq

Ali Thamer Hameed
Department of Dermatology and Venereology, Baghdad Teaching Hospital, Medical City, Baghdad, Iraq

Gérald Chene, Vincent Baillif and Emeline Van Goethem
Ambiotis SAS, Cana Biotech 2, Toulouse, France

Jean-Eric Branka
EPHYSCIENCE, Nantes, France

Toni Ionescu, Géraldine Robert and Luc Lefeuvre
Laboratoires Dermatologiques d'Uriage, Siège Social, Courbevoie, France

Yumi Murakami-Yoneda, Yoshie Shirahige, Kozo Nakai and Yasuo Kubota
Department of Dermatology, Faculty of Medicine, Kagawa University, Kagawa, Japan

Mieko Hata
Department of Dermatology, Nippon Medical School, Tokyo, Japan

Hayder R. Al-Hamamy
Scientific Council of Dermatology and Venereology-Iraqi Board for Medical Specializations, Baghdad, Iraq

Adil A. Noaimi and Ihsan A. Al-Turfy
Department of Dermatology, College of Medicine, University of Baghdad, Baghdad, Iraq

Adil A. Noaimi
Arab Board for Dermatology and Venereology, Baghdad Teaching Hospital, Medical City, Baghdad, Iraq

Adil Ibrahim Rajab
Department of Dermatology, Baghdad Teaching Hospital, Baghdad, Iraq

Isabelle Rousseaux
Cabinet de Dermatologie Esthétique, Lille Côté Sud, Loos, France

Brandon Goodwin and Richard Wagner
Department of Dermatology, The University of Texas Medical Branch, Galveston, TX, USA

Adeline Jeudy, Thomas Lihoreau, Ferial Fanian, Rafat Messikh, Christine Lafforgue and Philippe Humbert
Research and Studies Center on the Integument (CERT), Department of Dermatology, Besançon University Hospital, Besançon, France
Clinical Investigation Center (CIC Inserm 1431), Besançon University Hospital, Besançon, France
Inserm UMR1098, FED4234 IBCT, Besançon University Hospital, Besançon, France

Francesco Scarci and Federico Mailland
Scientific Department, Polichem S.A., Lugano, Switzerland

Gallant Kar Lun Chan, Zack Chun Fai Wong, Kelly Yin Ching Lam and Lily Kwan Wai Cheng
Laura Minglu Zhang, Huangquan Lin, Tina Tingxia Dong and Karl Wah Keung Tsim
Division of Life Science and Center for Chinese Medicine R&D, The Hong Kong University of Science and Technology, Kowloon, Hong Kong, China

Michael H. Gold
Tennessee Clinical Research Center, Nashville, USA

Hela Goren
Home Skinovation Ltd., Yokneam, Israel

Khalifa E. Sharquie and Adil A. Noaimi
Scientific Council of Dermatology and Venereology-Iraqi and Arab Board for Medical Specializations, Department of Dermatology and Venereology, College of Medicine, University of Baghdad, Baghdad, Iraq

Raad M. Helmi
Department of Oral Medicine, College of Dentistry, Al-Mustansiriya University, Baghdad, Iraq

Mohand A. A. Kadhom
School of Dentistry, Faculty of Medical Science, University of Duhok, Duhok, Iraq

Raafa K. Al-Hayani
Department of Dermatology and Venereology, Baghdad Teaching Hospital, Baghdad, Iraq

R. López-García and A. Ganem-Rondero
División de Estudios de Posgrado (Tecnología Farmacéutica), Facultad de Estudios Superiores Cuautitlán, Universidad Nacional Autónoma de México, Cuautitlán Izcalli, Mexico

Hayder R. Al-Hamamy
Scientific Council of Dermatology & Venereology, Iraqi Board for Medical Specializations, Baghdad, Iraq

Ihsan A. Al-Turfy
College of Medicine University of Baghdad, Baghdad, Iraq

Farah S. Abdul-Reda
Department of Dermatology & Venereology, Baghdad Teaching Hospital, Baghdad, Iraq

Judith Hellman
New York, USA

Hela Goren
Yokneam, Israel

R. Stephen Mulholland
Private Plastic Surgery Practice, Toronto, Canada

H. M. Osman
Department of Biochemistry, Faculty of Pharmacy, University of National Ribat, Khartoum, Sudan

M. E. Shayoub
Department of Pharmaceutics, Faculty of Pharmacy, University of Khartoum, Khartoum, Sudan

Munzir M. E. Ahmed
Department of Biochemistry, Faculty of Medicine, AL-Gadarif University, Gadarif, Sudan

E. M. Babiker
Department of Zoology, Faculty of Sciences, University of Khartoum, Khartoum, Sudan
James K. M. Chan
DR JAMES CLINIC, Hong Kong, China

Inna Belenky
Viora Inc., Jersey City, NJ, USA

Monica Elman
Elman Medical Services Ltd., Tel Aviv, Israel

Khalifa E. Sharquie and Adil A. Noaimi
Department of Dermatology, College of Medicine, University of Baghdad, Baghdad, Iraq
Arab Board for Dermatology & Venereology, Baghdad Teaching Hospital, Medical City, Baghdad, Iraq

Halla G. Mahmood
Department of Clinical Biochemistry, College of Medicine, University of Baghdad, Baghdad, Iraq

Sameerah M. Al-Ogaily
Department of Dermatology, Baghdad Teaching Hospital, Medical City, Baghdad, Iraq

Khalifa E. Sharquie and Adil A. Noaimi
Department of Dermatology, College of Medicine, University of Baghdad Iraqi and Arabic Board of Dermatology, Baghdad, Iraq

Mohammad S. Al-Zoubaidi
Department of Dermatology, Baghdad Teaching Hospital, Medical City, Iraq

Khalifa E. Sharquie, Raafa K. Al-Hayani, Waqas S. Abdulwahhab and Abd-Allah S. Mohammed
The Scientific Council of Dermatology and Venereology-Iraqi and Arab Board for Medical Specializations, Department of Dermatology and Venereology, Baghdad Teaching Hospital, College of Medicine, University of Baghdad, Baghdad, Iraq

Atsushi Noguchi, Mitsutoshi Tominaga, Kyi Chan Ko, Hironori Matsuda, Hideoki Ogawa and Kenji Takamori
Institute for Environmental and Gender Specific Medicine, Juntendo University Graduate School of Medicine, Urayasu, Japan

Yasushi Suga and Kenji Takamori
Department of Dermatology, Juntendo University Urayasu Hospital, Urayasu, Japan

Alexander Levenberg
Department of Plastic Surgery, Tel Aviv Sourasky
Medical Center, Tel Aviv, Israel

Mickey Scheinowitz and Orna Sharabani-Yosef
Department of Biomedical Engineering, Faculty of
Engineering, Tel Aviv University, Tel Aviv, Israel

**Pedro Valerón-Almazán, Anselmo J. Gómez-Duaso,
Néstor Santana-Molina and Gregorio Carretero**
Dermatology Service, Hospital Universitario de Gran
Canaria Dr. Negrin, Las Palmas, Spain

Miguel A. García-Bello
Research Unit, Hospital Universitario de Gran Canaria
Dr. Negrin, Las Palmas, Spain

Chung-Pin Liang
Department of Dermatology, Chung-Shan University
Hospital, Taiwan

Haw-Yueh Thong
Department of Dermatology, Shin-Kong Wu Ho-Su
Memorial Hospital, Taiwan

Judith Hellman
Mt. Sinai Hospital, New York, USA

Ruzhi Zhang and Yuhua Yang
Department of Dermatology, The Third Affiliated
Hospital of Suzhou University, Changzhou, China

Wenyuan Zhu
Department of Dermatology, The First Affiliated Hospital
of Nanjing Medical University, Nanjing, China

www.ingramcontent.com/pod-product-compliance
Lightning Source LLC
Chambersburg PA
CBHW080506200326
41458CB00012B/4103